Handbook for Health Care Ethics Committees

Handbook for Health Care Ethics Committees

SECOND EDITION

Linda Farber Post
and Jeffrey Blustein

Johns Hopkins University Press

Baltimore

© 2007, 2015 Johns Hopkins University Press
All rights reserved. Published 2007, 2015
Printed in the United States of America on acid-free paper
9 8 7 6 5 4 3 2

Johns Hopkins University Press
2715 North Charles Street
Baltimore, Maryland 21218-4363
www.press.jhu.edu

Library of Congress Cataloging-in-Publication Data

Post, Linda Farber, author.
    Handbook for health care ethics committees / Linda Farber Post and Jeffrey Blustein.
—Second edition.
        p. ; cm.
    Includes bibliographical references and index.
    ISBN 978-1-4214-1657-1 (pbk. : alk. paper) — ISBN 1-4214-1657-3 (pbk. : alk.
paper) — ISBN 978-1-4214-1658-8 (electronic) — ISBN 1-4214-1658-1 (electronic)
    I. Blustein, Jeffrey, author.   II. Title.
    [DNLM: 1. Ethics Committees, Clinical—ethics.   2. Bioethical Issues.   3. Ethics,
Clinical. WB 60]
    R725.3
    610—dc23   2014027016

A catalog record for this book is available from the British Library.

*Special discounts are available for bulk purchases of this book. For more information, please
contact Special Sales at 410-516-6936 or specialsales@press.jhu.edu.*

Johns Hopkins University Press uses environmentally friendly book materials, including
recycled text paper that is composed of at least 30 percent post-consumer waste, whenever
possible.

*To all the health care ethics committees whose work
continually enhances the quality of health care*

Contents

Preface

The advantage of a second edition is the opportunity to revise, update, and amplify the material from the first edition. The disadvantage of a second edition is the temptation to include everything that we felt was left out of the first. Mindful of this danger, we have tried to impose restraint. But the limitations of the first edition, plus the evolution of bioethics and the significant events affecting the field, require a broader and deeper discussion of matters that come before health care ethics committees.

Handbook for Health Care Ethics Committees was conceived and published in 2007 to meet the needs of ethics committees, ubiquitous institutional resources that were increasingly relied on to play an essential role in education, clinical case consultation, and policy development and review. Anyone who had been paying attention to health care—patient, family member, professional care provider, policy maker, or interested observer—appreciated the profound changes during the past decades. Major advances in scientific knowledge, clinical skill, and technology had been paralleled by significant developments in how and by whom health care decisions are made and implemented. Decision making that used to be confined to the patient and family doctor now included treating and consulting clinicians, relatives, health care proxy agents, risk managers, attorneys, judges, ethicists, organizational administrators, and other interested parties.

Among the most effective and increasingly valued resources in the health care decision-making process was the institutional ethics committee. As health care was becoming more complex, fiscal and bureaucratic pressures mounted, and governmental regulations expanded, clinicians and administrators were increasingly looking to committees like yours for analysis and guidance in resolving health care problems. Depending on the size and needs of the institution, the ethics committee typically was serving as moral analyst, information clearinghouse, dispute mediator, educator, policy reviewer, and clinical ethics consultant. The importance and scope of these responsibilities suggested that committees should be familiar and comfortable with bioethical theory and analysis, clinical consultation skills, institutional policies, legal precedents, organizational function, and resource allocation.

At that point, we could hear committee members saying, "Are you kidding? Our committee is made up of clinicians and administrators who volunteer our time because we are interested in the ethical issues in health care. But it's all we can do to keep up with what we need to know to meet our clinical and administrative responsibilities. Don't ask us to take a course in bioethics."

Your very legitimate concern is what prompted the first edition of *Handbook for Health Care Ethics Committees*—a handbook, not a textbook—that filled the need for an accessible, informative, useful guide for members of health care ethics committees, especially those who lacked a formal background in bioethics. Because bioethics raises complex questions that require essays rather than short answers, we packed a great deal into that volume, distilling a basic foundation of bioethical theory and its practical application in clinical and organizational settings. To make the material more accessible and useful, we provided illustrative vignettes, discussion questions, suggested strategies, and sample cases with ethical analyses to explain how the principles and concepts apply to what you do.

Almost from the moment of publication, however, opportunities for enhancement were apparent. We realized that the book would be strengthened and relevant to a wider audience by more attention to ethics committees in settings other than acute care hospitals or large medical centers, including long-term care facilities, small community hospitals, hospices, and facilities for specialized care, such as rehabilitation centers and psychiatric hospitals.

In addition to updating the curriculum chapters in part I, we have added three entirely new chapters addressing reproduction, disability, and the special needs of the elder population; rather than combining justice and organizational ethics in one chapter, we have given each a chapter of its own. These changes reflect the fact that bioethics is a dynamic and evolving field. Scientific and technological advances, especially at the beginning and end of life, continue to create new and difficult ethical dilemmas about the proper uses of medicine, surgery, and other therapeutic technologies. The ethical obligations of health care organizations, apart from those of individual professionals, are also attracting increasing attention by organizational leaders and ethics committees, And framing these issues, major changes in health care delivery, most notably the Patient Protection and Affordable Care Act, call for new approaches to access, reimbursement, measures of quality, and allocation of scarce resources. These and other equally important developments will benefit from the deliberations of knowledgeable ethics committees.

Responding to the growing need for ethics committees to provide their members with a solid foundation of knowledge about bioethics and its practical application, this book builds on the format and content of the first edition with the following expanded sections, each of which examines one or more ethics committee functions and suggests ways in which your committee can be a most effective asset to your institution:

- Part I is a 12-chapter ethics curriculum, organized according to the issues that arise in health care.
- Part II addresses the creation, nature, and functioning of an ethics committee, including its typical responsibilities of education, case consultation, and policy development and review, supplemented with sample educational materials and strategies, cases and analyses, and policies.
- Part III provides examples of organizational codes of ethics.
- Part IV presents summaries of key legal cases in bioethics.
- Part V provides the transcript of a hypothetical ethics committee meeting that demonstrates the foregoing principles, concepts, analyses, and strategies in action.

An exciting new feature that we have added to the second edition is supplemental material for chapter 17. Readers can find additional sample policies and procedures at jhupbooks.press.jhu.edu, by searching for the second edition of *Handbook for Health Care Ethics Committees*. Readers should also check the website periodically for any updated materials, such as new legal cases.

Acknowledgments

This handbook owes its existence and utility to numerous individuals and groups, whose contributions, assistance, and support must be acknowledged. We wish to thank our two wonderful research assistants, Georgina Campelia and Chloe Cooper-Jones, for their invaluable help with this second edition. They reviewed and commented on drafts of all the chapters, updated legal cases, and combed the bioethics literature to provide us with the most up-do-date reference material. We are grateful to Nancy Neveloff Dubler, Kenneth Berkowitz, Tia Powell, and Jack Kilcullen for allowing us to reprint all or portions of their contributions to the first edition. Professionals, including Dr. Jamie Beversdorf, Dr. José Contreras, Sunni Herman, Timothy Kirk, Barbara Reich, and Dr. Lisa Tank, generously shared their expertise by reading and providing important commentary on selected sections of the manuscript. Dr. Kalmon Post reviewed the manuscript and contributed valuable clinical insights. Maria E. denBoer provided helpful manuscript review, and Becky Hornyak prepared the comprehensive index. Our extraordinary editors, Kelley Squazzo and Deborah Bors, shepherded the book from first draft to finished product with skill, enthusiasm, creativity, support, and surpassing patience, and managing editor Juliana McCarthy expertly oversaw the entire process.

The insights and perspectives of the ethics committees at Hackensack University Medical Center, Montefiore Medical Center, Jewish Home at Rockleigh, and Visiting Nurse Service of New York provided the authenticity that kept this handbook grounded in the real world of health care ethics. Several institutions generously shared their policies and codes of ethics for discussion in chapter 17 and part III, including Bronx Psychiatric Center, Cleveland Clinic, Hackensack University Medical Center, Henepin County Medical Center, Jewish Home at Rockleigh, Lenox Hill Hospital, Long Island Jewish Medical Center, Methodist Hospital, Montefiore Medical Center, Mount Sinai Medical Center, Oregon Health and Science University, University of California at San Diego Healthcare, Visiting Nurse Service of New York, and Wycoff Heights Medical Center.

Finally, this second edition, like its predecessor, would not have been possible without the encouragement, critical commentary, and general forbearance of our families and friends.

PART I

CURRICULUM FOR ETHICS COMMITTEES

Part I comprises a 12-chapter curriculum designed to introduce the fundamentals of bioethics, explain the key concepts, and provide a basic analytic framework for addressing and resolving ethical dilemmas. As in the first edition, each chapter highlights a set of ethical issues that commonly arise in the clinical setting and generate requests for ethics committee attention. While the curriculum has been expanded with four new chapters, it is still beyond the scope of this handbook to provide a comprehensive treatment of these topics, and our discussion of the basic ethical principles and concepts draws on the work of expert theorists and practitioners who have contributed to the vast scholarly and clinical literature.

We encourage you to consult the selected but by no means exhaustive references listed at the end of each chapter. Any ethics committee's library should include classic texts, such as Beauchamp and Childress's *Principles of Biomedical Ethics*; anthologies, such as Arras, Steinbock, and London's *Ethical Issues in Modern Medicine*; newsletters, such as *Medical Ethics Advisor*; as well as journals, such as the *Hastings Center Report*, the *Journal of Law, Medicine & Ethics*, the *American Journal of Bioethics*, and the *Journal of Clinical Ethics*. The American Society for Bioethics and Humanities' publication *Improving Competence in Ethics Consultation: A Learner's Guide*, as well as the second edition of *Core Competencies for Ethics Consultation*, will be indispensable resources for individuals and organizations providing clinical ethics consultation and education. Finally, websites, such as www.asbh .org (American Society for Bioethics and Humanities) and www.ethicsweb.ca /resources/bioethics/institutes.html (a comprehensive list of resources with links to ethics institutes and organizations), are valuable sources of current information about what is happening in bioethics. These references are essential, providing ready access to the relevant research and in-depth analysis applicable to the cases and issues that committees consider.

CHAPTER 1

Ethical Foundations of Clinical Practice

The role of ethics in clinical medicine
Ethics committees in the health care setting
Fundamental ethical principles
Principlism and alternative approaches
The role of culture, race, and ethnicity in health care
Conflicting obligations and ethical dilemmas

As a member of your hospital's ethics committee, you have been called by Dr. Thomas, a second-year surgical resident who was paged for the following consult: Ms. Lawrence is a 23-year-old woman who was returning home from her bridal shower when her car skidded on the ice and hit an oncoming truck. Although her multiple injuries are serious, with immediate surgery and replacement of lost blood, her chances of full recovery are excellent.

Ms. Lawrence is in considerable pain, but she appears coherent and her answers to Dr. Thomas's questions reflect understanding of her condition, the treatment options, and their consequences. Because of her beliefs as a Jehovah's Witness, however, she will not accept blood or blood products and will not consider surgery unless she is promised that it will be done without transfusions.

Dr. Thomas knows that surgical and hemodynamic intervention can prevent this patient's almost certain death. He also knows that saving her life in this way will violate Ms. Lawrence's deeply held religious convictions. What are the conflicting professional, legal, and ethical obligations? What is the role of the ethics committee in resolving this dilemma? What resources are available to help you?

Perhaps the threshold question that should begin our discussion is, What is health care ethics and why does it matter? The short answer is that *health care ethics* is an umbrella term that encompasses a number of subspecialties that address the ethical issues that arise in the health care setting, including clinical ethics, organizational ethics, and research ethics. As will become clear in the following pages, however, the issues do not lend themselves to short answers, and further clarification and analysis are necessary. The concerns of health care ethics include the well-being and dignity of the patient; matters of choice and decision making; rights and responsibilities of the patient, family, and care team; the responsibilities of health care organizations; access to care; and fairness and justice in health policy.

These matters are neither new nor exotic, but they have become more prominent. Health care has traditionally dealt with the profound moral issues of human existence, including life, self-determination, suffering, and mortality. What has changed are the complexity of medicine; the increased range of choices; and the way care is accessed, delivered, and financed. The ethical implications of these matters have attracted heightened attention, not only from those who make clinical and policy decisions but, especially recently, from those who make legislative and judicial decisions, as well. As ethics has become an integral part of the health care setting, institutional ethics committees have become increasingly visible and active in clinical and organizational decision making. The goal of this handbook is to help your committee be a knowledgeable, skillful, and effective ethics resource for your institution.

THE ROLE OF ETHICS IN CLINICAL MEDICINE

Ethics has a long and distinguished history, grounding both the practice of medicine and the laws related to it. Society considers ethical principles so important that it gives them legal sanction in statutory and case law. Thus, ethical principles, such as respect for autonomy and privacy, are translated into laws about informed consent and confidentiality. Issues related to providing and forgoing health care are governed almost exclusively by state law, however, creating wide variation in the way these matters are handled. For example, decisions about withholding or withdrawing life-sustaining measures might be very different if the patient were being treated in New York or Texas. For this reason, your ethics committee should have some familiarity with how your state laws and regulations address these issues.

While ethics informs all worthy endeavors, it has special significance in the health care professions because of the fiduciary relationship between practitioners and patients. A fiduciary relationship exists when one party, because of superior knowledge, skill, and authority, assumes responsibility for the welfare of another party who is in a position of reliance. In this trust-based relationship, fiduciaries have heightened obligations, including the moral imperative to put the interests of reliant parties ahead of their own interests. Patients, whose illness, injury, disability, pain, or suffering make them vulnerable, place themselves in the hands of health care professionals, based on the confidence that their well-being is the practitioner's highest priority.

Ironically, it is the very technological and medical advances, as well as their promise and potential, which have generated some of the most difficult ethical problems. In critical, acute, and long-term care settings, the very existence of new therapies often creates demand for their use, whether or not they are medically indicated or ethically appropriate. Stage and screen portrayals of brilliant diagnoses and dramatic recoveries have convinced the lay public and, often, clinicians, that everything is curable if enough money and expertise are thrown at it. When that does not happen, when the disease or injury is overwhelming and irreversible, patients and families feel betrayed and practitioners often feel as though they have failed. Likewise, the Internet has become both a help and a hindrance. Patients sometimes come to the therapeutic interaction armed with reams of information about therapies reported to cure their ailments, insisting that they should be tried. In the domain of clinical research, expectations of dramatic breakthroughs are also high, despite the fact that more clinical research results in failure and disappointment than success (Leaf 2013; Bains 2004).

Standing at the intersection of medicine, ethics, and law, health care ethics provides a useful analytic framework for committees charged with thinking through the ethical dilemmas of modern medicine in a rational and responsible manner.

ETHICS COMMITTEES IN THE HEALTH CARE SETTING

The development of bioethics as a powerful influence on the way health care is perceived and practiced was part of a larger social transformation. A hallmark of the latter half of the twentieth century was the heightened notion of individual rights. Virtually every social sphere was affected by the effort to promote equality and redress inequities in race, gender, class, and education. In the context of the various rights movements, including civil, women's, and gay rights, the ethical principle of autonomy became the major support for individual empowerment and self-determination in health care, most prominently in the doctrine of informed consent and the right of refusal. In the process, to a much greater extent than previously, patients became both partners in health care decision making and informed health care consumers.

Ethical, legal, and scientific developments created an obligation to evaluate critically the process of gathering scientific information, translating it into therapeutic applications, and using it responsibly. Advances in medical knowledge and skills generated a new array of treatment options, as well as the concern that the *ability* to intervene could become the *obligation* to intervene. For the first time, questions were raised not only about *how* and *when*, but *whether* to treat. Under what circumstances should therapies be withheld or withdrawn? When does the burden of an intervention outweigh its benefit? How should decisions be made about the allocation of limited medical resources? At the same time, the law was becoming involved in life-and-death matters that used to be confined to the doctor-patient interaction.

Bioethics as a discipline is generally considered to have developed between the 1960s and the 1980s as it became apparent that emerging issues could benefit from thoughtful analysis by people with both clinical and nonclinical perspectives. Philosophers, social scientists, theologians, legal scholars, and biomedical scientists increasingly focused their attention on clinical research, allocation of limited resources, organ transplantation, reproductive technologies, genetic testing and treatment, terminal illness and end-of-life care, and the obligations in the clinical interaction. Clinicians too turned their attention to these matters. These deliberations revealed that ethical analysis had practical application in the research and clinical settings.

The hospital ethics committee was an early institutional effort to bring a formal ethical perspective to the clinical setting, otherwise described as "a politically attractive way for moral controversies to be procedurally accommodated" (Moreno 1995, pp. 93–94). In the early 1980s, hospitals increasingly began to establish ethics committees to answer questions and help make decisions about health care issues with ethical dimensions. These committees had their roots in several types of small decision-making groups, each intended to address specific ethical problems. Sterilization committees, composed mainly of physicians with expertise in psychiatry and psychology, functioned mainly during the 1920s and 1930s to determine which individuals with mental disabilities should be involuntarily sterilized. Abortion selection committees functioned in many hospitals before the 1973 U.S. Supreme Court decision in *Roe v. Wade* legalized abortion. Beginning in 1945, their purpose was to evaluate the requests of women who wished to terminate their pregnancies and determine whether therapeutic abortions were indicated to preserve maternal life or health. Dialysis selection committees emerged during the early 1960s in response to the development of the dialysis machine, the first publicly recognized life-sustaining technology. Made up of lay members of the community, they were charged with choosing among the candidates with end-stage renal disease and determining who would receive chronic hemodialysis.

Beginning in the 1970s, institutional review boards (IRBs) responded to revelations of abuse in medical experimentation by reviewing all government-funded research using human subjects. The 1974 federal mandating of IRBs represented the first codified suggestion of institutional obligation to address ethical concerns. Prognosis committees were occasionally convened by the mid-1970s to assess the projected course of patients' illnesses. In its 1976 ruling in *In re Quinlan*, the New Jersey Supreme Court referred to an article by Dr. Karen Teel and recommended that hospitals have an ethics committee to deal with termination of life-sustaining treatment for incapacitated patients. Although the court used the term *ethics committee*, it was actually suggesting a *prognosis committee* that would render opinions on the likely benefits of continued treatment for patients with grave and irreversible illness.

Infant care review committees began appearing in the wake of the 1982 "Baby Doe" ruling that permitted parents to approve withholding life-saving treatment from a neonate with Down syndrome. These committees, which were intended to review care plans for severely disabled newborns, were also recommended by the President's Commission for the Study of Ethical Problems in Medicine and Behavioral Research in 1983 and endorsed by the U.S. Department of Health and Human Services and the American Academy of Pediatrics. Medical-morals committees met in Catholic hospitals to address sensitive issues, including those related to reproduction, analgesia, and extraordinary interventions at the end of life, in terms of Church doctrine.

Against this backdrop, clinical and administrative staffs began to meet for interdisciplinary deliberations about issues of high-tech care, undertook self-education, and exhibited a growing professional awareness of ethical issues and their implications. During the 1970s and 1980s, hospitals began to establish ethics committees to provide guidance about health care issues with ethical dimensions. Over time, these committees have taken on the additional functions of staff education, clinical guideline development, institutional policy advisement, and clinical case review. Some ethics committees also advise on resource allocation and express or reinforce the institution's commitment to certain values.

Since 1992, the Joint Commission (formerly known as the Joint Commission on Accreditation of Healthcare Organizations, or JCAHO) has required as a condition of accreditation that every health care institution have a standing mechanism to address ethical issues and resolve disputes. In addition, several states, including

Massachusetts, New Jersey, Colorado, Maryland, New York, and Texas, have passed statutes requiring hospitals to have ethics committees (Pope 2011). According to a 2007 report of U.S. hospitals, 100% of hospitals with 400 or more beds also have an ethics consultation service, which is commonly part of or allied with an ethics committee (Fox, Myers, and Pearlman 2007). The result is that almost all acute care hospitals, long-term care facilities, hospices, psychiatric institutions, facilities for the developmentally disabled, and other care-providing centers in the United States have ethics committees that meet on a regular or ad hoc basis.

Just as there are different care-providing institutions serving different needs, there are different models of health care ethics committees, based on the size, resources, patient base, type of care delivered, geographic location, community demographics, budget, consultation needs, and other resources of each facility. Large academic medical centers typically have a multidisciplinary ethics committee that meets monthly and some have additional committees that focus on ethical issues in specific clinical settings, such as pediatrics or neonatology. Many large centers supplement their committees with a full-time bioethicist, who directs the ethics service; conducts or participates in clinical ethics consultation; teaches medical and nursing students, residents, and other staff; and serves as the frontline bioethics resource. Ethics committees in small community hospitals, nursing homes, hospices, and facilities for the developmentally disabled may meet quarterly for education, case review, and policy development, relying on subcommittees or specified individuals to address ethical issues and clinical consultations as the need arises.

Hospice and long-term care ethics committees may be on-site and specific to one institution or provide off-site resources to multiple institutions. These committees typically focus on ethical issues and decisions at the end of life. Ethics committees at psychiatric institutions and facilities for the disabled are also often off-site and serve several facilities.

Ethics consortium committees are off-site resources for multiple institutions that share one or more characteristics or needs. Some focus on specific research, such as stem cell studies, conducted at several centers, while others focus on clinical issues. Some consortium committees address the educational and networking needs of organizations and individuals without offering consultation services, while others provide clinical consultations for practitioners, administrative staff, and the general public. Consortiums may cover a wide range of health care organizations and issues, or they may focus on specific areas, such as research, non-acute care, long-term care, hospice, or particular disease entities or disabilities.

As you read though this handbook, bear in mind that your committee does not own ethics in your institution. As discussed in chapter 13, the committee should strive to develop ethics expertise, but it would be counterproductive to encourage the notion of ethics exclusivity and the perception that ethics resides only in a select group. Rather, one of your most valuable roles is that of a resource, which, through education, policy development, and consultation, helps clinical and administrative staff to integrate ethics knowledge and skills into their daily practice.

Accordingly, an important committee function is helping staff to identify or anticipate ethical issues and conflicts, develop the skills to handle routine cases in ways that you have modeled in consultation on similar cases, and distinguish complex cases that require the attention of your consultation service. One mark of a successful ethics consultation is when you are stopped in the hall by someone who says, "Remember that case you consulted on two weeks ago? Well, we had another one just like it and we *didn't* have to call you. But now, we've got one that really has us stumped and we need your involvement again."

A crucial task is to make ethics and your committee relevant to the clinical and organizational functioning of your institution. Your clinical consultation and educational strengths will not be solicited if people do not appreciate how what you do can enhance what they do. Make your committee visible by having each interested member regularly attend morning rounds on a particular unit to contribute observations about ethical issues that arise during case discussions. Other members might join select committees—patient safety, institutional review board, conflict of interest—to provide an ethics lens to the deliberations. At the same time, while your committee retains the responsibility to provide ethics expertise, education, and guidance, it is important to reinforce the notions that bioethics is an integral part of the work that health care professionals do every day, and that the health care organization and all those who practice in it are moral agents with ethical obligations that cannot be delegated.

FUNDAMENTAL ETHICAL PRINCIPLES

As you no doubt expected, any discussion of applied bioethics must begin with a review of its theoretical underpinnings. Understanding the key concepts and how they relate to clinical practice is essential to the effective functioning of ethics committees.

The core ethical principles that support the therapeutic relationship and give rise to clinician obligations include

- respecting patient autonomy—supporting and facilitating the capable patient's exercise of self-determination in health care decision making;
- beneficence—promoting the patient's best interest and protecting the patient from harm;
- nonmaleficence—avoiding actions likely to cause the patient harm; and
- justice—allocating fairly the benefits and burdens related to health care delivery.

Respecting Patient Autonomy

Autonomy is the ethical principle widely considered most central to health care decision making. Its prominence here and in other bioethics literature reflects the heightened emphasis typically accorded patient rights, self-governance, and individual choice. Autonomy includes determination of health care goals, power over what is done to one's body, and control of personal information. Only when the individual cannot make decisions are others asked to choose. Autonomy gives priority to personal values and wishes, supporting choices that are informed and uncoerced, and confers the professional obligation to respect patient privacy and confidentiality.

The significance of autonomy to health care decision making is seen in the ethical concepts of decisional capacity, informed consent and refusal, and truth telling. Patients exercise autonomy by making informed care decisions that reflect their goals, values, and preferences. Clinicians demonstrate respect for autonomy by providing information and guidance that enable patients to make knowledgeable decisions, honoring patient choices and implementing them in care plans, preserving patient confidentiality, and protecting the security of patient information.

The notion of autonomy encompasses a range of conceptions, some highly individualistic and somewhat isolating, others more relational and compatible with communitarian values. Criticisms of some versions of the principle of respect for patient autonomy do not invalidate the principle since other versions might be immune to those objections. The search for a full understanding of autonomy has spawned a vast literature and is beyond the scope of this handbook but, for an ethics committee, the role of autonomy has applied as well as theoretical importance. For example, when considering patient rights and decision making, it is crucial to distinguish autonomy as self-governance according to one's values and principles from the unrestricted liberty to behave entirely according to one's preferences (Gaylin and Jennings 2003). There is also a distinction between negative and positive rights, the former being the right not to have one's self-chosen plan controlled or interfered with, and the latter being a claim on others to behave in certain ways (Takala 2007). This distinction has important implications for patient decisions and clinician obligations, which are the focus of chapter 2. Likewise, while an individualistic conception of autonomy emphasizes each patient's capacity for self-advocacy and self-governance, a relational conception focuses on the conditions, including organizational structure, policy, and process, which either promote or inhibit the exercise of autonomy (Nedelsky 2011).

The heightened emphasis our society customarily places on individualism and independence is a largely Western, and some feminists have argued gendered, phenomenon that is not shared across all cultures or even by all within our culture. Some patients may come from cultures that favor decision making by the family rather than the individual. Even in a culture that prizes self-governance, not everyone is comfortable with or capable of independent decision making. For many patients, authentic decision making is an exercise shared with trusted others and reflects *supported* or *delegated* autonomy. Patients with diminished or fluctuating cognition are likely to rely on spouses or adult children for help in care planning, and even those who are cognitively capable may elect to have others make decisions for them or to consult with them before deciding on a course of action.

Ultimately, respecting patient autonomy does not mean elevating it to a position where it trumps all other considerations. While it is legally and ethically appropriate to honor the wishes of capable patients, it is also necessary to consider the ethical principles that give rise to other, often competing, obligations.

Beneficence

The principle of beneficence underlies obligations to provide the best care for the patient and balance the risks and burdens of care against the benefits. Promoted goods typically include prolonging life, restoring function, relieving pain and suffering, and preventing harm. Beneficence is the principle with arguably the greatest resonance for caregivers, whose traditional mission is to heal and comfort, and notions of nurturing and protecting are reflected in heightened care for those who are most vulnerable. Assessing the patient's "good" is a complex process, however, since perceptions of benefit and best interest are not purely scientific or medical, but involve the patient's expectations, goals, and value judgments. Recognition that patients and their doctors may differ in these assessments has been at least partly responsible for the noticeable shift from physician paternalism to greater emphasis on patient choice and shared decision making.

Nonmaleficence

At the very core of the healing professions is the principle of nonmaleficence, captured in the ancient maxim, "First, do no harm." This principle grounds obligations to avoid the unnecessary infliction of harm or suffering, recognizing that conceptions of harm, as of good, are inextricably tied to individual values and interests. Most, if not all, therapies carry the potential for some risk as well as benefit, and it would not be feasible to limit the therapeutic arsenal to treatments that are entirely benign. Nevertheless, the benefits of recommended treatments are expected to outweigh the possible harms and physicians are required to discuss that calculus with their patients, comparing the burdens and risks to the anticipated goods, being mindful that patients differ in their tolerance of risk. Likewise, the duty to prevent foreseeable harm requires investigators to disclose the benefits and risks of proposed research to potential subjects and IRBs.

Justice

Justice, or equity, refers to those principles of social cooperation that define what each person in the society or member of a group is due or owed. The several types of justice, including distributive, punitive, and compensatory justice, all share the basic notion of treating similar cases similarly and dissimilar cases dissimilarly. In the domain of health care, justice demands that care decisions be based on clinical need rather than ethically irrelevant characteristics, such as race, religion, or socioeconomic status. Most relevant to medical ethics is distributive justice, which concerns the norms and standards for allocating benefits and burdens across a given population. Distributive justice demands that the benefits, risks, and costs of actions—in this case, access to resources related to physical and mental health—be apportioned fairly and without discrimination on both societal and institutional levels. According to the principle of distributive justice, there should be ethically defensible reasons why certain individuals or groups receive benefits or endure burdens that other individuals or groups do not.

PRINCIPLISM AND ALTERNATIVE APPROACHES

The four ethical principles discussed above—autonomy, beneficence, nonmaleficence, and justice—have assumed a central place in much of bioethics literature, theory, and clinical analysis. They are used in an attempt to render our moral convictions and the reasons for them coherent. Our very brief tour just touches the surface and you are encouraged to consult Beauchamp and Childress for an in-depth treatment. Because these principles have validity and can be useful in thinking through ethical issues, they are referred to frequently in the following chapters. As a cautionary note, however, it is important to resist the temptation to employ principles in a mechanical fashion. If used with judgment and sensitivity, they can provide structure and inform sound ethical reasoning. Used rigidly without reference to context and narrative, however, principlist ethics can lead to a distorted and unhelpful analysis.

Challenges to principlist ethics use different theoretical and analytical frameworks in considering ethical issues. Narrative ethics employs the methods and techniques of narrative analysis to provide a richer characterization of ethical problems as a supplement to the dominant principlist approach. Feminist ethics is committed to the view that the moral experience of women, in particular their history of sexual oppression, must be taken seriously in the identification, analysis, and resolution of ethical problems. Virtue ethics gives matters of character, such as courage, loyalty, and compassion, a preeminent place in ethical analysis. Pragmatic ethics stresses the continuity between the methods of problem solving in science and ethics.

It is equally useful in doing ethical analysis to consider clinical situations in terms other than that of ethical principles or analytic frameworks, referring to concepts such as decisional capacity and authority, power imbalances, pain and suffering, confidentiality, truth telling, informed consent, the family's role in decision making, the patient's best interest, forgoing treatment, and quality of life and death. Ethical principles have a foundational role in justifying decisions, but they are given meaning and application by additional considerations. These and other ethical issues will be referred to in analyzing clinical situations throughout the curriculum in part I and in discussing the clinical cases in part II.

THE ROLE OF CULTURE, RACE, AND ETHNICITY IN HEALTH CARE

How people confront decisions about health care is shaped in large part by the beliefs, attitudes, and values inherent in the cultures with the greatest formative influence on them. Choices about advance care planning, approaches to decision making, disclosure of information, life-sustaining interventions, and palliation are often informed by culturally determined notions of self-governance and destiny, truth telling and protection from harm, the power of language to reflect or create reality, filial obligation, the meaning of suffering, religion and spirituality, historical discrimination, and mistrust of health care or the health care system.

The following brief examples are offered to illustrate how culture, race, and ethnicity can influence health care. Studies have found that European Americans, who tend to value independence and self-empowerment, are more likely than others to favor advance directives, full disclosure of health information, and limited treatment at the end of life. In contrast, African Americans have demonstrated reluctance to delegate decision-making authority through advance directives; objection to limiting treatment; and preference for aggressive life-sustaining technology, including cardiopulmonary resuscitation. Hispanics have been shown to defer to physician judgment, value decision making by the family rather than an appointed health care agent, and place great importance on how the family is affected by the patient's illness. Asian and Middle Eastern cultures typically prefer to protect patients from knowledge about serious illness or impending death, and favor family rather than individual decision making. Native American cultures tend to reject advance care discussions because they might bring on the envisioned health problems (Major, Mendes, and Dovidio 2013; Sorkin, Ngo-Metzger, and DeAlba 2010). Similarly, race, culture, ethnicity, and gender inform how pain is experienced, expressed, perceived, and treated, with women receiving less analgesia and more sedation than men, and Hispanics less likely to receive pain management than non-Hispanic white patients. Reports of these studies emphasize the need for balance in interpreting them. Overreliance on the findings risks cultural stereotyping, while failure to attend to cultural distinctions risks assuming that all patients share Western attitudes and values (Morrison and Meier 2004; Kagawa-Singer and Blackhall 2001; Hopp and Duffy 2000; Blackhall et al. 1999; Shepardson et al. 1999; Morrison et al. 1998; Berger 1998; Post et al. 1996; Pellegrino et al. 1992). The same commentators also point out that cultural determinants influence the values and attitudes of physicians as well as those of their patients. The result is the potential for misperception and miscommunication when the parties to the clinical interaction come from different cultural backgrounds.

The extensive literature on cultural influences on health care delivery indicates that, in an increasingly diverse population, multiplicity of languages, socioeconomic inequities, and differing religious beliefs, community values, and cultural traditions may inhibit the provision of clinical services, resulting in widespread disparities in access to and quality of care. These inequities present across the age, geographic, ethnic, nationalistic, and religious spectrums. Increasing the cultural competence of practitioners and care-providing organizations is repeatedly offered as an effective way to diminish these disparities and enhance the quality of care delivered (Aseltine, Katz, and Holmes 2011; Boone 2011; Padela, Imran, and Punekar 2009; Giger et al. 2007; Flores and Lin 2013; Lau et al. 2012).

A valuable ethics committee function is educating care providers about the personal and cultural differences that influence the clinical dynamic and affect patient care. Consider, for example, a series of grand rounds or in-service presentations on how cultural background can inform patient and provider comfort with notions of autonomy, privacy, advance directives, informed consent, and disclosure.

CONFLICTING OBLIGATIONS AND ETHICAL DILEMMAS

The several ethical principles discussed above confer on clinicians multiple ethical obligations—duties that are grounded in moral norms and must be fulfilled unless there are competing and more compelling obligations. Not surprisingly, these obligations frequently collide, and this is often responsible for the complex character of ethical decision making in health care.

The tension between and among ethical principles may create dilemmas for clinicians when their obligations are in conflict. Ethical dilemmas usually occur in two types of situations. In some instances, an act can be seen as both morally justified and unjustified, but the arguments supporting each position are inconclusive. This makes it difficult for the individual to determine the appropriate course of action. Many commentators have said this about abortion and assisted death, where broad-based social consensus on the ethics of each is lacking. In other instances, an individual may be required to respond to different moral imperatives, each of which is clear, but both of which cannot be discharged at the same time. For example, care professionals are required to respect and promote the autonomy of their patients *and* to protect and enhance their well-being, to provide care to those who need it *and* to be responsible stewards of limited resources, to protect patient confidentiality *and* to alert vulnerable third parties who do not know they are at risk. Resolving these dilemmas requires clinicians and ethics committees to scrutinize carefully the competing interests and obligations, identify the likely consequences of the available choices, and weigh the benefits and risks to those involved.

Let's return to Ms. Lawrence, the patient who is refusing blood transfusion. The dilemma here concerns the tension between Dr. Thomas's obligation to honor his patient's autonomous decision about blood transfusion and his obligations to prevent harm and promote her best interests by providing what he believes is the most beneficial care. On the surface, it seems that he cannot possibly meet one obligation without violating the others, yet he must act. Because both of the principles involved are so central to professional practice and the consequences in this case so profound, the goal must be to protect both Ms. Lawrence's rights and her well-being. The members of your ethics committee can function usefully in a consultative role as these issues are considered.

The first responsibility is to confirm that Ms. Lawrence is capable of making decisions about her care and to ensure that she and Dr. Thomas have clarified the clinical situation, the care goals, the therapeutic options, and their likely consequences. As discussed in chapters 2 and 3, the exercise of patient autonomy through informed consent and refusal depends on the patient's decisional capacity, the quality of the information provided by the physician, and the trust underlying the therapeutic relationship. An ethics consultation can create the opportunity for the patient and appropriate members of the care team to engage in these important discussions.

The next step is to consider the ethical issues, including Ms. Lawrence's right to make care decisions based on her goals and values, and to confirm that her refusal is the product of her deeply held religious convictions rather than coercion or misinformation about blood transfusions. The discussion should explore alternative options and resources, including nonblood therapies and transfer to other institutions that specialize in treatment without transfusion, and their relative risks and benefits. Ms. Lawrence, her family, and the clinical team must be reassured that her refusal will in no way compromise the rest of her care.

Resolving the conflict between the obligation to respect the patient's autonomy and the obligations to promote her best interest and protect her from harm will require a careful collaborative assessment of her decision making, including how she weights the benefits and burdens of the proposed treatment. While it is neither necessary nor appropriate to argue her out of her religious beliefs, the ethics consultant is obliged to be certain that her decision to forgo a life-saving intervention is informed, carefully considered, voluntary, and settled. If Ms. Lawrence genuinely believes that surviving with a blood transfusion would be morally unacceptable, then, for her, the benefits of the intervention would be significantly outweighed by the burdens of the outcome. Under those conditions, her refusal of transfusion should be honored while she receives all other appropriate care and support. In this time-consuming and exacting process, the ethics consultant is a valuable resource, providing all parties with information, ethical analysis, practical guidance, and support.

The patient's autonomy is not the only thing at stake, however. Dr. Thomas and his colleagues also bring to this situation their professional obligations and personal values. Not unreasonably, surgeons and anesthesiologists in this circumstance are likely to be very uneasy about attempting surgery under conditions that restrict their ability to provide optimal care. Even though the patient has agreed to and assumed the risks of surgery without blood transfusions, the doctors will argue that they would be knowingly putting her at what they consider unacceptable risk. Doing so would erode both their competence and professional integrity. Under these restrictive conditions, many surgeons and anesthesiologists may decline to provide care, but they cannot simply abandon the patient. Instead, they must make reasonable efforts to transfer Ms. Lawrence to colleagues or other institutions more comfortable with her limitations, agreeing to operate only if life-saving alternatives were not available.

REFERENCES

Ahronheim J, Moreno JC, Zuckerman C. 2000. *Ethics in Clinical Practice.* 2nd ed. Gaithersburg, MD: Aspen Publishers.

Annas GJ. 1991. Ethics committees: From ethical comfort to ethical cover. *Hastings Center Report* 21(3):18–21.

Arras JD, Steinbock B, London AJ. 1999. Moral reasoning in the medical context. In Arras JD, Steinbock B, eds. *Ethical Issues in Modern Medicine.* 5th ed. Mountain View, CA: Mayfield Publishing Co., pp. 1–40.

Aseltine RH, Katz MC, Holmes C. 2011. Providing medical care to diverse populations: Findings from a follow-up survey of Connecticut physicians. *Connecticut Medicine* 75(6):337–44.

Bains W. 2004. Failure rates in drug discovery and development: Will we ever get any better? *Business:* 9–18.

Beauchamp TL, Childress JF. 2001. *Principles of Biomedical Ethics.* 5th ed. New York: Oxford University Press.

Beauchamp TL, Walters L, eds. 2003. *Contemporary Issues in Bioethics.* 6th ed. Belmont, CA: Wadsworth-Thomson Learning.

Berger JT. 1998. Culture and ethnicity in clinical care. *Archives of Internal Medicine* 158:2085–90.

Blackhall LJ, Frank G, Murphy ST, Michel V, Palmer JM, Azen SP. 1999. Ethnicity and attitudes towards life sustaining technology. *Social Science & Medicine* 48:1779–89.

Boone S. 2011. A case for diversity, cultural competency and ending disparities in the 21st-century medical practice. *Connecticut Medicine* 75(6):345–46.

Childress, J. 1990. The place of autonomy in bioethics. *Hastings Center Report* 20(1):12–17.

Fletcher JC. 1991. The bioethics movement and hospital ethics committees. *Maryland Law Review* 50:859–94.

Flores G, Lin H. 2013. Trends in racial/ethnic disparities in medical and oral health, access to care, and use of services in U.S. children: Has anything changed over the years? *International Journal for Equity in Health* 12(1):1–16.

Fox E, Myers S, Pearlman RA. 2007. Ethics consultations in United States hospitals: A national survey. *American Journal of Bioethics* 7(2):13–25.

Gaylin W, Jennings, B. 2003. *The Perversion of Autonomy: The Proper Uses of Coercion and Constraints in a Liberal Society.* Washington, DC: Georgetown University Press.

Giger J, et al. 2007. American Academy of Nursing Expert Panel report: Developing cultural competence to eliminate health disparities in ethnic minorities and other vulnerable populations. *Journal of Transcultural Nursing* 18(2):95–102.

Hopp FP, Duffy SA. 2000. Racial variations in end-of-life care. *Journal of the American Geriatrics Society* 48(6):658–63.

In re Quinlan, 70 N.J. 10, 355 A.2d 647 (1976).

Joint Commission on Accreditation of Healthcare Organizations. 1999. *Comprehensive Accreditation Manual for Hospitals.* Oakbrook Terrace, IL: Joint Commission on Accreditation of Healthcare Organizations.

Jonsen AR. 1998. *The Birth of Bioethics.* New York: Oxford University Press.

Kagawa-Singer M, Blackhall LJ. 2001. Negotiating cross-cultural issues at the end of life: "You've got to go where he lives." *Journal of the American Medical Association* 286(23):2992–3001.

Lau M, Lin H, Flores G. 2012. Racial/ethnic disparities in health and health care among U.S. adolescents. *Health Services Research* 47(5):2031–59.

Leaf C. 2013. Do clinical trials work? *The New York Times Sunday Review*, July 13.

Levine RJ. 2003. Informed consent: Some challenges to the universal validity of the Western world. In Beauchamp TL, Walters L, eds. *Contemporary Issues in Bioethics.* 6th ed. Belmont, CA: Wadsworth-Thomson Learning, pp. 150–55.

Lo B. 2000. *Resolving Ethical Dilemmas: A Guide for Clinicians.* 2nd ed. Philadelphia: Lippincott Williams & Wilkins, pp. 140–46.

Major B, Mendes WB, Dovidio JF. 2013. Intergroup relations and health disparities: A social psychological perspective. *Health Psychology* 32(5):514–24.

Mappes TA, Degrazia D. 2001. *Biomedical Ethics.* 5th ed. Boston: McGraw-Hill, pp. 1–55.

May L, Hua L, Glenn F. 2012. Racial/ethnic disparities in health and health care among US adolescents. *Health Services Research* 47(5):2031–59.

Miller B. 1995. Autonomy and the refusal of life-sustaining treatment. In Arras JD, Steinbock B, eds. *Ethical Issues in Modern Medicine.* 4th ed. Mountain View, CA: Mayfield Publishing Co., pp. 202–11.

Moreno JD. 1995. *Deciding Together: Bioethics and Moral Consensus.* New York: Oxford University Press.

Moreno JD. 1998. Ethics committees and ethics consultants. In Kuhse H, Singer P, eds. *A Companion to Bioethics.* Malden, MA: Blackwell Publishers, pp. 475–84.

Morrison RS, Meier DE. 2004. High rates of advance care planning in New York City's elderly population. *Archives of Internal Medicine* 164(22):2421–26.

Morrison RS, Zayas LH, Mulvihill M, Baskin SA, Meier DE. 1998. Barriers to completion of health care proxies: An examination of ethnic differences. *Archives of Internal Medicine* 158(22):2493–97.

Nedelsky J. 2011. *Law's Relations: A Relational Theory of Self, Autonomy, and Law.* New York: Oxford University Press.

O'Neill O. 2002. *Autonomy and Trust in Bioethics.* Cambridge: Cambridge University Press.

Padela AI, Imran RA, Punekar BS. 2009. Emergency medical practice: Advancing cultural competence and reducing healthcare disparities. *Academic Emergency Medicine* 16(1):69–75.

Pearson SD, Sabin J, Emanuel EJ. 2003. *No Margin, No Mission: Health-Care Organizations and the Quest for Ethical Excellence.* New York: Oxford University Press.

Pellegrino ED. 1992. Intersections of Western biomedical ethics and world culture. In Pellegrino ED, Mazzarella P, Corsi P, eds. *Transcultural Dimensions in Medical Ethics.* Frederick, MD: University Publishing Group.

Pope TM. 2011. Legal briefing: Healthcare ethics committees. *Journal of Clinical Ethics* 22(1):74–93.

Post LF, Blustein J, Gordon E, Dubler NN. 1996. Pain: Ethics, culture, and informed consent to relief. *Journal of Law, Medicine & Ethics* 24:348–59.

Powell T, Lowenstein B. 1996. Refusing life-sustaining treatment after catastrophic injury: Ethical implications. *Journal of Law, Medicine & Ethics* 24:54–61.

Protection of Human Subjects, 45 CFR 47.107; see also 45 CFR 46.112 (1990).

Rosner F. 1985. Hospital medical ethics committees: A review of their development. *Journal of the American Medical Association* 253(18):2693–97.

Ross JW, Glaser JW, Rasinski-Gregory D, Gibson JM, Bayley C. 1993. *Health Care Ethics Committees: The Next Generation.* Chicago: American Hospital Publishing.

Ross JW, Michel V, Pugh D. 1986. *Handbook for Hospital Ethics Committees.* Chicago: American Hospital Publishing.

Rothman DJ. 1991. *Strangers at the Bedside: A History of How Law and Bioethics Transformed Medical Decision Making.* New York: Basic Books.

Schneider CE. 1998. *The Practice of Autonomy: Patients, Doctors, and Medical Decisions.* New York: Oxford University Press.

Shepardson LB, Gordon HS, Ibrahim SA, Harper DL, Rosenthal GE. 1999. Racial variation in the use of do-not-resuscitate orders. *Journal of General Internal Medicine* 14(1):15–20.

Solomon MZ. 2005. Realizing bioethics goals in practice: Ten ways "is" can help "ought." *Hastings Center Report* 35:40–47.

Sorkin DH, Ngo-Metzger Q, DeAlba I. 2010. Racial/ethnic discrimination in health care: Impact on perceived quality of care. *Journal of General Internal Medicine* 25(5):390–96.

Spencer EM, Mills AE, Rorty MV, Werhane PH. 2000. *Organization Ethics in Health Care.* New York: Oxford University Press.

Takala T. 2007. Concepts of "person" and "liberty," and their implications to our fading notions of autonomy. *Journal of Medical Ethics* 33(4):225–28.

Teel K. 1975. The physician's dilemma: A doctor's view. What the law should be. *Baylor Law Review* 27:6–9.

Thomasma DC. 1993. Assessing bioethics today. *Cambridge Quarterly of Healthcare Ethics* 2:519–27.

Thomasma DC, Monagle JF. 1998. Hospital ethics committees: Roles, membership, structure, and difficulties. In Monagle JF, Thomasma DC, eds. *Health Care Ethics: Critical Issues for the 21st Century.* Gaithersburg, MD: Aspen Publishers, pp. 460–70.

Toulmin S. 1981. The tyranny of principles. *Hastings Center Report*: 31–39.

Wear S, Katz P, Andrzejewski B, Haryadi T. 1990. The development of an ethics consultation service. *HEC Forum* 2:75–87.

Wolf SM. 1991. Ethics committees and due process: Nesting rights in a community of caring. *Maryland Law Review* 50:798–858.

CHAPTER 2

Decision Making and Decisional Capacity in Adults

Health care decisions and decision making
Decision-making capacity
Assessment and determination of capacity
Deciding for patients without capacity

Mrs. Klein is an 89-year-old woman admitted from home 5 days ago with cellulitis of the legs. Despite her discomfort, she has cooperated with her diagnostic work-up and treatment and consented to all interventions related to the cellulitis. She was able to provide accurate information about her medical history, which was corroborated by her niece. According to both women, Mrs. Klein has been very healthy and self-sufficient all her life, a state she attributes largely to "keeping my distance from doctors and hospitals." Her goal, expressed repeatedly since admission, is "to go home to my cats."

Mrs. Klein's admission blood tests revealed anemia that suggests slow internal bleeding. Despite repeated attempts to explain the dangers of unchecked bleeding and the importance of identifying the source, she has consistently refused consent for a GI series. When asked why she is opposed to a diagnostic work-up, she replies, "Darling, you look, you'll find. No more tests or treatments. Just get me back on my feet so I can go home to my cats."

After several days, the attending physician requests a psychiatric consult to do a capacity assessment, suggesting that the patient is not capable of making decisions in her best interest and cannot be discharged under these circumstances.

Why does no one question Mrs. Klein's capacity to consent to treatment, only her capacity to refuse?

We now embark on a discussion of one of the issues most frequently brought to ethics committee attention—who is morally authorized to make health care decisions for a patient. Ethical principles of respect for patient autonomy, beneficence, and nonmaleficence normally require that decisions about care and treatment be made by the decisionally capable patient and honored by her caretakers, following adequate discussion of the benefits, burdens, and risks of the therapeutic options. When the patient is not able to participate in this process, the responsibility for making care decisions must be assumed by others.

The quality of the decision-making process and the moral validity of the resulting consent or refusal are dependent on the clarity of physician-patient communications;

the patient's understanding of the information presented and her ability to give due weight to this information in making a decision; the physician's attention to patient values and preferences; and the patient's trust in the physician that encourages questions and full discussion. Although decisional capacity is required for morally valid consent, and capacity and consent are inextricably linked, for logistical purposes they are discussed separately in this curriculum. This chapter examines decision making and capacity, while chapter 3 sets out the ethical basis and significance of the consent process.

HEALTH CARE DECISIONS AND DECISION MAKING

Health care in general and bioethics in particular deal with decisions requiring attention to patient needs and preferences in the context of medicine's capabilities and limitations. These decisions involve deeply personal ideas about life and death; the meaning of health, illness, and disability; and the importance of self-image, self-determination, and trust. While the patient has the greatest stake in these decisions, and so should be the ultimate decision maker, others, including family members and care professionals, bring their perceptions and concerns to the discussion and influence the patient's assessment of information. Indeed, it is the value- and interest-based nature of care decisions, and the multiple parties who have a stake in them, that makes these decisions so complex and often difficult to negotiate.

DECISION-MAKING CAPACITY

It is tempting to suggest that, like obscenity, decisional capacity is something that cannot be precisely defined but we know it when we see it. While we may sense that a patient is or is not able to make decisions, intuition is not enough to guide an evaluation with such crucial implications. In the health care setting, the exercise of autonomy is promoted or hindered by the assessment of decisional capacity, which effectively includes or excludes patients from making decisions about their care. Determining the patient's ability to understand the issues, consider the consequences of different options, and communicate these thoughts to professionals is necessary to supporting autonomy. Without this set of cognitive capacities, patients will need assistance in making and articulating choices, or others must decide for them. Indeed, as noted below, even capable patients can benefit from assistance in making autonomous decisions.

Here, it may be useful to distinguish the principle of respect for *autonomy* from another with which it is often elided, the principle of respect for *personhood*. We ought to respect the personhood of all patients, regardless of their ability to make capable decisions, and this includes newborns, people with profound cognitive impairment, and patients who are comatose. But, they cannot, nor do we expect them to, make autonomous decisions because autonomy is a product of maturity, values, information, experience, and judgment. If a 5-year-old insists that he doesn't want to be vaccinated, and he's very sincere about this, no one should mistake his statement as expressing an autonomous decision. Someone will vaccinate him over his very vigorous objections because we care about him and don't want him to be the victim of his own non-autonomous choice. Excluding a decisionally capable patient from making choices violates the principle of respect for patient autonomy; treating an incapacitated patient "as if" he were capable makes him vulnerable to the consequences of deficient decision making. Thus, the importance of the clinical assessment of decisional capacity is chiefly explained by its relationship to safeguarding and supporting the autonomy of patients. This assessment is critical to determining whether the patient can participate in care decisions and provide informed consent or refusal.

Capacity and Competence

Although the terms *capacity* and *competence* are often used interchangeably, in the health care setting there are important distinctions that go beyond semantics. Competence is a *legal* presumption that a person who has reached the age of majority has the requisite cognition and judgment to negotiate *legal* tasks, such as entering into a contract, making a will, or standing for trial. Incompetence is a functional assessment and determination by a court that, because the individual lacks this ability, she should not be permitted to do certain things. Because the legal system is and should rarely be involved in medical decisions, in a clinical context it is customary to refer to the patient's decisional capacity, a *clinical* determination of the ability to make decisions about *treatment* or *health care*.

Elements of Decisional Capacity

Decisional capacity refers to the patient's ability to perform a set of cognitive tasks, including

- understanding and processing information about diagnosis, prognosis, and treatment options;
- weighing the relative benefits, burdens, and risks of the therapeutic options;
- applying a set of values to the analysis;
- arriving at a decision that is consistent over time; and
- communicating the decision.

Decisional capacity thus encompasses several skills, including understanding, assessing, valuing, reasoning, and articulating the factors relevant to a choice. Capacity can be seen as an index of a person's *ability* to exercise autonomy by making decisions that reflect personal preferences, values, and judgments at a given time. This is not the same, however, as the person's *willingness* to make autonomous decisions. Having capacity *enables* but does not *obligate* patients to act independently. Despite our good intentions, we cannot force people who are unwilling to exercise their capacity for self-determination to do so. In many instances, insisting that patients make decisions when they are unwilling to do so is a form of patient abandonment that may be psychologically harmful and medically counterproductive.

Frequently, capacitated patients look to family, friends, and trusted others to help them exercise autonomous decision making. Patients demonstrate *supported* autonomy when they rely on others for advice in making choices ("I want my son to help make the decision"). Some patients, especially those who are elderly or from cultures in which self-determination is not a central value, demonstrate *delegated* autonomy. These patients often entrust to others the authority to make decisions on their behalf ("Talk to my daughter and do whatever she thinks is right"). Here, autonomy is expressed in the voluntary choice to delegate rather than independently exercise decision-making authority. Patients with capacity who benefit from the advice, guidance, and support of clinicians and trusted others can be said to demonstrate *assisted* autonomy.

The take-away message is that patients bring to the clinical setting the decision-making dynamics they are accustomed to using and these should not be overridden in the belief that there is one and only one morally proper way for decisions about their care to be made. Rather than insisting on the necessity of independent decision making, patient-centered care planning recognizes and supports the decision-making strategies that most effectively promote each patient's interests, choices, and abilities. The ethics committee can perform a useful service by clarifying for the care team—through clinical consultations, in-service presentations, or informal conversations—the several ways in which patients can make autonomous decisions.

Decision-Specific and Fluctuating Capacity

Capacity is not global, but decision-specific, referring to the ability to make *particular* decisions. A patient may have the ability to decide what to have for lunch but may be incapable of weighing the pros and cons of surgery. For this reason, nothing is less helpful than a chart note that says, "Patient lacks capacity to make decisions." The misleading implication is that the patient lacks the capacity to make *all* decisions, effectively excluding her from making *any* decisions.

In fact, many patients have the capacity to make some decisions and not others. For example, a lower level of capacity is required to appoint a health care proxy agent (appreciation of the likelihood that someone will have to make decisions on her behalf and consistent designation of the same person) than to make the often complex decisions the proxy agent will eventually make. Thus, the appropriate response to the question, "Does this patient have capacity?" is "For what decision?" Likewise, a request for a capacity assessment is most helpful when it specifies the decision(s) at issue, such as "Please evaluate the patient's capacity to make decisions about discharge." Distinguishing among the specific decisions facing the patient and assessing her capacity to make them offers her the opportunity to make the widest range of choices within her ability.

Just as capacity is not global in its application to all decisions, it is not always constant. Depending on their age, cognitive abilities, clinical condition, and treatment regimen, patients may exhibit fluctuating capacity, demonstrating greater ability to make decisions at some times than others. For example, elderly patients, who are especially prone to "sundowning," often exhibit greater alertness, sharper reasoning, and clearer communication earlier in the day. Recognizing this tendency allows care providers to approach patients for discussion and decisions when they are at their most capacitated, thereby increasing their opportunities for autonomous action. Ethics committees in long-term care facilities, where decisional capacity issues arise regularly, can be very helpful to care teams balancing the relevant interests and obligations.

To return to the case of Mrs. Klein, the 89-year-old patient with cellulitis of the legs, a critical threshold question is whether, in making a decision to refuse the diagnostic work-up and return to her home against medical advice, the patient is demonstrating decisional capacity. If she appreciates the implications and accepts the consequences of her decision and if, moreover, her decision is a voluntary one, it should be honored, despite the caregivers' concerns that it is not in her best interest. Nevertheless, efforts to persuade her to reconsider and consent to suggested treatments are still appropriate, especially if the potential risks of nontreatment and the benefits of treatment are significant. In this way, her caregivers seek to honor their professional obligations of beneficence and nonmaleficence, as well as respecting her autonomy.

Disagreement with medical recommendations is not by itself evidence of a lack of decisional capacity. Mrs. Klein's decision may be foolish and ill advised, but it is not necessarily the product of misunderstanding, delusion, or confusion. Continued discussion will be necessary to confirm her understanding and the consistency of her decision with characteristic behavior and prior choices. She has led an independent life that she attributes partly to avoiding doctors and hospitals. Her present decision to refuse the work-up, therefore, conforms to a pattern of life choices that, until now, have served her relatively well.

Practitioners and health care institutions have an ethical and legal obligation to arrange for a safe discharge for their patients. Ethical concerns arise when capable patients make decisions that run counter to their best medical interests. Here, clinicians' obligations to respect patient autonomy are in tension with their obligation to promote Mrs. Klein's well-being and protect her from harm.

One way to address these conflicting obligations is to ensure that, when capable patients are discharged, especially under less-than-optimal circumstances, they are encouraged to accept appropriate nursing and other home care services. In contrast, allowing patients who lack capacity to elect an unsafe discharge is a form of patient abandonment. Whatever the patient's level of decisional capacity, concerned family or other supporters should be encouraged to participate in discharge planning, follow-up care, and advance care planning for future health care decision making. Involving Mrs. Klein's niece in discussions and decisions would bring the security, support, and perspective of a trusted person to the deliberations.

Intervention by the ethics consultation service or ethics committee is often requested in cases of uncertain patient capacity, usually when questions arise about consent to or refusal of recommended treatment. These issues and the role of ethics intervention in resolving them are discussed further in chapter 3.

ASSESSMENT AND DETERMINATION OF CAPACITY

Mr. Herbert is back again. He is a 38-year-old man who is confined to a wheelchair because of bilateral amputations resulting from untreated leg ulcers. Mr. Herbert has had multiple admissions to treat his repeatedly infected areas of skin breakdown. Once the wounds have been cleaned and repaired and the infection is under control, however, he signs himself out against medical advice (AMA) to return to his fifth-floor walk-up apartment, where he has a thriving business dealing street drugs. He insists that, with his buddies to carry him up and down and his girlfriend to help him with meals and activities of daily living (ADLs), he can manage just fine. He acknowledges that his recovery might be better if he remained in the hospital longer or if he came to the clinic regularly but, if he is not home, his business will be picked up by other dealers. He insists that he is willing to risk future infections, although he is confident that "you guys will always get me back on my game." Nevertheless, each time he returns, he is in worse shape and it is harder to resolve his medical problems.

The Importance of Determining Capacity

Decisional capacity requires more than the ability to articulate choices. As discussed in chapter 5, young children can be very vocal and sincere in expressing their wishes, but their choices would not be considered thoughtful judgments. The exercise of autonomy and the integrity of the informed consent process depend on the patient's ability to understand the facts and appreciate the consequences of treatment options. The presumption is that adult patients have the requisite capacity and, absent contrary evidence, decisions about treatment and nontreatment defer to patient preferences. Moreover, this deference usually extends to all capacitated decisions, including those that providers may think reflect poor judgment or are not in the patient's best interest. Yet troubling and potentially harmful decisions, such as patient rejection of recommended care, must be carefully explored because they may well reflect misunderstanding, lack of trust, or extreme fear and anxiety.

Mrs. Rodriguez is a 69-year-old woman transferred from a nursing home in a semi-comatose state and respiratory failure. She was admitted to the intensive care unit (ICU) and intubated to provide ventilatory support. Her multiple medical problems include congestive heart failure, non-insulin-dependent diabetes, and several prior episodes of pneumonia.

After several weeks, the care team recognized that Mrs. Rodriguez would not be able to breathe without ventilatory assistance and recommended that a tracheostomy be done to promote safety and comfort. Because she was still unresponsive, the procedure was explained to her daughter, who provided consent. The following day, Mrs. Rodriguez unexpectedly became more alert and responsive. The critical care resident expressed concern because he believed the patient was indicating opposition to the tracheotomy.

The ear, nose, and throat (ENT) attending argued that the endotracheal tube made it impossible to determine what, if anything, the patient was trying to communicate and, in any event, she did not have the capacity to make decisions about her care. He insisted that the trach, which would be in the patient's best interest, be performed in accordance with the daughter's consent. The critical care attending asked Mrs. Rodriguez a series of yes-no questions that she could answer by nodding or shaking her head. Her nonverbal but consistent responses, which indicated that she understood the purpose of the tracheostomy and agreed that it should be performed, were considered a ratification of the consent provided by her daughter.

Would Mrs. Rodriguez's capacity have been considered sufficient for her to consent to the tracheostomy without her daughter's involvement? Why might a higher level of capacity be required for her to refuse the procedure?

One widely used strategy for approaching decisional capacity employs a sliding scale, which weighs the required level of capacity against the seriousness of the decision. This takes a flexible approach to capacity assessment. As the risks associated with a decision increase, and as these are not offset by the likelihood of greater benefits, the level of capacity needed for the decision to be honored should also increase. For example, a decision about whether to go to physical therapy before or after lunch carries a low risk of harm. This decision could safely be made by a patient with diminished capacity because the consequences of either choice are relatively benign. In contrast, a decision about whether to undergo a life-saving amputation or enroll in an experimental trial of chemotherapy, requires that a higher and stricter capacity threshold be met. Asking a patient with uncertain capacity to take responsibility for a choice this serious would abandon her to the consequences of her deficient decisional ability. Clinically, the sliding scale provides heightened scrutiny when the potential outcomes of decisions require clinicians to be confident that patients fully appreciate the benefits, burdens, and risks of their choices. Mrs. Rodriguez's low level of capacity was considered sufficient to ratify her daughter's consent because she concurred with the plan her care professionals and family agreed would benefit her. If she had refused the recommended procedure, however, it is likely that further assessment of her decisional capacity would have been indicated.

The danger in the sliding scale approach is that of paternalism, the tendency to treat otherwise capable adults as though they were children in need of others to make decisions for them. While it is not necessary that the family and care team agree with the patient's decision, choices considered irrational or harmful to the patient are likely to be challenged or at least closely scrutinized to protect incapable and, therefore, vulnerable patients from making decisions not in their best interest.

The fact is, we only question the capacity of people who do not agree with us. Think about it—when was the last time you saw a capacity consult called to evaluate a patient who had just agreed with the doctor? It is equally important, however, to beware of agreement. If the patient is nodding enthusiastically during discussion, it may signify that he understands and endorses what is being said or it may just mean that he wants to be agreeable. Not uncommonly, a patient who has nodded and said, "Uh huh" during an informed consent discussion turns to the nurse after the doctor has left and asks, "What did he say?"

Capacity assessments require a conscious effort to look beyond the decision we would make for ourselves or even recommend for the patient. If we focus exclusively on the *content* or the *outcome* of the decision rather than the decision-making *process*, we risk disempowering capable people who make risky or idiosyncratic choices. An important safeguard against this is assessing *how* the decision is made, evaluating the patient's ability to manage the several skills required for capable decision making. Likewise, it is necessary to distinguish *questioning capacity* and *finding incapacity*. While treatment refusals or other questionable decisions may and often should *trigger* a capacity assessment, they do not automatically *confirm* incapacity.

How and by Whom Is Decisional Capacity Assessed?

Especially because the elder population is expected to double during the next 20 years, capacity assessments are likely to be requested and relied on with increasing frequency. Given the importance of assessing decision-making capacity, the desire for a precise method of measurement is understandable. Unfortunately, it is not that simple. Decisional capacity is an index of patient ability to make decisions and, therefore, involves cognitive processes. Nevertheless, its assessment requires more than a test of mental acuity or a psychiatric exam.

In the search for a reliable and easily administered method of determining capacity, various instruments have been developed and tested, with varying results. Ideally, an instrument would be accurate and consistent in evaluating capacity, as well as efficient and uncomplicated to use. Predictably, most scales fail to meet both sets of criteria. For example, the Mini Mental Status Exam (MMSE), designed to assess cognition, is often employed by clinicians to evaluate capacity. While the MMSE has been found useful in gauging "orientation of the subject to person, place, and time, attention span, immediate recall, short-term and long-term memory, ability to perform simple calculations, and language skills" (Lo 2000, pp. 84–85), it is less helpful in assessing an individual's ability to grasp situations, weigh alternatives, and appreciate consequences—the skills required for capable decision making. At best, very high and low MMSE scores have been found to correlate highly with decisional capacity, making the test most useful as a screening tool rather than a predictor in capacity assessment.

A comprehensive review of several additional capacity assessment instruments (Racine and Billick 2012) concluded that sensitivity and specificity tend to be in tension with efficiency and ease of use. Some can be administered in less than 30 minutes but may be more general, while others, which are more specific and in-depth, require considerably more time and complicated scoring systems. While none of the instruments is considered to be the gold standard, the literature indicates that their use in clinical practice could improve accuracy in capacity determination. Especially in the elder population, where capacity issues may be complex and multifactorial, these tools may be useful adjuncts to clinical interviews, medical record reviews, interviews, neuropsychological testing, and functional assessment.

Calling for a "psych consult" to assess capacity may sometimes be helpful in assessing decisional capacity, but it is not always necessary or sufficient. To be sure, psychiatric intervention can be invaluable in engaging patients in discussion; eliciting and interpreting their concerns; and identifying mental illness, cognitive impairments, and interpersonal conflicts that can mask or interfere with decisional capacity. Even a skillful psychiatric consultation, however, captures only a snapshot of the patient's thinking at a specific moment rather than over time.

Ultimately, the clinicians who observe and interact with the patient day to day—especially attending physicians, nurses, residents, as well as medical and nursing students—may be in a better position to evaluate the quality and consistency of the patient's decision-making ability, particularly if they are assisted by reliable and accurate capacity assessment tools. This is especially important in nursing homes, psychiatric hospitals, and facilities for those with developmental delays, where long-term patients and residents are well known to the care team. For this reason, assessing decisional capacity should be considered part of the clinical skill set of care professionals and the responsibility of the medical team. Reinforcing this aspect of the caregiver role can be a valuable ethics committee function in all care-providing facilities, especially those in which decisional capacity assessment is frequently requested.

DECIDING FOR PATIENTS WITHOUT CAPACITY

Usually, health care decisions are made by capable patients with the advice and support of their caregivers, families, and friends. Frequently, however, treatment decisions must be made for patients who lack the capacity to make decisions for themselves. These may be persons who were formerly but are no longer capacitated because of illness, injury, age, or other factors. Or they may be patients, such as newborns and those with profound cognitive impairment, who have never had or have not yet had an opportunity to form values or preferences.

Making medical decisions for others raises a series of questions involving the patient's clinical needs and treatment options, what is known of the patient's care wishes, and the appropriate delegation of decision-making authority. Answering these difficult questions is often complicated by disagreements between and among the patient's family and care providers. Mediating these conflicts and facilitating decision making for incapacitated patients are among the most frequent and effective interventions by health care ethics committee and ethics consultation services. The theory and skills important to clinical consultation are discussed at greater length in chapter 14.

Standards of Surrogate Decision Making

The standards of health care decision making typically rely on the patient's voice as the central and most authentic source. When that voice is temporarily or permanently unavailable, those who act on behalf of the patient have only indirect access to her wishes and values. Three standards are customarily invoked in attempting to make decisions as the patient would have made them. They vary according to how much direct information the surrogate has from the patient.

- Prior explicit articulation, possibly in the form of an instructional advance directive or a recalled explicit conversation, is the previous expression of a capacitated person's wishes, the most reliable information about her preferences. "*What do we know* about this person's wishes based on what she has said or written?"

- Substituted judgment is a decision by others based on the formerly capacitated person's inferred wishes or preferences. "What can we *infer* about what *the patient* would choose in these circumstances, based on what we know about her past behavior, values, and prior decisions?" Substituted judgment is commonly thought of as a way to respect the value of patient self-determination, using a constellation of durable and characteristic cues rather than explicit communication as guidance.
- Best interest standard is used to arrive at a judgment based on what a reasonable person in the patient's situation would want. This standard is invoked when the incapacitated person never had or made known treatment wishes and her preferences cannot be inferred. Others weigh the benefits and burdens to the patient of a proposed intervention or care plan. "*What do we believe* would best promote this person's well-being in these circumstances?"

According to the standard approach, a patient's verbal or written statements of preference reflect autonomous decisions and should be honored whenever feasible, but they may be interpreted in the light of current circumstances that the patient may not have been able to anticipate. There is also consensus that the substituted judgment standard is the most problematic because, as commonly formulated, it requires the intellectually convoluted task of imagining what the now-incapacitated patient would choose if she were magically capable and in possession of all the relevant clinical facts. This has led some commentators to adopt an interpretation of the substituted judgment standard that focuses on a notion of *authenticity* rather than self-determination. Authenticity expresses the value of having one's life be a coherent narrative, and surrogate decisions guided by this value seek to maintain the coherence of the patient's life through the decisions that are made on her behalf, rather than to honor her hypothetical choices (Dworkin 1993; Blustein 1999; Brudney 2009).

Surrogate decision making is a complex process that requires attending to and balancing a number of different factors, and it may not be entirely clear what the surrogate should choose on the patient's behalf. Surrogate decision making is often a weighty moral responsibility because it happens under conditions of uncertainty and has serious, possibly life-altering, consequences for the patient. Yet decisions must be made and these standards, conscientiously applied, can help surrogates identify the care plan that will most effectively and authentically promote the interests of the incapacitated patient.

Decision Making for the Formerly Capacitated

The notion that only the explicit statement of a capable patient can inform treatment decisions has proved to be double-edged—both a protection of the patient's right to consent or refuse and a barrier to decision making when the patient has lost the capacity to make decisions. Among the clinical setting's greatest challenges is the patient who was formerly but is no longer capable and communicative, making it difficult to determine or honor her wishes or to promote authenticity. In this category are the elderly demented and patients of any age with terminal illness or irreversible injury that has impaired their decision-making ability. In order to protect the interests of the formerly capacitated, reliance on some type of advance directive has become the preferred method of surrogate decision making.

Advance Directives

Mrs. Stern is a 74-year-old woman admitted from home for surgical repair of a hip fracture. Although she is in the early stages of dementia and has mild coronary artery disease, she has been healthy and fairly independent until her recent fall. She has lived alone since her husband's death three years ago, but her daughter, Mrs. Keller, lives nearby and they either visit or speak daily.

On admission, despite her considerable discomfort, Mrs. Stern was alert, understood her medical condition, and was able to provide consent for the surgery. During the postoperative period, however, she has been increasingly agitated and confused. When recent blood tests indicated anemia, she was unable to discuss the need for a transfusion. She asked that the doctors talk to her daughter, who provided the necessary consent.

Mrs. Stern is scheduled to be discharged to a nursing home for rehabilitation in preparation for her eventual return home. She is expected to make a good recovery from her surgery and should be able to resume her normal activities with some assistance. Her doctors anticipate that, once she is in familiar surroundings, she will be less agitated and confused. Because her dementia is likely to progress, however, she will find it increasingly difficult to make independent decisions, including those related to her health care. For that reason, the care team is encouraging the execution of an advance directive that will enable care decisions to be made on her behalf when she is no longer able to make them herself.

If Mrs. Stern is determined to lack the capacity to make care decisions, is she capable of executing an advance directive? Would different levels of capacity be required to execute a living will and appoint a health care proxy agent?

Advance directives are legal instruments intended to secure an individual's ability to set out prospective instructions regarding health care. Conceived during the 1970s, they responded to the concern that patients who were unable to speak for themselves might be subjected to unwanted medical interventions, especially at the end of life. The 1990 federal Patient Self-Determination Act (PSDA) requires any health care facility receiving federal funds to offer patients the opportunity to execute advance directives and assistance in doing so. Although all 50 states and the District of Columbia have statutory and/or case law governing advance directives and all states honor them, their standards and restrictions differ (Olick 2012). While advance directives are helpful whenever substitute decision making is required, they are most often invoked in making decisions at the end of life. For that reason, they are discussed further in chapter 9.

Advance directives commonly come in two varieties—instruction directives, also known as living wills, and appointment directives, also known as health care proxies or powers of attorney for health care. In different ways, they provide direct expression of the patient's wishes, enabling caregivers to rely on the most immediate of the decision-making standards. The living will is a written set of value-neutral instructions about the particular medical, surgical, or diagnostic interventions the individual *does* or *does not* want under particular circumstances, usually at the end of life. The structure of the document generally has a trigger phrase, such as, "If I am ever in an irreversible coma, . . ." or "If I am ever unable to recognize or relate to my loved ones and my doctors say that I will not regain those abilities . . . ," followed by the list of instructions related to the specified circumstances.

Patient wishes may also be communicated orally when the patient is unable to execute a written document. In these instances, the patient's verbally expressed instructions can be documented by a health care provider or other individual. If properly documented and witnessed, these statements are considered formal advance directives in several states.

Because the living will presents explicit articulation of the patient's prior capacitated wishes, it can provide helpful guidance to family and clinicians about what she would or would not want in current circumstances. It is significantly limited by the fact that it is a static document, written when the person could not accurately anticipate her future medical condition. Individual beliefs and preferences change over time, and it is not unusual for patients to change their minds about medical interventions that they thought they would or would never be able to tolerate. In addition, these documents do not always mean what they say. The person whose living will says, "I don't ever want to be on a respirator" probably does not mean, "I don't want to be on a respirator for 4 hours if it gives me 10 more years on the tennis court." What she probably means is, "I don't want to live out the rest of my life on a respirator." But living wills typically do not provide for that kind of nuance. Finally, this type of advance directive usually refers only to end-of-life care. The result is a set of instructions that reflect what the patient *believed* and *tried to communicate* at a particular time about what she *thought she would want* under different circumstances at a later time. Because of their limitations, living wills are most useful for someone who does not have trusted friends or family to make decisions in the event of her incapacity.

The preferred advance directive is the appointment directive, also known as a health care proxy or a durable power of attorney for health care. This document enables a capable individual to legally appoint another person—an agent or proxy—to make health care decisions on her behalf after capacity has been lost. The agent is authorized to make any and all health care decisions the individual would make, not just those about end-of-life treatment.

The appointment directive is recommended over the instruction directive because it authorizes decision making in the event of temporary or permanent incapacity and permits greater flexibility in responding to unanticipated or rapidly changing medical conditions. The agent is generally required to honor the patient's previously expressed wishes in making care decisions. If those instructions do not apply to or are inconsistent with the patient's current health needs, however, the agent is empowered to use his knowledge of the patient's wishes, values, and decision history to exercise judgment in making choices that promote the patient's best interest. The agent has the same decisional authority as the patient and may make any and all care decisions the patient could make if capable. Moreover, the authority of the agent supersedes that of anyone else, including next of kin. This scope of authority presupposes a patient-proxy relationship characterized by trust, familiarity with the patient's wishes and values, and the agent's willingness to exercise judgment and make hard decisions in the patient's interest.

There are two important but often misunderstood conditions that your ethics committee can usefully reinforce with your clinicians: (1) As noted earlier, patients deemed incapable of making medical decisions may still have the capacity to appoint an agent to assume this responsibility. (2) The term *power of attorney* (POA), when applied to advance directives can cause confusion. Powers of attorney are the delegation of authority for specified tasks. Not uncommonly, a well-meaning person will show up in the clinical setting, clutching a document and saying, "I'm the POA so I'm responsible for making decisions." Encourage the staff to read the document. Very often, it will be a POA for banking or real estate or some other nonmedical responsibilities. Unless the document includes "health care decisions" or other similar language, the document should be returned to the person with the explanation that the delegated powers do not include health care decision making.

A hybrid advance directive, Five Wishes, provides the opportunity to communicate decisions about (1) the person I want to make care decisions for me when I can't; (2) the kind of medical treatment I want or don't want; (3) how comfortable I want to be; (4) how I want people to treat me; and (5) what I want my loved ones to know. For many people, this frames the issues in an accessible and nonthreatening way. Five Wishes is currently recognized in 42 states (Five Wishes, Aging with Dignity 2013).

Advance directives are statements of patient intention about health care, not medical orders. These statements must be translated by physicians into medical orders in the patient's medical record before they become operational. Thus, an advance directive that says, "If I am ever terminally ill or permanently unconscious and my doctors do not expect my condition to improve, I do not want resuscitation attempted if my heart stops," will require the patient's physicians to determine whether she meets the specified clinical criteria. Only under clinically appropriate circumstances may a do-not-resuscitate (DNR) order be entered in the medical record, which will preclude cardiopulmonary resuscitation.

Mrs. Stern is a good example of a patient who lacks the capacity to make health care decisions, yet is capable of appointing a trusted person to make decisions for her. Her current illness and hospitalization have exacerbated the agitation and confusion of her early-stage dementia, making it difficult or impossible for her to understand and decide about her medical treatment adequately. Moreover, she does not want to assume this responsibility, preferring to delegate decision-making authority to her daughter. Thus, while she may not have the capacity to make decisions about her current treatment or articulate instructions about future care, she does understand the notion that someone will have to make decisions for her and she consistently designates the same trusted person for that task, meeting the criteria for appointing a health care agent.

Deciding for Patients without Capacity or Advance Directives

Advance directives appear to provide all the authorization and safeguards necessary to communicate and implement prior care wishes effectively. You might reasonably think that every capable person would have one. Unfortunately, you would be wrong. Even though people are encouraged to express their health care preferences prospectively through the designation of a health care agent or the execution of a living will, only one-third of adults in the United States have an advance directive (American Bar Association Commission on Law and Aging 2014). Thus, decisions for most patients who lack capacity are made by unofficial or informal surrogates—people who assume the decision-making role without specific legal appointment or the guidance of documented patient wishes. In some states, a surrogate's authority to make health care decisions for someone else may be based on statutory or case law. More often, an informal surrogate is asked by the medical team to participate in making treatment decisions. The people who fill this void and act on behalf of incapacitated patients include family, close friends, and trusted others. Many states have approved hierarchies, setting out potential surrogates in order of their relationship to the patient, providing guidance to staff working to identify an appropriate surrogate decision maker. A sample policy in chapter 17 includes such a framework. In the absence of unofficial surrogates, care providers and courts, which are essentially strangers to the patient, may assume this responsibility.

Without the patient's explicit instructions in an advance directive, health care decisions made by surrogates have traditionally been based on the remaining two decision-making standards—either substituted judgment (when the patient's wishes can be inferred) or the best interest standard (when the patient did not have or did not articulate treatment preferences). Clinicians and families of patients unable to participate in care discussions or decisions work to determine a course that meets medical, legal, and ethical imperatives.

Goals and plans of care are considered in light of the patient's condition and prognosis; the benefits, burdens, and risks of the therapeutic options; and what is known about her wishes or best interests. Depending on the laws of the state in which the patient is treated, family and trusted others may have greater or lesser latitude in drawing on their knowledge of and concern for the patient in making decisions on her behalf. In helping to guide substitute decision making, ethics committees and consultants need to be familiar with the scope of authority that their states accord informal surrogates.

Decision Making for Patients Who Never Had Capacity

Those who never had the opportunity or ability to form values or preferences include newborns and adults with severe cognitive impairment. As discussed in chapter 5, decisions for the endangered or profoundly disabled newborn are almost always made by the parents who are presumed, by tradition and law, to act in the best interests of their child. However, the child's health care providers may disagree with the parents' decisions, favoring either less or more aggressive life-sustaining treatment, as the case may be. Whenever possible, these disagreements should be mediated without court involvement, but that is not always feasible. Courts tend to override parental refusals of specific life-saving interventions, especially if the child can be returned to reasonable health.

Adults with profound cognitive impairment, much like infants and young children, are considered to need decision making by others because they are and have always been incapable of reasoned judgment. As in the case of salvageable newborns, courts tend to overrule requests to withhold or terminate beneficial treatment.

Addressing the needs of never-capacitated patients does not raise the question, "What would this person want in these circumstances?" Sometimes, in an attempt to represent the patient's interests, care providers and surrogates create what amounts to a fiction of substituted judgment. For example, they might ask, "What would this imperiled newborn or profoundly impaired adult want if he could want anything?" Careful review of the decision-making standards reveals the fallacy in this approach. Precisely because this patient has no history of expressed preferences or known values that would permit inference about his wishes, substituted judgments cannot be made. Rather, decisions on his behalf must be based on the best interest standard, drawing on what *others* believe would be best for him.

In these instances, the analysis is based on the objective assessment of what would be most likely to benefit or promote the well-being of a generalized patient in the same circumstances, similar to the legal reasonable person standard discussed in chapter 3. In the clinical setting, the best interest standard might consider mitigating pain and suffering, prolonging life, restoring and enhancing comfort, and maximizing the potential for independent functioning.

REFERENCES

American Bar Association Commission on Law and Aging. 2014. Myths and facts about health care advance directives, www.americanbar.org/content/dam/aba/administra tive/law_aging/2011/2011_aging_bk_myths_factshcad.authcheckdam.pdf (accessed May 22, 2014).

American Hospital Association. 1985. *Values in Conflict: Resolving Issues in Hospital Care. Report of the Special Committee on Biomedical Ethics.* Chicago: American Hospital Association.

Beauchamp TL, Childress JF. 2001. *Principles of Biomedical Ethics.* 5th ed. New York: Oxford University Press, pp. 98–103.

Berger JT. 2005. Patients' interests in their family members' well-being: An overlooked fundamental consideration within substituted judgment. *Journal of Clinical Ethics* 16(1):3–10.

Blustein J 1999. Choosing for others as continuing a life story: The problem of personal identity revisited. *Journal of Law, Medicine & Ethics* 27:20–31.

Braun M, Moye J. 2010. Decisional capacity assessment: Optimizing safety and autonomy for older adults. *Generations* 34(2):102–5.

Breslin JM. 2005. Autonomy and the role of the family in making decisions at the end of life. *Journal of Clinical Ethics* 16(1):11–19.

Brudney D. 2009. Choosing for another: Beyond autonomy and best interest. *Hastings Center Report*: 31–37.

Buchanan AE, Brock DW. 1989. *Deciding for Others: The Ethics of Surrogate Decision Making.* Cambridge: Cambridge University Press.

DeRenzo EG, Panzarella P, Selinger S, Schwartz J. 2005. Emancipation, capacity, and the difference between law and ethics. *Journal of Clinical Ethics* 16(2):144–50.

Drane J. 1984. Competency to give an informed consent: A model for making clinical assessments. *Journal of the American Medical Association* 252(7):925–27.

Dresser R. 2009. Substituting authenticity for autonomy. *Hastings Center Report* 39(2):3.

Dworkin R. 1993. *Life's Dominion.* Cambridge, MA: Harvard University Press.

Emanuel EJ, Emanuel LL. 1992. Four models of the physician-patient relationship. *Journal of the American Medical Association* 267(16):2221–26.

Five Wishes, Aging with dignity. 2013. www.agingwithdignity.org/catalog/product_info.php?products_id=28 (accessed August 2014).

Gillick MR. 2004. Advance care planning. *New England Journal of Medicine* 350(1):7–8.

Kennedy GL. 2000. Legal and ethical issues. In *Geriatric Mental Health Care*. New York: Guilford Press, pp. 282–317.

Lo B. 1990. Assessing decision-making capacity. *Journal of Law, Medicine & Ethics* 18(3): 193–203.

Lo B. 2000. Decision-making capacity. In *Resolving Ethical Dilemmas: A Guide for Clinicians*. 2nd ed. Philadelphia: Lippincott Williams & Wilkins, pp. 80–87.

Lo B, Steinbrook R. 2004. Resuscitating advance directives. *Archives of Internal Medicine* 164:1501–6.

Mezey M, Teresi J, Ramsey G, Mitty E, Dubrowitz T. 2000. Decision-making capacity to execute a health care proxy: Development and testing of guidelines. *Journal of the American Geriatrics Society* 48(2):179–87.

Olick RS. 2012. Defining features of health care advance directives in law and clinical practice. *Chest* 141(1):232–38.

Patient Self-Determination Act, 1990. 42 U.S.C. §1395 cc(a).

Post LF. 2007. Substituted decision making. In Capezuti E, Siegler G, Mezey MD, eds. *The Encyclopedia of Elder Care*. 2nd ed. New York: Springer Publishing Co.

Post LF, Blustein J, Dubler NN. 1999. The doctor-proxy relationship: An untapped resource. *Journal of Law, Medicine & Ethics* 27:5–12.

Powell T. 2005. Voice: Cognitive impairment and medical decision making. *Journal of Clinical Ethics* 16(4):303–13.

Powell T, Lowenstein B. 1996. Refusing life-sustaining treatment after catastrophic injury: Ethical implications. *Journal of Law, Medicine & Ethics* 24:54–61.

Racine CW, Billick SB. 2012. Assessment instruments of decision-making capacity. *Journal of Psychiatry & Law* 40(2):243–63.

Sabatino CP. 2010. ABA Commission on Legal Problems of the Elderly, 5 legal myths about advance medical directives, www.abanet.org/aging/myths.html (accessed 2014).

Schneider CE. 1998. *The Practice of Autonomy: Patients, Doctors, and Medical Decisions*. New York: Oxford University Press.

Sulmasy DP, Snyder L. 2010. Substituted interests and best judgments: An integrated model of surrogate decision making. *Journal of the American Medical Association* 304(17):1946–47.

Torke AM, et al. 2008. Rethinking the ethical framework for surrogate decision making: A qualitative study of physicians. *Journal of Clinical Ethics* 19(2):110–19.

CHAPTER 3

Informed Consent and Refusal

Mrs. Stack is a 67-year-old woman admitted with rectal bleeding, chronic renal insufficiency, diabetes, and blindness. On admission, she was alert and capacitated. Two weeks later, she suffered a cardiopulmonary arrest, was resuscitated and intubated, and was transferred to the medical intensive care unit (MICU) in an unresponsive and unstable state. Consent for emergency dialysis was obtained from her son, who is also her health care agent. Dialysis was repeated two days later.

During the past several years, Mrs. Stack has consistently stated to her family and her primary care doctor that she would never want to be on chronic dialysis and she has refused it numerous times when it was recommended. The physician, who has known and treated Mrs. Stack for many years, also treated her daughter who had been on chronic dialysis for some time and had died after suffering a heart attack. According to the physician and the patient's family, Mrs. Stack's refusal of dialysis has been based on her conviction that her daughter died as a result of the dialysis treatments.

Mrs. Stack's mental status has cleared considerably and, despite the ventilator, she is able to communicate nonverbally. Although she appears to understand the benefits of dialysis and the consequences of refusing it, including deterioration and eventual death, she has consistently and vehemently refused further treatments. Her capacity to make this decision is not now in question. Her son, however, wants her to undergo dialysis and insists, "She's feisty and I just have to be tough with her. It's for her own good." He has told his mother, "If you don't have dialysis, I'll put you in a nursing home." Finally, after several extended interactions with her son, the patient reluctantly agrees to undergo dialysis. How should her consent be interpreted? What are the care team's obligations?

Let's face it—many clinicians and administrators are less interested than you are in the principle of autonomy or the concept of decisional capacity. What concerns them is the fact that, unless the patient or a surrogate can authorize treatment, the clinical process comes to a screeching halt. Ethics committee involvement is frequently requested in the hope that clarifying and allocating decisional authority will get the process moving again. This brings us to the practical application of this authority.

In the clinical setting, the doctrine of informed consent is generally justified by appeal to the principle of respect for patient autonomy; as such, it is the legal and ethical embodiment of the right to self-determination in health care. Indeed, the right to determine what is done to one's body, including the right to consent to and refuse medical treatment, is considered so fundamental that it is protected by the U.S. Constitution and state constitutions, and supported by decisions of the U.S. Supreme Court. In the informed consent process, a decisionally capable individual who understands the benefits, burdens, and risks of a proposed treatment grants explicit permission for or rejects a particular intervention.

EVOLUTION OF THE DOCTRINE OF INFORMED CONSENT

The legal doctrine of informed consent was initially based on the law of battery, holding that any unconsented-to touching, even to promote the patient's well-being, constituted an unlawful act. In time, courts came to reject the rather crude notion that consent either did or did not occur. Considered more useful was the standard of negligence, which permits a more nuanced examination of whether a physician-patient discussion revealed the risks and benefits material to the patient's decision about treatment.

By the latter part of the twentieth century, the new dynamic of more robust patient participation had introduced a somewhat adversarial tone. Some patients came to see informed consent as their offensive security against physician overreaching, while some physicians saw it as their defensive protection against charges that they provided inadequate information and an opportunity to secure liability waivers— the medical equivalent of a prenuptial agreement. As a result of liability concerns, the critical role of informed consent as the expression and protection of patient self-determination in health care decision making has been somewhat modified by its risk management function.

ELEMENTS OF INFORMED CONSENT AND REFUSAL

The basic elements of informed consent and refusal include

- patient decisional capacity;
- disclosure by physician(s) of sufficient information relevant to the decision in question;
- understanding of the disclosed information;
- voluntariness (in acting without compulsion or coercion), and, on the basis of these;
- communication of consent to or refusal of the proposed medical intervention.

Each of these elements is essential to the integrity of the process. For example, disclosing information about the proposed treatment is necessary but not sufficient unless the information is both adequate and understood. Likewise, consent that is informed but coerced is invalid.

These elements come together in the following definition: "One can confidently presume that an act is an informed consent if a patient or subject agrees to an intervention on the basis of an understanding of relevant information, the consent is not controlled by influences that engineer the outcome, and the consent given was intended to be a consent and therefore qualified as a permission for an intervention" (Beauchamp 1997, p. 185). A more elaborated formulation includes *recommendation*, the physician's obligation to go beyond mere disclosure, and *authorization*, the patient's active ratification of the consent or refusal (Beauchamp and Childress 2001, p. 80). Indeed, it may be helpful and more accurate to think in terms of *assisted* or *advised consent* as the dynamic that links the physician's disclosure and guidance with the patient's understanding and decision making.

Capacity and Consent

As discussed in chapter 2, meaningful informed consent can only be provided by patients who are capable of making a decision about accepting or refusing the proposed intervention. Consent is more than permission to treat; it can be seen as the compact by which a capable patient voluntarily entrusts his care to a clinical professional. Capacity is the set of cognitive, volitional, and affective patient abilities that makes authentic and valid consent possible, and consent authorizes the professional to enter into and maintain the care-providing compact.

Disclosure of Information

Mr. Porter is a 52-year-old man whose advanced diabetes has resulted in decreased peripheral circulation and gangrene in his lower extremities, particularly severe in his left foot. He has worked as a mail carrier for 31 years and, he says proudly, "never missed a day." According to his family, he has resisted seeking medical attention because of his fear that amputation would be recommended, a course he would unquestionably refuse.

It is clear to the surgeon that only amputation of Mr. Porter's left foot will save his life, but that aggressive deep debridement (removal of dead or diseased tissue) of his right foot might possibly prevent the spread of gangrene on that side. When she approaches the patient for consent to surgery, she says, "Mr. Porter, we need to take you to the operating room to clean away all the dead tissue on your feet. If we don't do this, the infection will continue to spread and you could die. Don't worry, we do this all the time in cases like yours."

What is the nature of the interaction? Has the surgeon met her professional obligation? What would be the quality of Mr. Porter's consent?

True informed consent is impossible unless the patient can adequately evaluate his condition and has received relevant and sufficient information about the purpose of the proposed treatment; its potential benefits, burdens, and risks; treatment alternatives; and the benefits and risks of the therapeutic options. This informational imperative gives rise to the professional obligation of disclosure. The challenge to the physician is determining *what* and *how much* information to provide, as well as how to communicate that information so that the patient understands it.

In assessing the quality of disclosure for purposes of informed consent, the courts have defined two standards—professional practice and reasonable person. A third standard—subjective—has also been advocated. These standards reflect both the legal criteria for disclosure and the underlying ethical distinctions about who determines the relevance and sufficiency of the information to be disclosed.

The traditional professional practice standard bases adequate disclosure on what the customary practice of professionals in the physician's community would deem appropriate. This standard presumes that the physician, acting in the patient's best interest, is in the best position to determine what information to provide. Because the determination lies with the physician, this standard, also known as the reasonable doctor standard, risks undercutting the patient's autonomous decision making.

In contrast, the reasonable person standard holds that disclosure should be based on what a reasonable person would consider material in making *this* decision. This standard, which has gained acceptance in more than half of the states in the United States (Beauchamp and Childress 2009), shifts the determination of what is pertinent from the physician to the patient. In so doing, it supports patient autonomy and elevates the physician's ethical obligation to respect it even over the obligations of beneficence.

The subjective standard looks at what *this* specific patient would consider material in making *this* decision. It is also possible to combine the reasonable person standard with the subjective standard by disclosing what a reasonable person would consider material to the decision, and then providing opportunity for *this* patient to ask questions of particular importance to his situation.

The core information that physicians are obligated to disclose is generally held to include

(a) the facts about the proposed diagnostic or therapeutic intervention that patients typically consider relevant in decision making, including information about the intervention and its purpose;

(b) information about the consequences of alternatives to the proposed intervention, including nontreatment; and

(c) the physician's recommendation about how the patient might consider the intervention's benefits and risks.

The point of the disclosure requirement for informed consent is that the patient's beliefs about the therapeutic interventions and their possible outcomes should be well founded. There is no simple or single formula, however, for what is necessary to make this happen in all informed consent interactions. For example, less demanding standards of disclosure may be reasonable in the context of a close and trusting doctor-patient relationship than in a relationship in which the patient and physician know little about each other (Kihlborn 2008).

Mr. Silver is a 39-year-old man with prostate cancer. Although the disease is confined to his prostate, Dr. Binder knows that, in a patient this young, the cancer is virulent and should be treated aggressively. For this reason, he strongly recommends that Mr. Silver undergo a radical prostatectomy. Mr. Silver has heard about the potential side effects of the surgery, including impotence and incontinence, and he insists that he prefers radiation.

Dr. Binder has explained that the chances of a long-term cure are 30% to 40% better with the prostatectomy and that any resulting problems can be surgically corrected later. Mr. Silver is adamant, however, saying, "Unless you can tell me that the odds are overwhelming that I will not be impotent or incontinent, I'll take my chances with the radiation." His wife has told Dr. Binder privately, "I don't care about the side effects and he'll get used to whatever happens. I just want him alive. We could have many good years ahead of us if he has the surgery."

What would be the quality of Mr. Silver's consent to the prostatectomy if he did not fully appreciate the risks? Does the physician have an obligation to Mrs. Silver that is in conflict with his obligation to his patient?

The notion of patient best interest is far from clear in this case. The conflicting potential outcomes appear to be surviving cancer with sexual and urinary dysfunction versus maintaining those functions at an increased risk of dying from cancer. Depending on their personalities, values, and notions of an acceptable quality of life, reasonable patients, families, and professionals may disagree about which option is preferable.

This case illustrates the tension between the physician's obligation to respect patient autonomy and the obligation to promote patient best interest. Because Mr. and Mrs. Silver define best interest differently, the information Dr. Binder provides will greatly influence how they think about treatment. Mrs. Silver has very real concerns about her husband's welfare and his decision will have a significant impact on her life, affecting the most intimate aspects of their relationship. She is hoping to influence her husband to make the choice that she believes will be better for both of them.

While Dr. Binder can and should try to convince his patient to choose the most beneficial option, he should not manipulate the decision process by withholding critical information. Ultimately, his obligation is to his patient, who, as a capable person, is in the best position to assess the facts and consequences according to his own values, beliefs, and goals, as long as he has the necessary information and recommendation. He can and should, however, encourage Mr. Silver to engage his wife in a thorough discussion of her concerns and the short- and long-term implications of his decision on his health and their relationship.

Understanding of Information

Because the content and process of informed consent should enhance the patient's capacity to make decisions, limiting the professional obligation to mere disclosure of facts is inadequate. In addition to the provision of appropriate information by the physician, informed consent requires that it be *understood* by the patient or surrogate decider. Thus, the obligation has not been met unless the information is presented in ways that are educationally, linguistically, and culturally accessible to the recipients, who demonstrate that they can use it to make important decisions.

Meeting this obligation requires that the physician actively determine that the patient has understood the disclosed information. Asking the patient to repeat, even in his own words, what has been said is insufficient because it tests memory alone. In contrast, "Please tell me why you have decided to (or not to) have this treatment" requires the patient to explain the reasoning behind his decision, revealing misunderstandings and unrealistic expectations that can be corrected. Finally, the patient is also entitled to the physician's clinical reasoning in the form of recommendations about the treatment options and their likely outcomes in light of the patient's goals and values.

As discussed further in chapter 4, the patient's understanding of the disclosed information is greatly enhanced if the discussion is conducted in his preferred language. Even patients who speak more than one language are likely to achieve greater understanding and security if they can use the language with which they are most comfortable. In these situations, it is important to secure the services of a trained interpreter, either in person or through a telephone language line, rather than relying on the patient's family or friends. First, those close to the patient may, consciously or unconsciously, edit or soften the information in an effort to protect the patient from distressing news or for other, less compassionate reasons. Second, it is difficult to accurately translate medical terms and concepts from English to English; the process is even more formidable when the information must traverse two languages. Lest informal translators become offended, explain that both Joint Commission standards and the policies of most care-providing institutions require the use of certified or trained interpreters to ensure completeness and accuracy.

In addition, recent work in cognitive psychology and neuroscience has shown that an individual's emotional states can affect how the information that he is given is received and processed. For example, how individuals perceive and evaluate risks associated with a particular course of action is strongly influenced by their affective reactions to the information they are given and to the person providing the information. In order to improve the quality of patient understanding, those who seek informed consent should be sensitive to the intertwined role of emotion and cognition. They should not manipulate patient emotions since this would undercut the patient's autonomy, but should take account of how emotions can enhance, as well as diminish, his decision-making capacities (Braude and Kimmelman 2012).

Voluntariness

Mr. Jenkins is a 28-year-old man with chronic renal disease who has been on hemodialysis for several years. Despite scrupulous attention to his medication, diet, and dialysis regimen, multiple complications have led to his deteriorating condition. Peritoneal dialysis has been ruled out because prior surgeries have left abdominal adhesions. At this point, his doctors believe his only chance for improvement or even survival is a kidney transplant.

Mr. Jenkins's immediate family consists of his pregnant wife and their 3-year-old son, his parents, his 26-year-old sister, and his 19-year-old brother. His parents and sister have been tissue typed and found to be incompatible as donors. His brother has said that, as much as he cares about the patient, he does not want to give up his football scholarship to college, which would be required if he had only one kidney.

At a family meeting, called to discuss options, Mr. Jenkins's parents, wife, and sister pressure his brother to be tested. After 45 minutes of "How can you be so heartless?" "What is your career compared to your brother's life?" "You're no better than a murderer!" he agrees to be typed. When he is found to be a suitable donor, he says to the physician, "Now I have no choice. I have to donate or I'll be killing my brother and my family will hate me."

Is Mr. Jenkins's consent the product of altruism, family persuasion, or coercion? Does the physician have obligations to Mr. Jenkins that are in conflict with his obligations to the patient? How might the ethical dilemma be resolved, and what might be the role of the ethics committee?

But wait, there's more to consent and refusal. Genuinely voluntary decision making is both adequately informed and free of undue influence that prevents the individual's choice from being an authentic expression of his own values and beliefs. Voluntariness refers to the individual's independence in making decisions that are the product of information, analysis, and personal values, not influenced by threat, force, or manipulation. *Independent* decision making, however, is not the same as *isolated* decision making, which would deprive the patient of physician and family recommendations and support. Problematic influences are those that subvert autonomous action by distorting individual choice through coercion or deception.

Influences with detrimental impact on the informed consent process can come from the patient's physician, family, or others in a position to exert compelling pressure. Voluntariness can be overtly sabotaged by relentless badgering, threats of family disruption, or emotional manipulation. An example would be, "Undergoing this treatment is the only way to save our marriage." Voluntariness can also be undermined when the physician says, "I won't continue to care for you if you don't do what I say."

What distinguishes morally problematic from morally acceptable influences is the manner in which the influence is exercised. As discussed in chapter 2, patients often turn to trusted others for assistance in making decisions, especially those with significant consequences. Interactions that provide additional information, insights, encouragement, and support may modify the patient's choice by enhancing his decision-making powers. If, however, the influence is the product of deception that withholds or distorts information, if it denies or diminishes choice, if it appeals to fear rather than reason, even if this is not the intent, it compromises the patient's autonomy. Continual attention to the purpose, process, and impact of external influences is necessary to preserve the integrity of the consent process.

THE NATURE OF INFORMED CONSENT
Informed Consent as an Interactive Process

The move in recent years to make consent documents more detailed and explicit is intended to make the patient better informed and avoid litigation. But their complexity often has the opposite effect, leaving patients confused, poorly informed, and alienated from the informed consent process. When it functions well, informed consent is not an event, a moment in time, a perfunctory discussion, or a signed document, but a process. Meaningful consent is voluntarily and knowledgeably *given* by the patient, not *secured* or *imposed* by the staff as part of an assignment. Consent is not something the physician *extracts from*—"You need to get consent from

Mrs. Simon"—or *does to*—"I consented Mr. Thomas"—the patient. This attitude violates the autonomy of the patient and makes the signed consent form a trophy rather than the documentation of a process of communication, education, understanding, and trust.

The physician should begin the process by determining what the patient knows and whether he wants to participate in decisions about his care. As noted above, language differences that may be barriers to communication should be identified and, as far as possible, corrected through the use of certified interpreters (Schenker et al. 2011; Clark et al. 2011). Lack of medical background should not be used as an excuse for withholding information from the patient but should lead to new approaches for conveying it. Ongoing discussion should confirm his decisional capacity, his preferences and values, his appreciation of his condition, and the implications of his choices. Unless and until the patient is found to lack the ability to make his own decisions or he makes a capacitated and *voluntary* delegation of his decision-making authority to someone else, the patient is the person with whom the physician communicates.

The informed consent process, thus, assumes greater significance than simple physician disclosure of information and patient permission for treatment. It is an interaction between patient and physician, often including the family or trusted others, which promotes the exchange of relevant information and the provision of guidance and support that facilitates effective decision making. While this process is necessary each time consent is required for an intervention, these discussions are not isolated events. As this chapter and the ones that follow demonstrate, the collaborative nature of the therapeutic relationship requires ongoing physician engagement in the decision-making process, including

- working with the patient and family to determine the goals of care based on the patient's condition, prognosis, and health care wishes;
- developing a plan of care based on the goals that meet the patient's medical needs and is consistent with the patient's known wishes or the family's informed understanding of what is best for the incapacitated patient;
- providing care that benefits the patient without imposing unnecessary suffering or prolonging the dying process, and discontinuing interventions that have not demonstrated clinical effectiveness and benefit;
- regularly providing the patient and family with sufficient information to enable them to understand the progress and purpose of treatment, and appropriately affirm or revise care goals in light of the patient's evolving condition; and
- determining what elements of the care plan present genuine choices for patient and family decision making, and guiding and supporting those decisions.

The informed consent process as described above is a time- and labor-intensive enterprise that may strike many physicians as unnecessarily burdensome, especially in the light of growing pressures in our health care system to increase physician productivity and limit the time spent on each individual patient. No doubt, having a patient simply read and sign a document is much less time consuming than engaging in the educational and communicative process that informed consent requires. An important function of your ethics committee is to reinforce the notion of authentic informed consent as a process of physician-patient engagement in pursuit of collaborative decision making.

Sharing the Burden of Decision Making

The prevailing emphasis on patient autonomy risks diminishing the importance of the caregiver role in making difficult decisions. Treatment decisions require a grasp of medical information that is often complex, as well as insight into the patient's personal goals and values. As discussed in chapter 9, decisions about end-of-life care, in particular, are emotionally wrenching and may leave painful memories for those who make them. Both professionalism and compassion dictate that the burden of these decisions should be shared by those responsible for the care.

The suggestion is sometimes made that the full disclosure necessary for informed consent requires that physicians offer all possible treatment options for consideration. We argue that respecting patient or surrogate choice also recognizes that *some* care decisions, namely those that involve false choices, *do not require and should not impose the burden of patient or family consent.* Presenting patients and families with false choices diminishes the exercise of their autonomy and abdicates the professional's responsibility to exercise clinical judgment. False choices are offered when patients and families are asked to approve interventions for which there are no medical alternatives or to reject interventions that have no clinical indication. For example, asking family members for consent to stop dialysis treatments for an unconscious patient who is imminently dying inappropriately shifts responsibility for clinical decision making from the treating team to the family.

Especially when reversal of or improvement in the patient's condition is no longer possible, it is appropriate to limit the therapeutic options to those that are likely to benefit the patient. Interventions that are physiologically impossible or outside the standards of medical practice should not be proposed. These distinctions are addressed further in the discussion of medical futility in chapter 9. When specific treatments, such as dialysis, antibiotics, or vasopressors, are no longer effective, it is disingenuous and possibly cruel to present them as options and hope that patients and families will be savvy enough to refuse them, thereby making the decisions that physicians want them to make. When there are *no real (i.e., medically appropriate) options*, physicians can and should determine *which interventions ought to be offered for consideration.* This does not mean disempowering patients and families. It means assuming responsibility for making the judgments only physicians can make and then promoting the authentic choices reserved for patients and families.

Reflecting the tension between respecting patient autonomy and promoting patient well-being, physicians walk a fine line between supporting and usurping health care decision making. Patients and families depend on professional guidance in making care decisions and depriving them of clinical judgment, advice, and support is a form of abandonment. Even real choices should not be presented as value-neutral when one approach is clearly better, and physicians should be encouraged to clearly recommend what they believe to be the most appropriate course.

Guiding patient decisions should not be confused with paternalism, which demeans the capable adult and constricts the exercise of self-determination. Yet, patients and their surrogates have different levels of comfort assuming responsibility for treatment choices and caring physicians provide more or less structure as needed. Recognizing this delicate balance, commentators have suggested various approaches to providing information and decision-making support. For example, Emanuel and Emanuel (1992) offer four models of physician-patient interaction, representing different degrees of control and collaboration. Ultimately, providing genuine choices and thoughtful recommendations enhances patients' capacity to act in ways that promote both their autonomy and their well-being.

EXCEPTIONS TO THE CONSENT REQUIREMENT

The requirement for informed consent before treatment may be suspended in three narrow circumstances.

1. *Emergency Care*—Informed consent is not required when patients are unable to participate in care decisions, information about their wishes is not available, and delaying treatment would place their lives or health in peril. No one would seriously suggest that surgery to stop bleeding wait until an unresponsive accident victim regains consciousness and is able to provide consent or a surrogate decision maker is located. In such circumstances, consent is presumed based on the assumption that patients would want emergency treatment.

2. *Therapeutic Exception*—In very rare instances, physicians may believe that the disclosure of information about diagnoses or prognoses will cause clinically unstable patients to suffer *imminent, direct, and significant harm. Only in these limited and extreme circumstances* are physicians justified in withholding potentially harmful information from patients until such time as their clinical condition permits disclosure. The reasons for withholding the information must be detailed in the medical record and, whenever possible, the information must be disclosed to the patient's family or other trusted surrogate. Justifications for nondisclosure on this basis must be carefully scrutinized to ensure that it is the patient's well-being, not the physician's or family's comfort, that is being protected. As noted in the discussion of truth telling in chapter 4, inappropriately invoking this exception to the disclosure obligation must be avoided because it threatens the trust so essential to the therapeutic relationship.

3. *Waiver of Consent*—Corresponding to the right of informed consent is the patient's right not to be burdened with unwanted information or the pressure to make decisions *if he understands the consequences of giving up the opportunity to make decisions about care.* Electing not to know and delegating decisional authority to another person can be an authentic exercise of autonomy. But there must be an affirmative declaration by a capacitated patient that he wishes not to be involved in treatment decisions, such as "Talk to my daughter and do whatever she thinks is right. She makes all my decisions for me." The fact that he asks few questions or says, "Don't bother me with this now" is not the same as explicitly saying that he does not want to know or decide. Delegation of decision-making authority is not

something that should be inferred, but something that must be confirmed. Patterns of decision making that have been established over time may continue in the hospital setting, and in some cases physicians may know enough about the patient and his family to feel confident that the patient's delegation is not an aberration. Even then, clinicians should be encouraged to periodically ask capable patients, "Do you have any questions?" leaving the door open to patient involvement in her care, however limited it might be. The right not to receive information is further addressed in the discussion of truth telling and disclosure in chapter 4.

Returning to the case of Mrs. Stack, the 67-year-old woman with chronic renal insufficiency, a critical element in the ethical analysis is the assessment of decisional capacity. In her immediate post-arrest and intubated state, she clearly lacked the ability to make decisions. Nevertheless, she was known to have had this capacity prior to admission and, during her hospitalization, she was found to have regained it sufficiently to understand the benefits of dialysis and the consequences of not receiving it. Because physicians are usually obligated to respect the wishes of capable patients, determining Mrs. Stack's decisional capacity and her wishes is of paramount importance.

In this case, Mrs. Stack's primary physician and family believe that her repeated refusal of dialysis has been based on her belief that her daughter died *because* of the treatments. Thus, it may legitimately be asked whether Mrs. Stack's reasons for refusing are based on an adequate comprehension of the risks and benefits of dialysis or on misunderstanding. Some have argued that a patient's decision to refuse treatment should be discounted if it is based on irrational or false beliefs. Even so, coercing or disregarding otherwise decisionally capable patients should be avoided and efforts should focus on assisting them to make decisions based on accurate information and comprehension of the medical risks and benefits.

When the patient's ability to understand her medical condition and make choices is uncertain, consistency and durability of decisions can often substitute for capacity. Mrs. Stack's refusal of dialysis has been consistent over time, an important factor in assessing the quality of her decision making. While her refusal may be based on a misunderstanding, this durability indicates that she is comfortable with her position and speaks in favor of respecting her choice.

The patient's son threatens her with nursing home placement if she refuses dialysis—an odd ploy because she is not likely to survive for long without the treatments. Despite the possibility that he has pressured her into accepting treatment, some types of influence are ethically acceptable because they do not rise to the level of coercion, or objectionable manipulation. Therefore, even if the son persuades his mother to change her mind, it does not necessarily invalidate her decision to accept dialysis unless his strategy appears to be more threat than persuasion. Caregivers should confirm the patient's change of mind and satisfy themselves that it is truly informed and voluntary. One approach is to observe discussions between the patient and her son, if they do not object. Another safeguard is to review Mrs. Stack's decision with her when her son is not present.

This chapter has discussed informed *consent* and its rationale in providing ethical as well as legal authorization for the physician to treat. In contrast, *assent*, a notion with particular relevance in pediatrics, reflects the patient's *agreement* with a treatment plan rather than *authorization* of it. Only when the conditions of informational disclosure, understanding, and voluntariness have been met in the context of decisional capacity can the patient's consent or refusal be considered truly informed and authentic.

REFERENCES

Ackerman TF. 2001. Why doctors should intervene. In Mappes TA, DeGrazia D, eds. *Biomedical Ethics*. 5th ed. Boston: McGraw-Hill, pp. 80–85.

Arnold R, Lidz C. 2001. Informed consent: Clinical aspects of consent in health care. In Levine C, ed. *Taking Sides: Clashing Views on Controversial Bioethical Issues*. 9th ed. Guilford, CT: Dushkin/McGraw-Hill, pp. 4–11.

Beauchamp TL. 1997. Informed consent. In Veatch R, ed. *Medical Ethics*. 2nd ed. Sudbury, MA: Jones and Bartlett Publishers, pp. 185–208.

Beauchamp TL, Childress JF. 2001. *Principles of Biomedical Ethics*. 5th ed. New York: Oxford University Press, pp. 77–98.

Beauchamp TL, Childress JF. 2009. *Principles of Biomedical Ethics*. 7th ed. New York: Oxford University Press, pp. 120–27.

Braude H, Kimmelman J. 2012. The ethics of managing affective and emotional states to improve informed consent: Autonomy, comprehension, and voluntariness. *Bioethics* 26(3):149–56.

Brenner LH, Brenner AT, Horowitz D. 2009. Beyond informed consent. *Clinical Orthopaedics and Related Research* 467:348–51.

Brock D. 1993. Informed consent. In *Life and Death: Philosophical Essays in Biomedical Ethics*. New York: Cambridge University Press, pp. 21–54.

Brody H. 1989. Transparency: Informed consent in primary care. *Hastings Center Report* 19(5):5–9.

Clark S, Mangram A, Ernest D, Lebron R., Peralta L. 2011. The informed consent: A study of the efficacy of informed consents and the associated role of language barriers. *Journal of Surgical Education* 68(2):143–47.

Emanuel EJ, Emanuel LL. 1992. Four models of the physician-patient relationship. *Journal of the American Medical Association* 267(16):2221–26.

Garrett TM, Baillie HW, Garrett RM. 2001. Principles of autonomy and informed consent. In *Health Care Ethics: Principles and Problems*. 4th ed. Upper Saddle River, NJ: Prentice Hall, pp. 29–56.

Katz J. 2003. Informed consent—must it remain a fairy tale? In Steinbock B, Arras JD, London AJ, eds. *Ethical Issues in Modern Medicine*. 6th ed. Boston: McGraw-Hill, pp. 92–100.

Kihlborn U. 2008. Autonomy and negatively informed consent. *Journal of Medical Ethics* 34:146–49.

Lo B. 2000. *Resolving Ethical Dilemmas: A Guide for Clinicians*. 2nd ed. Philadelphia: Lippincott Williams & Wilkins, pp. 19–29.

Manson NC., O'Neill O. 2007. *Rethinking Informed Consent in Bioethics*. Cambridge: Cambridge University Press.

Meisel A, Kuczewski M. 1996. Legal and ethical myths about informed consent. *Archives of Internal Medicine* 156:2521–26.

O'Neill O. 2001. Informed consent and genetic information. *Studies in History, Philosophy, & Biomedical Science* 32(4):689–704.

President's Commission for the Study of Ethical Problems in Medicine and Biomedical and Behavioral Research. 1982. *Making Health Care Decisions: The Ethical and Legal*

Implications of Informed Consent in the Patient-Practitioner Relationship (Vol. 1: Report). Washington, DC.

Schenker Y, Fernandez A, Sudore R, Schillinger D. 2011. Interventions to improve patient comprehension in informed consent for medical and surgical procedures: A systematic review. *Medical Decision Making* 31(1):151–73.

Schneider CE. 1998. *The Practice of Autonomy: Patients, Doctors, and Medical Decisions.* New York: Oxford University Press.

Shalowitz KI, Wolf MS. 2004. Shared decision-making and the lower literate patient. *Journal of Law, Medicine & Ethics* 32(4):759–64.

State of Tennessee Department of Human Service v. Mary C. Northern, Court of Appeals of Tennessee, Middle Section, Feb. 7, 1978. In Steinbock B, Arras JD, London AJ. 2003. *Ethical Issues in Modern Medicine.* 6th ed. Boston: McGraw-Hill, pp. 283–87.

Transcript of proceedings: Testimony of Mary C. Northern. In Steinbock B, Arras JD, London AJ. 2003. *Ethical Issues in Modern Medicine.* 6th ed. Boston: McGraw-Hill, pp. 287–90.

Veatch RM. 2001. Abandoning informed consent. In Levine C, ed. *Taking Sides: Clashing Views on Controversial Bioethical Issues.* 9th ed. Guildford, CT: Dushkin/McGraw-Hill, pp. 12–18.

CHAPTER 4

Truth Telling
Disclosure, Privacy, and Confidentiality

Arguably, the most valuable health care resource is information. Clinicians depend on its accuracy in making their diagnoses and prognoses. Patients rely on its adequacy in evaluating their options and arriving at their decisions about care. Families wait for news of their loved ones' changing conditions. But beyond lab data and examination findings, how clinical information is elicited, protected, and shared is bound up with the very nature of the therapeutic relationship. It is, therefore, a matter of ethical concern for professionals and patients alike.

The idea that care professionals should tell their patients the truth seems self-evident and uncontroversial. Chapters 1 through 3 have devoted considerable space to discussing the importance of *informed* decision making and the trust that is so central to the therapeutic relationship. Like most other aspects of the clinical interaction, however, obligations of truth telling are complex. How do we determine the "truth"? To whom is the truth owed? When does withholding the truth, or massaging information, shade into deliberate deception? The ethics of truth telling is also complicated when patient autonomy, beneficence, nonmaleficence, and justice collide.

Mr. Nunez is a 46-year-old Hispanic man suffering from terminal esophageal cancer. He speaks no English, but his wife, who is bilingual and constantly at his bedside, translates for the care providers. This way of relating to Mr. Nunez—through his wife—is not recent. For the nine months that Mr. Nunez has been coming to the hospital for treatment, Mrs. Nunez has essentially directed his care and determined what he is to be told. Believing that she is acting in his best interest, his care providers have honored her wishes, but they are increasingly uncomfortable.

It has become clear that Mrs. Nunez is not translating everything that she is being told. In particular, she seems to be censoring information about the seriousness of Mr. Nunez's condition. When asked about this, Mrs. Nunez has made it very clear that she does not want her husband told that he is dying of cancer. He knows that he has a "growth" on his esophagus but not that he has cancer. Indeed, according to her, he does not even understand what cancer is. Mr. Nunez has also recently been enrolled in a phase I/II cancer research protocol, consent for which has been given by his wife.

Mrs. Nunez is adamant that her husband not be told about his diagnosis or prognosis. She seems to believe sincerely that, if he were to find out the truth, he would do violence to himself and possibly to her. When asked why she thinks this, she cites an incident in which the patient threatened to harm himself if his condition were found to be more serious than he thought. Although she has been assured that patients usually benefit from understanding their conditions, she insists that nothing can be gained for Mr. Nunez by telling him the truth. She concedes that he occasionally asks questions, but claims that she has been able to satisfy him with evasive or deceitful answers. When asked whether she would agree to have Mr. Nunez told the truth when he is finally too weak to harm himself, she emphatically replied, "No! Never! I can't imagine what it would be like for him to know that he is dying. I won't have this!" Although she describes her husband as "like a baby," there is no reason to believe that the patient could not comprehend the nature and seriousness of his condition. His cognitive status cannot be confirmed, however, because Mrs. Nunez has forbidden a psychiatric evaluation.

Members of the care team are conflicted about the limits on their ability to interact with Mr. Nunez. Several strongly believe that he is being deprived of his rights to information, while others suggest that his wife knows him better than they do. The oncology fellow notes that "in certain countries, such as Japan, patients are not routinely told the truth about their diagnoses as a way of protecting them from stress, but at least they are not tortured by being enrolled in research that is not likely to benefit them."

How and by whom should this patient's best interests be defined? Do Mr. Nunez's rights conflict with his best interest? What arguments support disclosure or non-disclosure in this case?

JUSTIFICATIONS

Truthfulness is a core interpersonal value in social life generally and it has particular significance in the clinician-patient relationship. Three justifications have been advanced to support the obligation of veracity in the clinical setting. They are "respect owed to persons . . . fidelity, promise-keeping, and contract . . . [and] the role of trust in relationships between health professionals and patients and subjects" (Beauchamp and Childress 2013, p. 303):

1. Respect for others is reflected in the ethical principle of autonomy. The capable individual's right to be self-determining imposes on clinicians the obligation to provide adequate information for informed health care decision making.
2. Fidelity and the keeping of promises are central elements in the trust-based relationship between patient and clinician. This fiduciary bond creates an

implicit contract that both parties will be honest and will honor their commitments.

3. Productive therapeutic interactions rely on the truthful management of information. The effective clinician-patient relationship depends on the exchange of accurate and complete information about symptoms, diagnoses, prognoses, and treatment options, as well as confidence that care plans will be followed and patient wishes will be honored.

In this context, the uneasiness of the professionals caring for Mr. Nunez is understandable if they believe that withholding information undercuts his autonomy, erodes their trusting relationship, and inhibits effective clinical management. Only the strong likelihood that disclosure would be genuinely *harmful* to the patient can justify withholding information about his condition. This very rare therapeutic exception to the disclosure obligation is discussed below.

DISCLOSURE

Ethical Obligation

As discussed in chapter 3, collaborative decision making and informed consent depend on the reasonable disclosure of necessary or material information. Capable patients or their authorized surrogates are ethically and legally entitled to information that enables them to understand the likely course of the medical condition, evaluate the therapeutic options, and make choices consistent with patient goals and values.

Disclosure invokes respect for the patient's right to information that promotes effective decision making and the ethical imperatives to maximize benefits and minimize harms. Yet, as the case of Mr. Nunez illustrates, these same principles create tension between and among professionals' obligations. The analysis weighs the benefits of disclosing information that enhances patient understanding and self-determination against the potential harms of anxiety and stress that disclosure may cause.

Because laboratory and examination findings are controlled by the care team, particularly the medical staff, disclosure of clinical information is at the discretion of the physician. Access to medical information is thus an inherently unequal process that places the patient at a potential disadvantage in decision making, although this is changing somewhat with the wide availability of the Internet and the marketing of direct-to-consumer tests. This imbalance confers on doctors the disclosure obligation.

Arguments for Disclosing Information

Ms. Kim, a 23-year-old woman, presents with an isolated case of first-bout optic neuritis. The ophthalmologist, Dr. Frank, is concerned about whether to inform her that multiple sclerosis (MS) may develop in the future. His dilemma arises because, at the time the optic neuritis presents, the likelihood of subsequent development of MS is uncertain. At one time, it was thought that the degree of association between optic neuritis and MS was around 11%. Increasing evidence, however, suggests that the association may be as high as 50% (Brodsky et al. 2008). In light of current evidence, what should Dr. Frank disclose to her? How does the degree of association between optic neuritis and MS affect Dr. Frank's disclosure obligation?

The arguments in favor of disclosure are both ethical and practical. To know the truth about one's current and future medical condition is, for many patients, essential to a sense of self-mastery, especially as that condition evolves and possibly deteriorates. In addition, the therapeutic value of patients maintaining a sense of control in such circumstances is promoted by information disclosure. Even when treatment options are limited, life plans may need to be altered, and knowing what to expect allows patients to understand and prepare for what lies ahead.

Dr. Frank's concern is that disclosing the possibility of MS could cause Ms. Kim needless anxiety about an illness that she may never develop. Moreover, because MS cannot be prevented or cured, the information will not afford her any protection against developing the disease. On the other hand, it can be argued that she has the right to prepare herself for the heightened likelihood that she may experience a debilitating condition that would inevitably affect her ability to function independently. This knowledge may be an important influence in making decisions about lifestyle, career, family, and finances, as well planning treatment that might potentially delay the onset or mitigate symptoms of MS. Finally, if Ms. Kim discovers this information independently, her trust in Dr. Frank may be damaged by the belief that he was not honest about her risks.

Evan Barry was 17 years old when he was diagnosed last year with renal cell carcinoma. His right kidney was removed and he began several rounds of chemotherapy. Earlier this year, he came to the emergency department (ED) complaining of shortness of breath and chest pain. He seemed to be unaware of his diagnosis and could not explain the scar from the kidney surgery. A chest x-ray showed metastases to his lungs.

Evan was transferred from the ED to the adolescent unit and given gamma interferon. The physicians on the adolescent floor were puzzled by his apparent ignorance of his condition. When they approached his mother, Mrs. Barry was equivocal about what her son had been told. She said that she had been candid with Evan when he was first diagnosed but, when the physicians encouraged further discussions during the current admission, she adamantly refused to allow anyone to talk with him about his diagnosis and treatment. She expressed fear that he would be devastated and become suicidal, although she acknowledged that he had never attempted or threatened to harm himself.

Staff on the adolescent unit believed that Evan was frightened and isolated by the lack of information and communication. One of the residents carefully asked questions to probe the extent of his knowledge about his cancer. Evan said tearfully that he did not know what was wrong with him and that the doctors always spoke with his mother, not with him. He also said, "My mom is very worried about me but it makes her sad to talk about my problems and I don't want to upset her even more."

The team agreed that, while the lack of information was probably very frightening for Evan, he seemed to be protecting his mother by not asking questions. Concern was expressed that, even though he was not yet an adult with legal rights to information, as a bright adolescent who appeared to want and need information and support, he should be told the truth.

What are the care providers' obligations in this situation and, if they conflict, how can they be resolved? What benefits and risks should be considered? Who should determine what Evan is told?

The assumption that truth will normally be told goes to the heart of trust-based relationships of all sorts, including relations among family members and between patients and care professionals. Shielding patients from the truth is generally an imperfect enterprise in any case, requiring the collusion of others, including staff, family, and friends, in a conspiracy of silence. Uncertainty about what the patient knows and discomfort with the deception often result in caregivers and even family avoiding contact with the patient. It is not unusual to hear, "I was so sure that I would give it away that I just didn't want to be around him."

Yet, patients—even children and adults with a history of not wanting to know—sense when things are being kept from them and may avoid discussion as a way of accommodating those protecting them. Evan, for example, is reluctant to ask questions about his condition because he knows that talking about it upsets his mother. The result is a cycle of increasingly difficult efforts for mother and son to protect each other from acknowledging their sadness and fear. The burden of the deception itself, thus, can be a barrier to communication. Paradoxically, withholding information from the patient in order to protect him ends up isolating the patient at precisely the time when close and supportive relationships are critical. In short, although the obligation of truth telling, like other obligations, is not an absolute, it is something that requires a compelling reason to disregard.

Conflicting Obligations

Tension arises when clinicians feel that their obligations require them to either disclose information that the patient may not want or withhold potentially problematic information, all in the name of promoting the patient's well-being. The challenge is determining what the patient should know about his care without causing him harm and without violating his right to make autonomous decisions.

As you might suspect at this point, disclosure is not simply a matter of rattling off the results of lab tests or physical examinations. Effective disclosure is a clinical skill that depends on physician judgment and communication, as well as knowledge. Too much information can be as harmful as too little. The difference between truth telling and truth dumping is the difference between providing specific material information that facilitates decision making and indiscriminately overloading the patient with facts in the interests of completeness. An unbroken monologue of clinical data can be counterproductive, leaving the patient with glazed eyes and little recollection of what was said. Far more useful is breaking up the explanation every few sentences with, "Does that make sense?" or "What else can I tell you that would be helpful?" or "Can you tell me what you have understood so far?" Patients often indicate what they want to know and perceptive clinicians can be guided by their spoken or unspoken signals.

Truth telling is also counterproductive when information is disclosed without the accompanying explanations or guidance that frame the decisions patients or surrogates must make. More helpful is something like, "Let me tell you what all this means and then we can figure out the reasonable choices you might consider." Finally, patients need to be reassured that they are not expected to absorb everything all at once. "I know that this is a lot to take in right now and we will talk again. When you think of questions, it might be a good idea to write them down so that we can address them next time."

Arguments for Not Disclosing Information

Patients have both the right to receive information and the right *not* to receive it. Some people, especially those who are elderly, anxious, easily confused, or from cultures that do not place a high premium on individual autonomy, find it burdensome and even frightening to learn about their conditions and be asked to make treatment decisions. For example, while persons from European American backgrounds typically value full disclosure of medical information, those from Asian and Middle Eastern cultures tend to protect patients from knowing about illness or impending death. For them, authentic decision making in the clinical setting is expressed in the capacitated request *not* to be informed and the voluntary delegation of decision-making authority to trusted others (Zahedi 2011). Implicit is a longstanding or culture-based comfort with the practice of decision making by surrogates. In that sense, Mr. and Mrs. Nunez may exemplify families that have their own decision-making patterns, which may be effective and comfortable, rather than paternalistic or coercive. Decision making, like other interpersonal dynamics, comes in assorted shapes and sizes entitled to respectful attention. But, as noted in chapter 3, a waiver of informed consent is something that must be explicitly confirmed, not inferred, to demonstrate respect for the patient and protect his autonomy.

The more common disclosure dilemmas concern withholding information from patients who have not waived their right to information, usually justified by notions of shielding them from harm (invoking the principle of nonmaleficence) and sometimes by notions of promoting their interests (invoking the principle of beneficence). Disclosure, especially of bad news, is one of the most difficult clinical tasks, and evasion or awkwardness is often the result of efforts to avoid inflicting pain. Physicians frequently protect themselves and—they think—their patients by softening the message and resorting to euphemism. "The patient has a grim prognosis" becomes "The patient is not doing well." "The patient is dying" becomes "The patient is failing." Sometimes it sounds as though, if only the patient and care team tried harder, she would not be dying.

Rather than comfort, however, deliberate vagueness creates confusion, anxiety, mistrust, and unrealistic expectations. It is not uncommon for a family to react with frustration and seemingly unreasonable demands when told that, although the patient is *not doing well*, aggressive cure-directed treatments should be limited. The family argues that she could be doing *better* if only the care team were doing *more* rather than *less*. The importance of compassionate candor is emphasized in chapter 9, in the discussion of medical futility and forgoing treatment at the end of life.

Sometimes, discomfort in discussing bad news with the patient persuades care professionals that disclosure would be *harmful*, when in fact it might only be *distressing*. The risk is that the therapeutic exception, noted in chapter 3, may be expanded beyond its strict definition (exception to the disclosure obligation when the information itself would cause *imminent, direct, and significant harm* to the patient) and applied to situations in which the information would be upsetting, but not dangerous. The principle of nonmaleficence is formulated in terms of *harm* and does not require physicians to shield their patients from upset or distress. Whenever clinicians consider withholding information, especially from capable patients, they need to question who is being protected, whether the protection is truly warranted, and what the cost will be to the trust between doctor and patient. This dilemma, which requires balancing the ethical obligations of respect for autonomy, beneficence, nonmaleficence, and justice, often triggers a clinical ethics consultation to explore the benefits and risks of disclosure to the patient.

Pressure also comes from families—parents of young children, grown children of aging parents, or concerned spouses like Mrs. Nunez—not to share information with the patient. These are typically concerned family members who want to protect their loved one, although sometimes their motives are less creditable. In other words, "If we can't prevent Papa from having cancer, at least we can keep him from feeling anxious or scared." The reasons given are usually "The news will kill him" or "You will take away all hope." The first objection indicates the need to reassure anxious relatives that disclosure is part of clinicians' skill set and the patient will not be burdened with information that he does not want or cannot safely assimilate.

The second objection speaks to expectations and the importance of hope. As further discussed in chapter 9, bad news or even a terminal diagnosis need not signal a future so bleak that deception is justified. Depriving patients and families of hope is never justified. It is frequently necessary, however, to redefine what can be hoped for—perhaps not long life or unlimited function, but rather increased comfort, attendance at a special celebration, or a peaceful death surrounded by loved ones. Helping patients and families adjust their goals to be achievable is an essential part of care professionals' responsibilities.

Let us consider how these issues relate to Mr. Nunez. His caregivers are faced with conflicting obligations in determining what he should be told about his condition. Because they have been prevented from interacting with him directly, they have no independent assessment of his capacity, emotional stability, or desire for information. All communications have been filtered through his wife, whose motives may be well meaning but overprotective, or possibly not in his best interest. As noted in chapter 3, for precisely this reason, the policies of most hospitals, as well as Joint Commission standards, require that trained and certified interpreters, rather than family, manage communications between the care team and patients who prefer to use a language other than English. Not only is this requirement a safeguard against deliberately distorted messages, it also relieves family members of the burden of trying to digest unfamiliar medical terms and clinical concepts and then translating them into another language in a way that is understandable to the patient. The care professionals need to clarify with Mrs. Nunez that providing her husband with good care requires that they interact with him directly. She should be reassured that harmful or unwanted information will not be forced on him but that his perceptions and wishes will be skillfully assessed as part of his clinical evaluation.

In addition to helping protective families appreciate the reasons supporting disclosure, it is also important to explain the risks of withholding or distorting information. They must understand that the care team will not lie to patients, that direct questions will require truthful answers. They must also realize that, given the number of people involved in patients' care and the ease with which information can be accessed from the Internet and other available sources, it will be difficult if not impossible to guarantee that they will not learn what is being kept from them. Potential damage to family relationships is another compelling argument for disclosure. "If your husband learns about his condition independently, he might begin to wonder what other things you've kept from him. Let's work together to figure out how to give him the information he needs in a way that is controlled and comfortable for both him and you."

When withholding information is suggested, it is necessary to determine the patient's capacity, understanding of the clinical situation, desire for information, and the degree to which he wants to be involved in care planning and decision making. Using the patient's preferred language, one approach might be, "Mr. Nunez, the examinations and tests will give us information about your condition and then some decisions will have to be made about your treatment. Some patients want to know all the information and others don't. What would make you comfortable? Do you want us to discuss these things with you or with someone else?" Capable patients can then elect to participate in the process or voluntarily delegate that responsibility to another person. Even if Mr. Nunez explicitly says, "I don't want to know and I want my wife to make decisions for me," he should be kept in the communication loop by being asked periodically, "Do you have any questions? Is there anything we can tell you?" A wish not to be burdened with information or decision making should not deprive patients of attention in other ways.

DISCLOSURE OF ADVERSE OUTCOMES AND MEDICAL ERROR

Mrs. Allen, a pregnant woman with diabetes, had been encouraged to undergo amniocentesis to determine the fetus's lung development in order to plan induction of her delivery. Because there is a window of safety in delivering diabetic patients, this procedure is considered standard of care. During the amnio, the umbilical cord was nicked, resulting in bleeding and requiring an immediate caesarean section.

The neonatology house staff has requested an ethics consult to discuss whether the parents should be told the reason for the emergency delivery and, if so, whether the information should come from the obstetric team or the neonatologists.

Adverse Outcomes and Medical Error

Disclosure of bad news is difficult under any circumstances. Disclosure of bad news when things go wrong is a clinician's worst nightmare, but it is one that must be confronted for the sake of patients and professionals. We begin with some important definitions. *Adverse outcomes* are undesired and unintended negative results of medical care that create actual or potential harm to the patient. These untoward occurrences may be the result of carelessness or ineptitude, or they may reflect foreseen but unavoidable risk even when standard of care was practiced. The former—*medical errors*—are considered avoidable, while the latter are generally seen as unavoidable, an inherent part of the imperfect art of medicine. Distinguishing between these types of adverse outcomes may be problematic, but standard of care is routinely used as an important criterion. The distinction is crucial in recognizing that unintended outcomes do not always mean that someone is to blame.

Other analyses distinguish between *system* and *individual or human errors*, attributing some adverse outcomes to problems in the health care delivery system and others to the actions of individual providers. This approach reflects the notion that "no one person [is] responsible, because it is virtually impossible for one mistake to kill a patient in the highly mechanized and backstopped world of a modern hospital" (Belkin 1997, p. 28). The 2000 Institute of Medicine report, *To Err is Human: Building a Safer Health System*, generated considerable interest in disclosure of information as a key to managing and preventing adverse outcomes. As a result, oversight and accrediting bodies, clinicians, and institutions are adopting the concept of health care delivery as a system-wide interlocking dynamic that can either allow or prevent error. In analyzing adverse events, this perspective focuses on *organizational processes* rather than *individual performance*, searching for systemic solutions rather than assigning blame.

Scope of Disclosure

Disclosure includes but is not limited to the requirements of informed consent that concern *prospective* analysis of proposed interventions. Armed with adequate information, the patient can proceed to make decisions about future care. Full disclosure that promotes patient self-determination and protection also includes *retrospective* analysis of unintended consequences, which involves informing patients that an adverse outcome has occurred and providing an explanation of why it happened. This aspect of disclosure recognizes that, in addition to patients' need for information to enhance care planning and decision making, they have a desire and a right to understand what did or will happen to them. Taken together, the *preview* and *review* aspects of the disclosure obligation can be grounded in the patient's need to *know* and *act* on the basis of adequate information.

Obligation of Disclosure

The obligation to disclose adverse outcomes rests on both ethical and legal foundations. Recognizing the need to ensure the provision of adequate information, courts have imposed fiduciary obligations of disclosure on physicians. Judicial reasoning is that these obligations exist when "one party is dependent on another for information or knowledge that only the first party possesses" (Vogel and Delgado 1980, pp. 66–67). In the clinical setting, the physician is the person most likely to have and control information about an untoward event or medical error, heightening the professional obligation of disclosure. The patient who has suffered an undisclosed adverse event is not only likely to be unaware of what happened and the actual or potential harm she faces, but she is also unable to prevent or mitigate the harm or to seek fair compensation for it. Her reliance on the physician for information that will minimize harm and help her cope with the consequences creates an ethical imperative for timely and full disclosure of the adverse event. This obligation has received explicit attention in the various codes and opinions that provide ethical guidance and analysis for physicians. In the name of transparency, health care organizations also have an obligation to promote disclosure of anticipated outcomes by their medical practitioners, and they should include this in their organizational codes of ethics.

A related basis for the disclosure obligation can be found in the values underlying informed consent. This analysis views informed consent as a compact entered into by physician and patient. The doctor says, in effect, "Here is the information you need, including the possible risks." The patient says, in effect, "I understand what you have said and I consent to the test or treatment *because I trust that you have told me everything I need to know* in order to make a decision." Implicit in the patient's response is, "I trust that you will exercise all due care in treating me. *I further trust that, if any foreseen or unforeseen harms should occur, you will disclose that information so that I can understand and manage the negative consequences.*" The informed patient is able to balance the benefits, burdens, and risks in advance of treatment and, if an untoward event occurs, mitigate any harm, protect herself from further harms, and seek appropriate compensation. Rather than a passive recipient of treatment, the patient becomes an active partner in planning for and managing the outcomes of care.

Barriers to Disclosure

Given the ethical and legal justifications, it seems hard to argue with the notion that information about untoward occurrences should be made available to patients or their surrogates. It will not be surprising, however, that physicians are very reluctant to discuss negative outcomes with patients and families. Reasons for avoiding disclosure include the difficulty of determining whether the event was medical error, the belief that the information will be needlessly upsetting, and the omnipresent fear of legal action. Additional barriers include the ideal of physician infallibility shared by patients as well as physicians, and the shame and guilt that physicians experience when admitting an untoward outcome, especially when it is a result of medical error.

Liability to medical malpractice suits is cited by physicians as the chief barrier to disclosure of unintended occurrences. Doctors' understandable risk aversion makes them uneasy about admitting error or other behavior that might have contributed to patient harm. Concerns about who assumes the duty of disclosure and bears responsibility are especially difficult in an academic medical center, with its multiple levels of interdisciplinary staff and different authority structures. That said, you should know and reinforce with physicians that legal action does not inevitably follow adverse events, including those caused by negligence. Instead, some evidence suggests that the pursuit of litigation by patients and families is related to how physicians handle discussions with them about untoward outcomes, including disclosure of information about actual or potential harm (Mastroianni et al. 2010; Liebman and Hyman 2004; Gallagher et al. 2003; Goldberg et al. 2002).

In an effort to encourage provider-patient communication about unanticipated clinical events, many states have passed "disclosure" or "apology" laws. These statutes are designed to protect communications that provide information about the event (disclosure) and expressions of sympathy and regret (apology) from being used as evidence of liability in malpractice litigation or administrative actions. As of 2010, 34 states and the District of Columbia had enacted some type of apology law; 9 had enacted mandatory disclosure laws requiring that patients or their surrogates be notified of adverse events; 6 states had enacted both types of laws; and 13 had neither (Mastroianni et al. 2010; Dresser 2008). One response to these statutory requirements and the potential that other states may enact similar legislation was the Project on Medical Liability in Pennsylvania, which used trained mediators to strengthen physicians' skills in communicating difficult news and established mediation as an alternative to litigation (Liebman and Hyman 2004).

Institutions have also developed promising initiatives that provide guidance and support to practitioners facing the daunting task of communicating bad news. These protective laws and institutional systems are still being studied to determine their impact on malpractice litigation, practitioner behavior, and organizational strategies. Your ethics committee can play an important role in educating clinical and administrative staff about these developments, as well as participating in the development of institutional systems that promote greater transparency and trust in the provider-patient relationship.

Perhaps even more threatening to physicians than the specter of malpractice litigation is the personal devaluation that accompanies acknowledging adverse events. This may include "a loss of personal confidence and self-esteem, diminished professional authority and reputation, as well as a loss of referrals and income" (Baylis 1997, p. 338). The inability to cope with untoward outcomes appears to stem less from blatant physician callousness or dishonesty than from belief in the widespread myth of infallibility and total control that define the perfect healer. This image, born in medical schools, nurtured throughout medical careers, and sold to the public, is shared by physicians and their patients, leading to unrealistic expectations, unreasonable disappointments, and unbridgeable gaps in communication.

PRIVACY AND CONFIDENTIALITY

Mr. Miller is a 42-year-old man who came to the emergency room with iritis and whose work-up was positive for syphilis. When Dr. David discussed the diagnosis with Mr. Miller, the patient requested that Dr. David not disclose the infection to his wife or report it to the state Department of Health. He said that he must have contracted the condition during a one-time extramarital encounter on a recent business trip. He also stated that he has not had sexual contact with his wife since that time and that he will undergo treatment before doing so.

Two other aspects of information management central to the therapeutic relationship are privacy and confidentiality. Privacy refers to "a state or condition of limited access," including "an agent's control over access to himself or herself" (Beauchamp and Childress 2013, p. 312). Privacy reflects the notion that one's self, whether the physical body, personal representations or identifiers, or personal information, should be guarded and under the control of the individual. The ethical obligation to protect patients' privacy recognizes that, in the clinical interaction, patients reveal sensitive physical or informational aspects of themselves, and they should retain the right to control who has access to these personal aspects.

Protecting physical privacy entails obvious measures, such as knocking before entering a patient's room; providing appropriate gowns, robes, and covers; and, during examinations, pulling the curtain, asking visitors to step outside, and admitting only those whose presence is necessary. Protecting informational privacy requires not discussing patient information in public areas and ensuring that written or electronic patient information is accessed only by those directly involved in a patient's care.

Closely related to privacy is confidentiality. "Confidentiality is present when one person discloses information to another, whether through words or an examination, and the person to whom the information is disclosed pledges not to divulge that information to a third party without the confider's permission" (Beauchamp and Childress 2001, pp. 305–6). In that sense, confidentiality, like truth telling and privacy, invokes the patient's trust in and reliance on the health care professional's integrity. When patients provide clinicians with access to their bodies and personal information, they do so with the trust-based understanding that these private aspects of themselves will be held in confidence by the professionals.

Privacy and confidentiality are associated with distinct but related ethical obligations. Although the common perception is that confidentiality binds only the patient and physician, the professional obligation also covers other clinicians, including chiropractors, clinical social workers, dentists, nurses, podiatrists, and psychologists. Moreover, with recent changes in the delivery of health care, these obligations do not only apply to the relationship between a patient and her primary practitioner. The circle of individuals who have necessary access to private information about the patient has expanded to include multiple care providers, and patients' rights to privacy are not violated simply because these individuals have access to this information. Nor has the primary practitioner failed to protect confidentiality simply because he shares patient information with other members of the care team. Obligations to respect privacy and protect confidentiality remain, but the relationships to which they apply have changed.

Justifications for Protecting Confidentiality

Mr. Gordon, a 43-year-old man, is picked up by the police on Saturday evening and rushed to the nearest emergency department after passing out on a mid-town sidewalk. ED physicians detect a high level of alcohol in his blood and a urine toxicology screen reveals opiates. Upon regaining consciousness, Mr. Gordon provides his past medical history, which is unremarkable, and says that his occupation is city sanitation truck driver. He acknowledges that he used alcohol and cocaine earlier in the evening, and reminds the physicians that they have a duty not to disclose to others confidential patient information.

What obligations do physicians have to Mr. Gordon and others, and how can they be reconciled? What ethical principles and additional factors should be considered?

The notion that the therapeutic interaction creates a zone of protected information can be supported by the same ethical considerations discussed earlier in connection with truthfulness. Respect for persons underlies patients' privacy, namely, their right to control who has access to their heath care information and the requirement that medical records and communications in the clinical setting be protected from unwarranted disclosure. If personal information can be seen as a reflection of the most intimate aspects of an individual's life, then control of that information can be seen as a form of self-determination that requires provider respect. Protecting confidentiality also prevents the harms that result from unauthorized disclosure of sensitive information, such as HIV status or psychiatric history.

Fidelity and promise keeping are reflected in the bond of trust that requires professionals to hold in confidence information learned in the clinical interaction. This justification is based on the moral imperative to honor a duty or promise regardless of the results. It holds that, without explicit patient waiver, the clinician is bound by the confidentiality inherent in the relationship. The argument also encompasses the notion of secrets, those pieces of our private selves we give in trust to others with the implicit or explicit understanding that they will be held in confidence.

The effectiveness of the clinical relationship and the resulting quality of the health care provided depend on an atmosphere of trust that promotes the candid and complete exchange of information. This justification rests on the need to encourage patients to provide all relevant facts about their medical history and symptoms, no matter how private or potentially embarrassing, to facilitate accurate diagnosis and effective treatment. This is a utilitarian rationale for protecting confidentiality since it appeals to the consequences for the patient and the practitioner-patient relationship of an obligation of nondisclosure. Without strict limits on what may be disclosed to others, patients would likely avoid seeking or fully cooperating in treatment.

Challenges to Privacy and Confidentiality

It would seem that nothing could be more ethically compelling than the promise to protect what patients reveal about themselves. Like truth telling and privacy, confidentiality seems a clear and simple duty that professionals owe their patients. But, like other ethical imperatives, the confidentiality obligation is neither absolute nor always easy to honor.

So what gets in the way of protecting patient confidences and personal health information? Medical information is generated in the health care setting as a product of the therapeutic interaction between clinician and patient; it is also generated in the pharmacy, the research lab, the autopsy room, the insurance office, the medical classroom, and the hospital elevator. It goes into reports, books, lectures, legal briefs, and computers, from which it is accessed by countless people for countless valid and not-so-valid reasons.

As noted above, the treating relationship is only one context in which medical confidentiality is raised. The dramatic change in health care delivery has altered what used to be a confidential relationship between patient and family doctor. Medical treatment has moved from the home to the institutional setting; multiple disciplines and subspecialties, legal and government bureaucracies, and third-party payers now converge on each case; and computers connect all parties to the clinical interaction. The result is that the number of people with legitimate and nonlegitimate access to medical information has increased geometrically. The growing use of e-medicine to provide medical services to patients, and to store, manage, and transmit patients' health information has exacerbated the problem. The contemporary clinical setting and technological developments have greatly enhanced the efficiency and efficacy of communication among care providers, but this is not an unmixed blessing: new worries arise about the extent to which the privacy of patients' medical information can actually be respected and protected. Concerns about the security of protected health information (PHI) prompted the inclusion of stringent regulations in the 1996 federal Health Insurance Portability and Accountability Act (HIPAA).

Consent to care with a loss of some measure of privacy is either explicitly obtained, through signed releases upon entering the care-providing institution, or presumed, but the consent is never to be considered unlimited. For example, although it should be explained upon admission, it is generally understood that treatment in a teaching hospital includes having one's records, examinations, and therapies available for observation and study by students and house staff. Most patients expect that their cases will be discussed formally and even informally to obtain the benefit of other opinions and to provide teaching examples. They neither expect nor deserve to have their personal or medical information shared in public hospital areas or social situations. Likewise, patients should have control over who has access to their medical information through updates in their clinical condition. As a precaution against inadvertent unwanted disclosure, it may be helpful to say early in the patient's hospital stay, "You seem to have a lot of family and friends who are concerned about you. Please know that we will not discuss your medical condition with anyone unless you specifically request that we do so."

In addition to those who use medical information for treatment purposes, such data are routinely used by medical researchers, law enforcement agencies, attorneys (requesting their own clients' records or those of other patients in connection with medical malpractice or personal injury litigation), insurers (life, health, disability, and liability), employers, and creditors. Although these secondary users are routinely required to access information through formal requests for patient record releases, they may not always follow procedure. Finally, there are other potential users of medical information who have nothing to do with the patient's health care, including those with commercial, political, and media interests.

So, are confidentiality and privacy obsolete or decrepit, as one commentator (Siegler 1982) suggested more than 30 years ago? Given the formidable barriers and incentives in the current health care setting, is it possible or even desirable to manage the flow of information?

The management of personal health information has been a concern since Hippocrates cautioned against indiscriminate disclosure. A new challenge is storing, transmitting, and selectively disclosing protected health information (PHI) in the context of e-medicine, including electronic medical records and online- and

Internet-based networks linking insurance companies, hospitals, providers, and patients (Bauer 2009). Reported incidents of intentional and unintentional breaches in security have demonstrated the real and potentially disastrous risks to individual and group medical records, provider-patient relationships, quality of care, administrative efficiency, and public confidence in the health care system. In short, e-medicine has the potential to both greatly enhance and seriously jeopardize health care.

The obligations of privacy and confidentiality are being reshaped and their boundaries are in flux. Yet, the ethical core remains intact and worth preserving. The contours may be redrawn, but the central values deserve protection through policies and regulations that respond to current clinical, ethical, and legal imperatives.

Justifications for Breaching Confidentiality

Even people with little experience in the health care setting know and rely on the sanctity of clinician-patient confidentiality. Based on well-established ethical and legal justifications, this obligation normally precludes professionals from disclosing information learned in the course of diagnosis or treatment. Precisely because this ethical mandate is so central to the clinical relationship, exceptions are justified only when disclosure of confidential information is essential to preventing significant harm to other vulnerable individuals, especially those at unsuspected risk. In these select instances, the patient's right to confidentiality is considered to be outweighed by the obligation to protect those who are not in a position to protect themselves.

The following two situations that justify breaching confidentiality illustrate that the obligation of fidelity to one's patients is not the only ethical obligation that practitioners have and that conflicts can arise as a result. In both circumstances, the needs of the non-patients are elevated because their vulnerability is heightened by their very ignorance of the risks they face.

1. Providing information that prevents harm to *identified* third parties at risk (e.g., partner notification). This exception reflects the opinion in *Tarasoff v. Regents of University of California*, a 1976 case in which the court held that a psychotherapist who had prior knowledge of a patient's intention to kill his unsuspecting girlfriend had a duty to warn her. This reasoning has been incorporated into the laws of many states in addressing the needs of those who have been unwittingly exposed to HIV/AIDS or other sexually transmitted disease (STD). When the infected patient refuses to inform sexual or needle-sharing partners, some states permit or require partner notification to enable those known to be at risk to be tested and treated. While most states recognize a duty to warn identified persons at risk of intended harm or exposure to other sexually transmitted or contagious diseases, there is no authority in most states for notifying persons exposed to HIV or AIDS (Hermann and Gagliano 1989). The *Tarasoff* ruling, which is also notable for expanding the scope of practitioner responsibility, is discussed further in part IV.

2. Providing information that prevents harm to *unidentified* others at risk (e.g., public health or public safety reporting). In some instances, the potential danger is to the general population, rather than to specified individuals. To protect the public health and safety, state laws commonly require that health care providers report

certain findings, including suspected cases of child abuse and neglect; wounds that are the result of gun shots, knives, or other pointed instruments; burn injuries of specified severity; and cases of reportable communicable diseases specified in state health laws.

In the case of Mr. Miller, Dr. David is in a difficult position. He knows that confidentiality is the bedrock of the patient-physician relationship, assuring the patient that he can share accurate and sensitive information with the doctor without fear of disclosure. Not only does the assurance of confidentiality promote trust, it facilitates full and candid communication that is vital to successful diagnosis and treatment. Fear that sensitive or embarrassing information, such as a diagnosis of STD, will be disclosed may dissuade Mr. Miller from providing critical facts or even seeking necessary treatment.

Sometimes, however, withholding information poses risks to others outside the physician-patient relationship. In this case, Mr. Miller's wife is at risk of contracting syphilis and she is especially vulnerable because she has no reason to suspect that she is at risk. By taking action early through testing and, if necessary, treatment, she may be able to avoid the dire consequences of syphilis and perhaps other STDs. To protect vulnerable persons, public health has traditionally intervened by contact tracing and partner notification. Clinicians are required by law to report most STDs by patient name to public health officials so that they can trace and notify partners at risk. Public officials try to maintain the anonymity of the index case as much as possible. But if Mrs. Miller's only sexual partner has been her husband, it may be difficult or impossible to prevent her from figuring out how she was exposed.

Despite pressure from Mr. Miller, it is ethically and legally unacceptable for Dr. David to cooperate with the request to withhold information that can prevent harm to an identified person at risk. Dr. David should counsel Mr. Miller about the importance of disclosure, including the legal requirements and the risks of nondisclosure, and encourage him to tell his wife. It may be helpful if he offers support in the disclosure process.

Mr. Gordon's case raises somewhat different issues. Here, the concern is whether the physicians have a responsibility to report the fact that a person who drives a sanitation truck for the city is known to have used alcohol and illegal drugs. In this analysis, the justifications underlying the confidentiality obligation would be weighed against the possible harms to unidentified persons—the public—who have no reason to believe that they are at risk. Relevant factors would include the potential for harm, the likelihood that it could be prevented, alternatives to breaching confidentiality, and the legal requirements of the state in which the situation occurs.

While no one would encourage Mr. Gordon to abuse alcohol or drugs, it can be argued that his behavior on this occasion does not place others at immediate or inevitable risk. In this case, the patient's substance-related loss of consciousness occurred on a weekend evening, not during work hours and not while he was driving a truck or any other vehicle. It would be important to know whether his use of alcohol and drugs is substantial or minimal, and whether it occurs daily or only occasionally. This information, which is relevant to his health care as well as the safety of others, is much more likely to be revealed to his caregivers if Mr. Gordon is assured that it will be kept confidential.

In terms of state law, the patient's only illegal behavior is his use of narcotics. Health care professionals should not be expected to compromise their obligations to their patients by functioning as agents of the law enforcement or judicial systems. Accordingly, all states presume a general rule of patient confidentiality, carving out selected specific instances when that obligation must be breached to protect others from harm.

If Mr. Gordon suffered from epilepsy, he would be required by all states to report his condition to the motor vehicle bureau and, if he worked as a school bus driver, his physicians would have a heightened incentive to discourage his driving. The argument might also be made that, if Mr. Gordon did not report his epilepsy, his doctors would have an ethical obligation to do so. None of those conditions apply here, however, and his care professionals are likely to respect his confidentiality, while counseling him about responsible behaviors.

GENOMIC TESTING AND CONTROL OF INFORMATION

The increasing use of and sophistication of genetic/genomic tests raise a variety of new ethical problems related to the control of personal health information. Consider the following:

Illana, a 20-year-old Orthodox Jewish woman, has been increasingly troubled about the fact that her grandmother and her mother had breast cancer. She recently read about a test for the BRCA2 gene that can provide information about the likelihood that she, her brother, or her children will develop the disease. While Illana wants to know her risk of breast cancer, she is afraid to take the test because, if the results are positive and her prospective marriage partner finds out, he may not want to marry her.

Lawrence is a 39-year-old man who works in a large manufacturing company that employs thousands of people. Recently, the management sent out a memo alerting employees to the opportunity to participate in a program of free and confidential testing for several genetic conditions. The memo strongly encouraged employees to be tested "to enhance your knowledge of your health risks and be able to make informed decisions." Lawrence is concerned because, even though the testing is supposed to be confidential, he does not want his employer to know about his family history of heart disease.

Alex and Lauren have been reading about direct-to-consumer (DTC) personal genomic testing (PGT) and they have decided to have full genomic profiles done of their 3-year-old, Hayden, and their 6-month old, Ian. When asked by their friends and family why they are having the testing done, they reply, "We want to know as much as possible about our children's health risks so that we can work with their pediatrician to keep them healthy."

Sophia, an 18-year-old college freshman, is an avid user of Facebook, Twitter, and YouTube. Especially now that she is away at school, her social networking enables her to stay in instant and constant contact with her large circle of friends and family. Prompted by her interest in Biology 101, she has decided to access information on her genetic profile through a DTC-PGT service. When asked, she says, "It's a high-tech way of learning more about myself and my genetic history. Gene mapping is the latest thing and I can't wait to tell my family and friends what I find out."

The remarkable has become commonplace. It seems that every newspaper, journal, news program, and blog features daily bulletins about wondrous technological advances and scientific discoveries, and how they will affect our lives. We have come to expect breakthroughs and wizardry.

Perhaps once or twice in every generation, however, something so momentous occurs that even the most jaded observer pauses to contemplate how the world has shifted. Such is the potential power of the genomic revolution. We have witnessed the deciphering of the human genome, which, while not yet revealing the genetic roots of disease and generating treatments, has opened a window onto who we are, where we come from, how we are constructed, and how we might ultimately enhance the quality of our lives. And, like Adam and Eve, we have also begun to glimpse some of the potential burdens and risks that attend such potent knowledge.

Genetic/genomic testing responds to our insatiable curiosity about ourselves and offers the seductive possibility that information about our genetic makeup could enable us to predict our medical future and empower us to protect ourselves and our children from undesirable medical conditions. Yet it remains unclear exactly what and how much we want or need to know. Information about the likelihood of developing a disease that can be prevented or treated is very different from discovering the inevitability of an illness that has no cure. Possessing information about family genetics begs the question of whether to alert siblings or other relatives to their potential risks. Knowledge may be power but it can also create anxiety and, once learned, it cannot be unlearned.

Some of the ethical questions that require careful attention include the following: What is the appropriate level of protection for genetic/genomic test information? Should access to genomic information be treated differently from access to other sorts of sensitive medical information? Is genetic/genomic test information exceptional with respect to permissible use? When are the risks to others revealed by genetic/genomic testing sufficient to justify breaching confidentiality? What are the ethical concerns related to DTC genetic tests that provide information without the explanation and counseling that are routinely part of medical testing? These are cutting-edge issues that give a very contemporary spin to some traditional bioethical problems.

For those who believe in what has been called "genetic exceptionalism," the type of information acquired by genetic testing is unique because of its implications for other persons who are genetically related to the tested individual, and the rules concerning privacy and confidentiality have to be modified accordingly. For those who reject this view, genetic data are not the only sort of information that has health implications for those related to the tested individual and, therefore, the normal rules concerning privacy and confidentiality apply. Widespread misconceptions about the meaning and significance of genetic information also raise concerns about its proper use and the marketing of genetic/genomic tests.

REFERENCES

Ahronheim JC, Moreno JD, Zuckerman C. 2000. *Ethics in Clinical Practice*. 2nd ed. Gaithersburg, MD: Aspen Publishers.

American College of Physicians. 1993. *Ethics Manual*. 3rd ed. Philadelphia: American College of Physicians. Cited in Witman AB, Park DM, Hardin SB. 1996. How do patients want physicians to handle mistakes? *Archives of Internal Medicine* 156(22):2565–69.

American Medical Association, Council on Ethical and Judicial Affairs. 1997. Patient information: Opinion E-8.12, issued March 1981, updated June 1994. *Code of Medical Ethics*. Chicago: American Medical Association.

Bauer KA. 2009. Privacy and confidentiality in the age of e-medicine. *Journal of Health Care Law & Policy* 12:47–62.

Baylis F. 1997. Errors in medicine: Nurturing truthfulness. *Journal of Clinical Ethics* 8(4):336–40.

Beauchamp TL, Childress JF. 2001. *Principles of Biomedical Ethics*. 5th ed. New York: Oxford University Press, pp. 283–319.

Beauchamp TL, Childress JF. 2013. *Principles of Biomedical Ethics*. 7th ed. New York: Oxford University Press, pp. 302–24.

Belkin L. 1997. How can we save the next victim? *The New York Times Magazine*, June 15, pp. 28–70.

Berger JT. 1998. Culture and ethnicity in clinical care. *Archives of Internal Medicine* 158(19):2085–90.

Bok S. 1983. The limits of confidentiality. *Hastings Center Report*: 24–31.

Brodsky M, et al. 2008. Multiple sclerosis risk after optic neuritis: Final optic neuritis trial follow-up. *Archives of Neurology* 65(6):727–32.

Cullen S, Klein M. 2000. Respect for patients, physicians and the truth. In Munson R, ed. *Intervention and Reflection: Basic Issues in Medical Ethics*. 6th ed. Belmont, CA: Wadsworth, pp. 435–42.

Dresser R. 2008. The limits of apology laws. *Hastings Center Report* 38(3):6–7.

Freedman B. 2003. Offering truth: One ethical approach to the uninformed cancer patient. In Steinbock B, Arras JD, London AJ, eds. *Ethical Issues in Modern Medicine*. 6th ed. Boston: McGraw-Hill, pp. 76–82.

Gallagher TH, Waterman AD, Ebers AG, Fraser VJ, Levinson W. 2003. Patients' and physicians' attitudes regarding the disclosure of medical errors. *Journal of the American Medical Association* 289(8):1001–7.

Goldberg RM, Kuhn G, Andrew LB, Thomas HA. 2002. Coping with medical mistakes and errors in judgment. *Annals of Emergency Medicine* 39(3):287–92.

Greenberg MA. 1991. The consequences of truth telling. *Journal of the American Medical Association* 266(1):66.

Hermann DHJ, Gagliano RD. 1989. AIDS, therapeutic confidentiality, and warning third parties. *Maryland Law Review* 48(1):55–76.

Institute of Medicine, Committee on Quality of Health Care in America. 2000. *To Err Is Human: Building a Safer Health System*. Washington, DC: National Academy Press.

Jansen LA, Ross LF. 2000. Patient confidentiality and the surrogate's right to know. *Journal of Law, Medicine & Ethics* 28:137–43.

Joint Commission on Accreditation of Healthcare Organizations. 2014. Patient Rights and Organization Ethics Chapter (RI), Standard RI.1.1.3; Intent of Standard RI.1.1.3. *Comprehensive Accreditation Manual for Hospitals*. Oakbrook, IL: Joint Commission on Accreditation of Healthcare Organizations.

Kagawa-Singer M, Blackhall LJ. 2001. Negotiating cross-cultural issues at the end of life: "You've got to go where he lives." *Journal of the American Medical Association* 286(23):2993–3001.

Kohn LT, Corrigan JM, Donaldson M, eds. 1999. *To Err Is Human: Building a Safer Health System*. A report from the Committee on Quality of Healthcare in America, Institute of Medicine, National Academy of Sciences. Washington, DC: National Academy Press.

Krumholz A, Fisher RS, Lesser RP, Hauser WA. 1991. Driving and epilepsy: A review and reappraisal. *Journal of the American Medical Association* 265(5):622–26.

Levinson W, Roter DL, Mullooly JP, et al. 1997. Physician-patient communication: The relationship with malpractice claims among primary care physicians and surgeons. *Journal of the American Medical Association* 277(7):553–59.

Liebman CB, Hyman CS. 2004. A mediation skills model to manage disclosure of errors and adverse events to patients. *Health Affairs* 23(4):22–32.

Liebman CB, Hyman CS. 2006. Prescription for improving the way health care and legal systems deal with unanticipated outcomes in medical care. Presentation, the Association of the Bar of the City of New York, May 24.

Mastroianni AC, et al. 2010. The flaws in state "apology" and "disclosure" laws dilute their intended impact on malpractice suits. *Health Affairs* 29(9):1611–19.

McDonnell WM, Guenther E. 2008. Narrative review: Do state laws make it easier to say "I'm sorry?" *Annals of Internal Medicine* 149:811–15.

McGuire AL, Fisher R, Cusenza P, Hudson K, Rothstein MA, McGraw D, Matteson S, Glasser J, Henley DE. 2008 July. Confidentiality, privacy, and security of genetic and genomic test information in electronic health records: Points to consider. *Genetic Medicine* 10(7):495–99.

Novack DH, Detering BJ, Arnold R, et al. 1989. Physicians' attitudes toward using deception to resolve difficult ethical problems. *Journal of the American Medical Association* 261(20):2980–85.

Pellegrino ED. 1992. Is truth telling to the patient a cultural artifact? *Journal of the American Medical Association* 268(13):1734–35.

Ptacek JT, Eberhardt T. 1996. Breaking bad news: A review of the literature. *Journal of the American Medical Association* 276(6):496–502.

Quill TE, Townsend P. 1991. Bad news: Delivery, dialogue, and dilemmas. *Archives of Internal Medicine* 151(3):463–68.

Ruddick W. 1999. Hope and deception. *Bioethics* 13(3/4):343–57.

Siegler M. 1982. Confidentiality in medicine—a decrepit concept. *New England Journal of Medicine* 307:1518–21.

Sigman GS, Kraut J, La Puma J. 2003. Disclosure of a diagnosis to children and adolescents when parents object. In Beauchamp TL, Walters L, eds. *Contemporary Issues in Bioethics*. 6th ed. Belmont, CA: Wadsworth-Thomson Learning, pp. 133–38.

Stein J. 2000. A fragile commodity. *Journal of the American Medical Association* 283(3):305–6.

Surbonne A. 1992. Truth telling to the patient. *Journal of the American Medical Association* 268(13):1661–62.

Tarasoff v. Regents of the University of California, 551 P.2d 334 (Cal. 1976).

Thomasma DC. 2003. Telling the truth to patients: A clinical ethics exploration. In Beauchamp TL, Walters L, eds. *Contemporary Issues in Bioethics*. 6th ed. Belmont, CA: Wadsworth-Thomson Learning, pp. 128–32.

Vincent C. 2003. Understanding and responding to adverse events. *New England Journal of Medicine* 348(11):1051–56.

Vogel J, Delgado R. 1980. To tell the truth: Physicians' duty to disclose medical mistakes. *UCLA Law Review* 28:52–94.

Wu AW, Cavanaugh TA, McPhee SJ, et al. 1997. To tell the truth: Ethical and practical issues in disclosing medical mistakes to patients. *Journal of General Internal Medicine* 12(12):770–75.

Zahedi F. 2011. The challenge of truth telling across cultures: A case study. *Journal of Medical Ethics and History of Medicine* 4:11.

CHAPTER 5

Special Decision-Making Concerns of Minors

Decisional capacity and minors
Consent for and by minors
Confidentiality and disclosure
Special problems of functionally alone adolescents

DECISIONAL CAPACITY AND MINORS

If you think that assessing adults' ability to make and take responsibility for decisions is challenging, keep reading. Minors, especially adolescents, present a whole other set of issues related to their emerging cognitive abilities, self-awareness, and moral authority. In addition, while very young children and newborns are generally regarded as the responsibility of their parents or guardians, there are limits to parental decision-making authority. Because minors are usually considered incapable of assuming responsibility for their health care, conflicts about treating this vulnerable population will likely come before your ethics committee.

As discussed in chapter 2, the concept of decision-making capacity involves notions of autonomy and moral responsibility. Autonomy refers to self-governance, which requires that, at the very least, the individual has a *self* to govern. In this sense, autonomy implies a more or less integrated set of personal values and preferences that are recognizable and generally well-established. Moral responsibility refers to a person's capacity to be accountable for his actions and suggests stability, consistency, and foresight. These qualities develop as part of the maturation process that begins in young childhood and continues through adolescence into adulthood, but there is usually no bright line separating immature from mature decision-making ability.

Children

Timmy, a healthy 3-year-old child, is scheduled for a tonsillectomy this morning. His parents have done everything they can to prepare him for the surgery, including reading him books about going to the hospital, "operating" on his stuffed rabbit, and packing all his favorite toys. Despite their presence and reassurance, however, Timmy becomes increasingly agitated. He resists all contact with any medical personnel, including the nurses, the surgeons, and Dr. Lewis, the anesthesiologist.

Although Dr. Lewis tries to explain what she is doing and what will happen, Timmy keeps screaming, "No! No!" He struggles to climb off the stretcher and spits out the Versed that the nurse tried to mask with apple juice. In order to proceed, Dr. Lewis must hold him down and sedate him with an injection. When Timmy is sufficiently sedated and offers no resistance, Dr. Lewis brings him to the operating room, where the surgery proceeds without incident.

Following surgery, Timmy is returned to the main recovery room and then to the pediatric ambulatory area, where his parents are waiting for him. He still screams when he sees clinical personnel but, except for continuous crying, there are no post-operative problems.

Anyone who has spent time with young children knows that they do and do not want things, sometimes loudly, often inconsistently, and almost always vehemently. The sincerity with which they voice their wishes, however, should not be confused with the judgment necessary for responsible decision making. Timmy genuinely does not want to be in the hospital and efforts by his caregivers or even his parents to reason with him will not change his mind. He is unable to appreciate the need for surgery or the prospect of feeling better once his tonsils are removed. He cannot be placated by promises of ice cream when the operation is over. He is incapable of thinking about anything except his current fear and his desperate desire to be elsewhere.

Because of their immaturity, young children lack the attributes associated with autonomy and self-governance, and cannot be held fully morally responsible for their actions. A shorthand way of putting this is that they do not have decision-making capacity. The same is largely true of older children, although they may have preferences that can and should be accommodated in treatment plans. The younger the child, the less problem we have in saying, "This is a person for whom most decisions must be made by others because he has not developed the cognitive ability, experience, or judgment necessary to reason or the opportunity to form values and preferences that will influence his decisions."

As noted in chapter 2, however, decisions run along a continuum from low to high risk. Certainly, even young children are able to make some choices—"Do you want to wear the red or the blue shirt today?"—and giving them opportunities to do so helps them develop decision-making skills. As the consequences of the decisions become more significant—selecting suitable television programs, eating nutritious food, using seat belts—the intervention of adults becomes increasingly important. The need for adults to act on behalf of young children becomes especially clear when the decisions have critical outcomes and long-lasting consequences, as in the health care setting.

Even if young children cannot provide morally valid or legally binding consent, *assent* can be a valuable means of involving them in treatment decisions. Assent sets a lower standard than consent because it does not require the depth of understanding or reasoning ability required for informed consent. Giving minors a say in their treatment not only promotes their cooperation and therapeutic goals, but also provides them with opportunities to gain practice in decision making. This, in turn, furthers their capacity to make autonomous decisions.

Adolescents

James Bell is a 16-year-old adolescent admitted to the hospital with pain in his right leg. He is a tall, good-looking young man who is an honor roll student and involved in numerous school and community activities. His main claim to fame is his prowess in several sports and he is hoping to get an athletic scholarship to college. He lives with his mother, with whom he appears to have a good relationship.

After examination and tests, a diagnosis of osteosarcoma of the right femur was made. The hematology-oncology and orthopedic doctors met with James and his mother two days ago to discuss the diagnosis, prognosis, and treatment options. All the professionals recommended amputation of the leg rather than local excision, because amputation has been shown to increase the survival rates. James and his mother were both shocked and distressed by the news. When the options were explained, Mrs. Bell asked many questions, but James was silent. Finally, she said to James, "There doesn't seem to be any question that amputation will give you the best chance to beat the cancer. I know it will be hard, but I think this is what we have to do." James replied, "No way! No way they're cutting off my leg! I'll agree to the local treatment, but that's it." When the doctors and his mother tried to persuade him, he said, "I'd rather die with my leg than live without it! You can't make me do this!" He has remained adamant, despite several attempts to explain the important benefits of amputation and the athletic successes other young amputees have achieved.

Can adolescents be considered to have the capacity to make health care decisions, especially those with serious consequences? Who does or should make health care decisions for adolescents? What else would be important to know about James's decision and reasoning? What is the relationship between consent and assent? Should surgery proceed over James's continued objections?

As anyone who has ever been or known an adolescent is aware, decision-making capacity and decisional authority become dramatically more complex during the teenage years. Along the decision-making continuum, adolescents occupy a position that is legally and ethically ambiguous. From a purely cognitive standpoint, by the age of 14, the typical child demonstrates a capacity to reason, including the ability to understand the causes and effects of illness, that is both as good and as flawed as it will be in adulthood. It will come as no surprise, however, that adolescent capacity to make autonomous decisions is enormously variable and that, even among adolescents of the same age, some are still extremely child-like in their behavior and thinking, whereas others are remarkably mature. This is partly because the young person's self-identity has not yet been consolidated and his values and commitments have not yet been fully formed, and these develop at different rates. As the individual matures in experience and judgment, he edges closer to assuming control of and responsibility for his own decisions and correspondingly greater weight is given to his values and preferences.

The challenge in evaluating this ability is to consider the relevant factors and skills in their appropriate context. The law, as a crude instrument, makes blunt distinctions necessarily based on somewhat rigid and arbitrary standards. Thus, we have those eagerly awaited milestone ages at which people are finally allowed to drive, vote, drink, and serve in the armed forces. Likewise, determining the ability to make decisions that provide *legally* binding consent is based on easily defined characteristics, such as the age of majority, marital or parental status, or economic self-sufficiency.

In contrast, the ethical analysis of adolescent decision-making capacity is more complex, multifactorial, and nuanced. In assessing the capacity of an adolescent to make decisions that will be given *moral* weight, it is necessary to consider a variety of factors, including

- biological and emotional maturity;
- appreciation of cause, effect, and consequences
- patterns of decision making and behavior, including risk taking;
- formation and execution of future-oriented plans;
- control of one's emotions;
- personal values; and
- voluntariness of choice.

An adolescent's decisional capacity is a function of both his stage of biological and psychological development and external factors, such as life experience, including health care and treatment experience. Adolescent decisional capacity is significantly influenced by ecological and experiential factors, and this accounts for much of its variability in comparison to most adult decision making. Adolescent decisions are typically the product of greater uncertainty and insecurity, less experience, more volatile emotions, immature self-image, unrealistic appraisal of risks and consequences, susceptibility to peer pressure and the desire to conform, and greater focus on the present than the future. These characteristics have direct implications for the capacity to make decisions, especially those with high-stakes consequences. For example, an adolescent patient with a chronic or serious illness may exhibit greater knowledge and more mature judgment about treatment decisions than would be displayed by a peer who has not had the same debilitating experience.

James has been presented with a prospect that would devastate a person twice his age. He is forced to confront his own mortality decades too soon. If that were not enough, he is asked to accept a drastic alteration in body image and the loss of what makes him special—his athletic prowess. No wonder he's reeling. As a newly diagnosed cancer patient, he is doing what many adults initially do in his situation— rejecting unwanted information.

At 16, James is approaching adulthood. He may very well have the cognitive ability to understand his situation and consider his treatment choices. What he may not have is the experience and judgment necessary to appreciate the long-term consequences of his decisions. Until now, he has not had the unthinkable happen and he cannot imagine that things may work out in positive ways he has not considered. To the extent possible, he should be given the opportunity to be an active participant in planning his care. His involvement will be critical to the success of his treatment and recuperation, as well as rebuilding his body image and sense of self-determination.

To assess his ability to participate, James's caregivers will need to know much more about his maturity, his ability to solve problems and consider alternatives, and his experience with illness and loss. It is not uncommon to hear people, especially adolescents, reject something by saying, "I'd rather die" as a way of expressing the strength of their feelings. Most often, however, they have little or no real sense of death or the implications of such a choice. It is also important to clarify James's reasons for refusing. If he does not understand or believe the seriousness of his condition, he needs further explanation. If he is looking at short-range issues, such as his appearance, his popularity with his friends, and his altered athletic ability, he may benefit from spending time with other adolescents in his situation.

A history of other illness and treatment will also affect James's ability to deal with his current situation. For example, a 16-year-old who has lived for years with chronic and debilitating illness, endured rounds of unsuccessful radiation and chemotherapy, or rejected one or more transplanted organs may be well positioned to say, "Enough. I know what this is about and it's not the way I want to live for whatever time I have left." In contrast, James is newly diagnosed with an illness that has the potential for remission or cure. Despite the significant burdens of the proposed amputation, they may be vastly outweighed by the long-term benefits. As a 16-year-old, however, he lacks the ability to envision himself as anything other than James-as-he-is, the person who has been and is expected to be successful in very specific ways that are now threatened.

Perhaps James has been exposed to others—his late father, other relatives, or even friends—in similar situations. If so, their clinical outcomes and successful or unsuccessful coping strategies will likely influence his response to his illness. If not, his lack of preparation for this unexpected assault will complicate his ability to absorb the implications of his diagnosis, prognosis, and treatment options.

Ideally, James, his mother, and his caregivers will be able to collaborate in a process of education and support while making these difficult decisions about his future. As discussed below, although he is unable to provide legally binding consent, his assent to treatment will be critically important. With skill, creativity, and persistence, it may be possible for his mother and the care team to introduce an alternate vision with another set of possibilities, goals, and achievements. If he remains unpersuaded by the benefit-burden analysis and adamantly opposed to amputation, however, it may be necessary to proceed with surgery over his objections. Ultimately, the gravity of his condition and the potential for life-saving treatment, the clinical judgment of his caregivers, and the experience and devotion of his mother will assume greater weight than his choice in making decisions with profound and lasting consequences of this magnitude.

As discussed in chapter 3, refusal of treatment is not simply the flip side of consent, a distinction with special relevance for minors. Just as a heightened level of capacity is required for adults to refuse treatment that is considered to be in their best interest, treatment refusal by or on behalf of minors triggers a heightened level of scrutiny to protect them from the consequences of deficient decision making. For example, courts in two cases (*In re Sampson*, 1970, and *In re Seiforth*, 1955) considered elective correction of facial deformities refused by parents and handed down very different rulings based on the degree to which the deformities affected the adolescents' intellectual, educational, emotional, and psychological development, and the fact that one young man strongly supported his father's refusal of treatment, which was considered likely to undermine his treatment. Additional concerns were raised about rupturing the father-son relationship. These cases are discussed further in part IV.

CONSENT FOR AND BY MINORS

How and by whom decisions are made has special significance in the health care setting. Because the law almost always considers minors to lack the judgment and experience necessary for responsible decision making, it generally denies them legal power and requires the consent of one or both parents or a legal guardian to authorize medical care. Sometimes, however, the law departs from this requirement when it appears that the young patient's best interests will be served by having others or, in selected instances, him assume decision-making authority.

Newborns

Baby Franklin was born at 34 weeks' gestation with Apgar scores of 0, 3, and 5 at 1, 5, and 10 minutes, respectively. His multiple medical problems included severe pulmonary hypertension and resulting ventilator dependence, frontal lobe hemorrhage, and one missing kidney. His chances of survival are uncertain. The decision was made to start him on peritoneal dialysis, which is more appropriate than hemodialysis for a child in his condition. A catheter was placed to facilitate the process, but it has now extruded and the doctors are considering whether they should take the baby to the OR under general anesthesia and replace the catheter. Though the prognosis for improvement in renal function is not good, it is possible that this will happen and that lifelong dialysis will not be necessary. As for Baby Franklin's neurological condition, if he does survive, he will likely be severely disabled. The baby's mother has made it clear that she wants "everything" done for him, although this may have been more of a reflexive statement than an informed directive. An ethics consult was requested, with the main question "Should Baby Franklin be taken to the OR and put under general anesthesia so that his catheter can be replaced?"

The neonatal intensive care unit (NICU) is the scene of both high drama and devastating choices. The care of newborns has changed enormously over the past few decades. Because of technological advances, substantial medical progress has been made in the care of very premature, seriously ill, and impaired neonates. In addition, decision making about the treatment of such infants has become more collaborative, including clinicians, parents, and other family members, and occasionally laypersons who work outside the NICU. Careful consideration of treatment options is increasingly important because, while new techniques enable health professionals to maintain the lives of infants who would otherwise not survive, this rescue is often at the cost of a significantly diminished quality of life.

These issues began to attract public attention and governmental regulation in 1982, when a baby born with Down syndrome and an opening between the esophagus and trachea was permitted to die without life-saving intervention. The parents' concern about the potential for some degree of mental retardation made them refuse the recommended surgical repair, a decision upheld by the state court. The case of Baby Doe generated considerable publicity, the outrage of right-to-life groups and advocates for the developmentally disabled, and a controversial response by the U.S. Department of Health and Human Services. This case and its regulatory results are discussed further in part IV.

Lantos and Meadow (2006) categorize the babies admitted to the NICU into three groups that raise different clinical and ethical challenges:

- Full- or near-term infants with acute illnesses, such as pneumonia or sepsis, that can be medically treated or anatomic abnormalities that can be surgically corrected require accurate diagnosis and immediate intervention. Because these babies have the potential for normal healthy lives once the acute problem is corrected, the moral obligation to treat is usually unquestioned.
- Neonates with congenital anomalies, such as Down syndrome, raise the question whether to address one or more life-threatening medical problems even though the underlying congenital syndrome cannot be cured. Deliberation about these situations tends to focus on the infants' projected quality of life rather than survival.
- Infants born very prematurely but with no medical problems other than prematurity raise the same ethical considerations as the other NICU patients but in the context of prognostic uncertainty. The spectrum of possibilities, which cannot be predicted with certainty, range from death to severe, moderate, or mild disability to no medical or developmental problems. Typically, decisions are based on the degree of prognostic certainty: parents may not refuse treatment when all indications support a good prognosis; life-sustaining treatment may be considered optional when clinical evidence points to poor outcomes; and treatment may be considered futile when birth is so premature that survival is unprecedented.

The ethical principles that guide neonatal intensive care decisions include beneficence, nonmaleficence, and justice. Also critically important is respect for parental choice, within limits. Beneficence and nonmaleficence create the professional obligation to provide care for the newborn that maximizes benefit and minimizes harm. Moreover, because the infant is the patient, his interests must be assessed independent of the interests of the family. Beneficence is a guiding principle for parents and professionals alike, obligating them to make decisions that will promote the welfare of the neonate. Conceptions of benefit and harm may be defined differently by health professionals and parents, however, creating conflicts in the NICU over how or even whether to treat. Justice requires that treatment decisions be based on the infant's best interests, without considerations of race, ethnicity, or ability to pay.

Taken together, these ethical principles create the obligation to provide newborns, who are especially vulnerable, with heightened protection. Decision making for critically ill and handicapped infants is complicated by two factors. First, uncertain prognostication in the early neonatal period may not be clarified until numerous aggressive life-sustaining measures have been instituted. Second, decisions to provide or forgo aggressive measures frequently involve quality-of-life judgments. Because parents and clinicians may have very different notions of what constitutes an acceptable or unacceptable quality of life for the child, consensus on these deeply personal issues is often difficult to achieve. The resulting collision of principled obligations can create painful conflict for those who care for and about the infant.

Our society's deference to parental decisions rests on respect for family integrity, the presumption that parents act in their children's best interests, and the need to have designated authority to make such decisions. Accordingly, parental decisions about the care of newborns are routinely honored unless they contradict the clinical judgments of the care team. Typically, when physicians recommend a course of treatment that is clearly in the newborn's best interests, parents agree. In rare cases, parents make decisions that are likely to harm their child and not provide compensating benefit. Decisions that put children at unjustified risk are considered abuse of parental authority and usually trigger outside intervention.

Between these two extremes, many decisions made by parents fall into a gray area, where it is not at all clear whether the choice will benefit their newborn. In these cases of uncertainty, parental decisions tend to be respected. The difficult issues that arise in the NICU place significant ethical responsibilities on caregivers, including

- putting the child's interests at the center of decision making;
- involving parents in the decision-making process;
- providing parents with full, accurate, and timely updates about their child's condition, prognosis, and treatment options;
- providing parents with guidance, support, and time to decide on care goals and plans that change as the infant's condition evolves;
- providing care recommendations, as well as information;
- letting parents know that it is appropriate to forgo treatment when the burdens to the infant clearly outweigh the benefits; and
- helping parents to modify their expectations in light of clinical realities without extinguishing their hopes.

In light of these factors, let's return to Baby Franklin, whose prognosis is the major factor in the ethical analysis. It may be tempting to argue that replacing the catheter is *medically futile* because, if he survives, his condition will be significantly compromised. But, as discussed further in chapter 9, there is no general consensus on the definition of medical futility, so appealing to that concept in a situation where the intervention may have some clinical benefit is unlikely to move the ethical analysis forward.

This is where prognostic uncertainty complicates the neonatal picture. Because there is a small chance that the baby will survive and the exact extent of his eventual neurological impairment cannot be known with certainty at this time, it can be argued that further aggressive treatment is *not* futile. Moreover, the baby's mother, who is the legally and ethically appropriate decision maker for her child, has requested that everything be done. While she may not have a complete understanding of what "everything" entails, as the parent of this imperiled neonate, her opinion ought to have considerable moral weight. At the same time, it would be critical for her to understand that her baby may not survive even if "everything" is done. This would be the case, for example, if the catheter could not be replaced or if the replacement catheter came out and the doctors were not able to reinsert it. Without badgering the mother with a steady stream of ominous predictions, it is important for her to be given clear, consistent, and candid updates so that if the proposed interventions are not effective, she will be prepared to make decisions that are consistent with clinical realities and in the best interests of her baby.

The following algorithm is often used in managing the care of critically ill newborns: if interventions can benefit the baby (e.g., fixing esophageal atresia in an infant with Down syndrome or providing a blood transfusion for a neonate whose parents are Jehovah's Witnesses), caregivers will likely intervene on the baby's behalf, even if doing so requires a court order. If, however, the consensus is that interventions will cause only suffering with no compensating benefit, the NICU team will provide supportive, palliative care only, as well as the offer of assistance in transferring the infant to another institution willing to provide the disputed care if the parents still request it. In the vast number of cases, which fall somewhere between these extremes on the continuum, caregivers will be guided by the treatment wishes of the parents, who are presumed to be acting in their child's best interest and will have to live with the consequences of their decision. At present, Baby Franklin seems to fall in this gray area of prognostic uncertainty, so his mother's preferences should be honored as long as it is medically possible and reasonable to do so. What is less clear at this time is whether it would be ethically appropriate to offer yet another catheter replacement if this one were to fail.

When conflicting values and interests complicate decisions about neonatal care, hospitals are increasingly referring these cases to infant bioethics review committees for special attention.

Children

Melissa is a 1-month-old infant admitted with a severe infection that has resulted in significant and irreversible brain damage. She is currently on a ventilator and cannot suck, so a tracheostomy and a gastrostomy will be necessary to support her respiration and nutrition. She responds only to painful stimuli, such as the frequent blood draws necessary to monitor her infection. According to the treating team, her condition will not improve because, as the intensivist explained to her mother, "the infection has destroyed Melissa's brain." The NICU care team's recommendation is a palliative care plan that will focus on Melissa's comfort without prolonging her suffering.

Melissa's mother, Ms. Green, is a 45-year-old deaf woman who has 11 children, most of whom are in foster care and several of whom are in the process of being adopted. It is not clear why the children have been taken from her, but she maintains contact with some of them. Melissa's father is reportedly a violent man with a drug problem and Ms. Green apparently left him because he abused her.

Ms. Green has told the sign language interpreter that this is her last chance to be a mother because she rarely has a chance to see her other children. She enjoys coming to visit Melissa anytime she pleases, "touching her, holding her, and feeling like a real mom." She does not want to let her baby go and she will not consent to anything, such as a recommended do-not-resuscitate (DNR) order, that would prevent the doctors from trying to keep Melissa alive. Even when the pain and lack of benefit to Melissa are explained, Ms. Green remains adamant that aggressive life-sustaining measures be continued.

How should Ms. Green's capacity to make decisions about Melissa's care be assessed? What factors might impair her ability to make decisions in Melissa's best interest? And how should Melissa's caregivers deal with Ms. Green's disagreement with their recommended care plan?

As in other instances of surrogate choice, care issues related to young children concern who makes decisions, according to what standards, and with what review. Legally, the first question is almost always resolved in favor of the parents, who are responsible for upbringing and welfare because they are presumed by tradition and law to act in their child's best interests.

Note that this presumption of parental authority distinguishes health care decision making for a minor from decision making on behalf of an incapacitated adult. In the latter case, the power to make treatment choices may be accorded to the patient's family or assumed by the court only when the adult patient has been *shown* to be incapable of choosing, and sometimes only when there has been some formal designation of a surrogate. In contrast, recognition that children lack the capacity to make their own health care decisions *presumptively* confers this authority on parents or guardians unless they are specifically disqualified by a determination of unfitness.

Ms. Green's capacity to make decisions for her daughter requires careful scrutiny because of her apparent inability to understand Melissa's medical condition, prognosis, and limited treatment options. While her impaired hearing may hinder her understanding of the clinical situation, her deafness can be accommodated with skilled sign language assistance and should not be the deciding factor. Her diminished capacity may be the result of several factors, including her deafness, possibly limited intelligence, years of abuse, and the stress of caring for a critically ill child.

These problems may be complicated by Ms. Green's apparent inability to appreciate her child's best interests or that they may be in conflict with her own interests. If her focus is on extending her opportunity to function as a mother rather than on what benefits her child, she may not be the best person to be making care decisions for Melissa.

Larry is a 12-year-old who was struck by a car and has been brought to the trauma ER. There, it was discovered that he has a severe renal injury with significant internal bleeding. When his parents arrive, they tell the physicians that, because they and Larry are Jehovah's Witnesses, transfusion of blood or blood products is out of the question.

How should the religious convictions of Larry's parents influence the decision about his receiving potentially life-saving blood transfusion? What weight should be given to Larry's religious beliefs?

The rights granted parents or guardians, as well as the restrictions placed on those rights, are rooted in an ethical perspective that assigns top priority to the interests of the child. In this view, widely shared in our culture, parents are entrusted with the well-being of their children and charged with specific duties, including the provision of food, clothing, shelter, basic education, and health care. Within the parameters set by these duties, parents may make choices based on their own values and beliefs about what is best for their children. So far, so good. Note, however, that parental authority is not unlimited because it is constrained by parental responsibility. When parents abuse their authority—for example, by refusing consent for clearly beneficial medical treatment—the child's interests trump even the well-established presumption of parental rights.

Accordingly, the law deviates from the almost automatic deference to parents in the context of decisions about health care when the child's welfare or life is at stake. In such cases, the law requires physicians to act on behalf of the child and permits the state to intervene in the protective role of *parens patriae*. For example, a standard exception to the requirement of parental consent for medical treatment is emergencies, when delaying treatment would threaten the child's life or health. Likewise, all states provide for removing children from abusive or harmful environments or situations in which they are deprived of necessary medical treatment. In addition, parents are prevented from interfering with needed medical care and can be criminally prosecuted for failing to provide that care.

Courts have agreed that parents may not withhold life-saving treatment from a child who is neither terminally ill nor permanently comatose. Treatment refusal has not been permitted even when the therapy is painful and only marginally effective if it is determined that the child will die without it. When the contested treatment is elective or carries substantial risks, however, courts are more likely to accede to parental refusal. Although decisions continue to vary, the trend appears to be limiting parents' authority when their decisions conflict with generally accepted medical judgment. Judicial intervention is less likely when parents are providing some kind of professionally accepted treatment. Several illustrative legal cases are summarized in part IV.

Court intervention usually involves authorization, at the request of health care providers, to perform a particular surgical procedure or course of medical treatment over parental objection. Because these cases focus on a specific, usually lifesaving, therapeutic objective, courts are likely to override parents' refusal, which is usually based on religious or philosophical belief. In these singular instances, traditional deference to parental decision-making authority gives way to the determination by others of what is best for the child. For example, courts have ordered children inoculated over their parents' religious objections.

Similarly, parents who are Jehovah's Witnesses are not permitted to refuse lifesaving blood transfusions for their children. Adherents to this faith believe that receiving blood or blood products places their souls in eternal jeopardy, making it worse to survive after transfusion than to die without having received the blood. This deeply held belief should be honored when it is expressed by capable adult patients who understand and accept the risks posed by their religious commitments. In contrast, a child who is too immature to have developed settled religious convictions or make autonomous decisions that place his life at risk cannot be permitted to assume this responsibility. Seen in this light, a child's agreement with his parents should not be considered conclusive evidence that he has made an autonomous and informed decision to refuse potentially life-saving treatment.

Given the extent of Larry's injuries and internal bleeding, he appears to be at risk of serious harm and possibly death if he is not transfused. The likelihood and magnitude of the harm if he does not receive blood mean that his parents' decision to withhold transfusion is not in his medical interest. Under most circumstances, this would justify overriding their refusal to consent to transfusion. In this case, however, Larry is approaching the age when he might be considered to have settled religious beliefs and values. If he is able to express an informed conviction about being a Jehovah's Witness, it becomes more complicated to support paternalistic intervention to transfuse over his objections. One recommendation would be to interview him without his parents present to evaluate his maturity, understanding, and the strength of his religious convictions.

Finally, courts tend not to order treatment for children who are comatose, for whom death is imminent, or for whom the marginal benefits of treatment are outweighed by its burdens. In these situations, courts have held that the decision to forgo treatment was in the children's best interest.

Just as there are limits to parental rights to refuse treatment, there are also limits to parental rights to insist on treatment. When specific interventions are determined by the care team to be medically inappropriate or ineffective, when the burdens and risks clearly outweigh the benefits, physicians have an obligation to protect their young and vulnerable patients from measures that are not clinically indicated.

It is important, however, to recognize and address the motivation behind much of what may appear to be unreasonable parental demands. The job of parents is to stand between their children and danger, to protect them from injury, illness, and other harms. When, despite their best efforts, their children are sick or hurt, parents may direct their efforts toward ensuring that everything possible is done to promote recovery. Whether the therapies they propose are standard of care or unconventional, they are likely to feel the obligation to advocate strongly for anything that holds out even the slimmest prospect of success. It is understandable, therefore, that they perceive refusal to provide requested treatments as yet another barrier to fulfilling their nurturing responsibilities.

As discussed further in chapter 9, demands for treatment should trigger a discussion with parents that begins by exploring what "everything" means, clarifying their expectations of the proposed therapies, and explaining the likely course with and without the treatment. The focus should be on the care that *will* be provided rather than what will not, emphasizing that the shared goal is to provide only care that will benefit the child and maximize comfort and quality of life. Whenever possible, parents should be involved as collaborators in care planning as a way of helping them retain their role as protectors against harm and guardians of their children's well-being.

Adolescents

Nora is a 17-year-old young woman initially seen in adolescent health clinic, referred by a pediatric nephrologist for primary care and contraceptive counseling. She has a history of urinary tract problems diagnosed two years ago after proteinuria was discovered on routine urinalysis. She has been taking Cozaar for the proteinuria.

Nora told the clinic physician, Dr. Gonzalez, that she became sexually active six months ago and has been intimate with the same male partner, Joe, who is 21 years old. She says they have always used condoms except once, which is when she became pregnant last year. At her mother's insistence, she terminated the pregnancy immediately.

During her clinic visit, Nora requested Depo Provera for contraception. Her last menstrual period had been six weeks earlier and she was awaiting her next menses. Routine blood work was ordered, including a test to rule out pregnancy before giving her the first Depo injection at her next period. Test results indicated an early pregnancy.

The clinic social worker made several unsuccessful attempts to schedule an appointment to discuss options, but Nora missed each appointment. Finally she came to the clinic 12 weeks after her last period. Dr. Gonzalez had a lengthy discussion with Nora about the potential risk to the fetus because she has been taking Cozaar, a medication contraindicated in pregnancy. Nora insisted that she understood the possibility of prematurity and birth defects, but said that she wanted to keep this pregnancy. She promised to discuss the situation with Joe over the weekend. She was explicit about not wanting her mother to know because "she made me have an abortion the last time." She was told to discontinue the Cozaar and return to the clinic on Monday.

When Nora and Joe met with the social worker, they communicated their decision to continue the pregnancy. Their plan is not to tell her mother until after Nora has moved in with Joe. It is also apparent that Nora has not told Joe about the risk of birth complications.

How should Nora's capacity to make decisions about this pregnancy be assessed? What factors should be considered? Is her mother required to be involved in these decisions?

Adolescents, who are neither children nor adults, stand with a foot in each world. Their intellectual and emotional development is greater than that of young children, yet most are not fully mature. While their cognitive skills are growing and they are likely to have a well-developed set of preferences and moral values, they still lack the experience and judgment of adults. Because the legal age of majority in almost all states is 18, adolescents are technically minors for most purposes. The few exceptions, provided for in state law, are the ability of the emancipated minor and the mature minor to make legally binding decisions. For example, a minor who has given birth may relinquish the child for adoption.

The age of and criteria for consent to health care vary by state, and the law has relaxed the customary requirement for parental consent by carving out specific situations in which adolescents may make decisions about their treatment. The trend began in 1976 with a line of cases in which the U.S. Supreme Court held that minors who are sufficiently mature should be able to authorize abortions without parental consent or notification. Subsequent cases permitted teens access to contraception and statutes provided access without parental consent to treatment for substance abuse and sexually transmitted diseases (STDs).

Why do courts carve out these particular decisions for minors to make without parental notification or consent? Does this trend reflect judicial recognition that minors are especially wise about these decisions? These pragmatic exceptions to the parental consent requirement apply in situations in which it is imperative that teens are treated for their own good and as a matter of public health. The underlying concept recognizes that some highly sensitive health care circumstances have serious implications for young patients and others. In these situations, adolescents are more likely to seek and, therefore, receive health care if they can consent to it without involving or notifying their parents. This utilitarian reasoning is often used in the justification of confidentiality, discussed in chapter 4.

The mature minor doctrine is based on the notion that some minors have the cognitive ability and maturity to make informed decisions about their care. This doctrine, given force in many states' case or statutory law, provides for minors to consent to care in the following circumstances:

- The minor is an older adolescent (e.g., older than 14 or 15 years).
- The minor is capable of giving an informed consent.
- The care is for the benefit of the minor.
- The care does not present a high level of risk.
- The care is within the range of established medical opinion (English 1999, p. 86).

Minor treatment statutes address the societal obligation to protect adolescents and provide access to care, rather than a societal recognition of adolescent maturity and decisional capability. The reasoning behind them is similar to that behind a sliding scale notion of decisional capacity. As discussed in chapter 2, the level of capacity required to make a decision depends on the seriousness of its consequences, with greater capacity required for decisions that have a unfavorable risk-benefit ratio for the patient and less capacity required for decisions that have a favorable risk-benefit ratio. Similar reasoning increases the likelihood that adolescents will be permitted to make care decisions that do not carry great risks. In this way, these laws reflect the goal of promoting minors' best interests.

Statutes in every state, known as minor consent statutes or medical emancipation statutes, authorize minors to consent to care based either on their *status* or on the specific *service* they are seeking. The categories of minors authorized by one or more states to consent to medical care based on their *status* are

- emancipated minors (often defined using one or more of the following criteria)
- married minors
- minors in the armed forces
- mature minors
- minors living apart from their parents
- minors over a certain age
- high school graduates
- pregnant minors
- minor parents (English 1999, p. 85)

Central to this legal framework is the notion that, because these minors are no longer under effective parental supervision, parental consent is not a sensible precondition to accessing care.

The categories of *service* for which one or more states authorize minors to give consent are

- emergency care
- pregnancy-related care
- contraceptive services
- abortion
- diagnosis or treatment of venereal or STDs
- diagnosis or treatment of reportable, infectious, contagious, or communicable diseases
- HIV/AIDS testing or treatment
- treatment or counseling for drug or alcohol problems
- collection of medical evidence or treatment for sexual assault
- inpatient mental health services
- outpatient mental health services (English 1999, p. 85)

Because these statues are state-specific and their provisions differ according to jurisdiction, clinicians treating adolescents should be very familiar with the laws of the jurisdiction in which they provide care. Likewise, if your ethics committee addresses issues of adolescent health care, knowledge of the relevant laws and regulations in your state would be important. For example, even states that do not carve out specific status or service provisions that permit adolescents to access care must have a judicial bypass. This mechanism provides for adolescents who believe they will be at risk if their parents know about their medical situations to appear before a judge who will determine whether care can be provided without parental involvement. The take-away message is that, given the range of adolescent decisional capacities, the range of health care issues confronting adolescents, and the range of risks and benefits associated with different treatment options, decisions involving this population demand a heightened level of scrutiny and a constant balancing of rights and interests.

CONFIDENTIALITY AND DISCLOSURE

Donna is a 15-year-old who has come to the clinic for her annual physical prior to the beginning of school. Her mother, who accompanied her, remains in the waiting room during the exam. Donna appears healthy and active. In addition to a demanding scholastic schedule, she is on the track team and participates in several extracurricular and community activities. Although she appears bright and pleasant, she is clearly uneasy about something. Finally, at the end of the examination, she tells Dr. Jin that she and her boyfriend have recently begun having sex and she feels it would be responsible for her to be on birth control pills. She asks for a prescription, but insists that the doctor not tell her mother about her sexual activity or her request for contraception. Dr. Jin's discussion with her about sexual relations and contraception indicates that her decision is not coerced and that she understands its implications.

When Dr. Jin leaves the exam room, Donna's mother approaches her in the hall and says, "Doctor, I suspect that Donna's boyfriend is pressuring her to have sex. She's just not ready for that and I need to know what is going on. Please tell me if she has discussed this with you."

What are Dr. Jin's obligations to Donna? What are Dr. Jin's obligations to her mother?

Remember when you were 15 and didn't want your parents to know about something in your life? Remember when you were afraid that your teenager was growing up too fast? Sorting out the boundaries of adolescent privacy and confidentiality is difficult under any circumstance; it can be especially challenging in the health care setting when so much more is at stake.

Maintaining the confidentiality of adolescents' health information serves many of the same important functions that it does for adults and some that are especially important to the adult-in-training. Patients are more likely to seek treatment, especially for conditions that are sensitive or socially stigmatizing, and, once in treatment, are likely to provide more complete and accurate histories if they know their confidences are secured. Protecting the privacy of adolescents also shields them from embarrassment, discrimination, and potential family disruption or even violence. Finally, honoring their privacy helps adolescents in their critical development of autonomy.

Adolescents' health care confidentiality is guarded by the protections built into federal and state constitutions, statutes and regulations, court decisions, and professional ethical standards. However, these safeguards are never absolute and the ambiguous status of adolescents adds to the difficulty of determining what information should be protected or disclosed, to whom, and under what circumstances. Some state statutes pair adolescents' right to consent to treatment with their right to confidentiality with respect to that treatment. Others require disclosure of health care information over the adolescent's objection in certain situations, including specific disclosure to parents, mandatory reporting of physical or sexual abuse, or disclosure when the adolescent poses a severe and imminent danger to herself or others.

Dr. Jin's obligations to Donna's mother are the same as they would be to the concerned family of any patient—to provide her daughter with the most appropriate health care in light of her medical needs, her appreciation of her condition, her options and their implications, and her wishes. Here, the ethical analysis would balance the likely benefits of protecting Donna's confidences (strengthening the trust in the therapeutic relationship and promoting further beneficial patient-physician interaction, preventing unwanted pregnancy, and facilitating autonomous decision making) against the likely risks (erroneously presuming that Donna is making a voluntary and mature decision about sexual activity, and inhibiting mother-daughter discussion about a sensitive topic that might benefit from parental guidance).

If Dr. Jin's clinical assessment indicates that maintaining Donna's confidentiality would promote her best interest, her ethical obligations would not include disclosure of information about contraception that Donna wishes to remain between herself and her doctor. It would be appropriate, however, for her to explore with Donna the potential advantages of confiding in her mother and the possible ways to do it.

Ellen Jordan is a bright, lively 14-year-old who comes to Dr. Singer for her first pre-school physical since her family moved to town 6 months ago. Her physical exam reveals a healthy, active adolescent. When asked whether she was sexually active, she shyly acknowledged that she and her boyfriend were "thinking about it" and she requested information about contraception. When Dr. Singer leaves the exam room, he is approached by Mr. and Mrs. Jordan, who explain that Ellen is adopted and has been HIV-positive since birth. She does not know her HIV status and they are adamant that she not be told until they believe she is ready. They assure Dr. Singer that Ellen takes antiretroviral medications, which she thinks are vitamins.

Confidentiality, discussed above, concerns protecting personal health information revealed *by* the adolescent patient to the practitioner. Disclosure concerns personal health information revealed *to* the adolescent patient, which raises many of the same issues as disclosure to the adult patient, discussed in chapter 4, as well as concerns specific to minors. In the pediatric setting, patients do not have the same legal rights to information as adult patients, although they do have ethical rights to be treated with respect and honesty. Moreover, the customary deference accorded parents derives from the presumption that they know their children best and are acting in their best interest.

Nevertheless, certain important factors must be considered when parents insist on withholding health information from their minor child, including the age and maturity of the patient, the risks that her behavior may present to her and others with whom she interacts, the potential for her to learn her medical situation in an unplanned and unsupported manner, and the risk of eroding trust in her parents and her caregivers.

Dr. Singer can help the Jordans by explaining to the parents the justifications for disclosing this information to their daughter. Caring for minors with chronic illnesses, such as HIV, is an important opportunity to help them learn how to manage their health care and make decisions that promote their best interest. Ellen is four years away from legally assuming these responsibilities. She is also at an age when she is or soon will be sexually active, which puts others at unanticipated risk and requires her to take special steps to protect her contacts. They must also understand that Dr. Singer will not lie to Ellen because of the irreparable harm that would do to their therapeutic relationship. Likewise, they must be helped to appreciate that, if Ellen learns her HIV status independently, she is likely to question the validity of other things her parents have told her, possibly eroding their trust-based relationship with Ellen, which they have worked so hard to establish and nurture. Mr. and Mrs. Jordan must be helped to understand these realities and to be assured of Dr. Singer's support and guidance in disclosing this information to Ellen in a safe, nonthreatening manner.

SPECIAL PROBLEMS OF FUNCTIONALLY ALONE ADOLESCENTS

Andy was 15 when he learned he had rhabdomyosarcoma of the spine. With his specific form of cancer, cure is highly unlikely. Andy's mother is an alcoholic who has been in and out of substance abuse treatment for years. Throughout his illness, she has not been available for support or help in decision making. Andy's father also has not been present in his life. Andy did rely heavily on a close friend of his mother who, unfortunately, is no longer available to him.

Before his illness, Andy was a bright, athletic young man who enjoyed many activities. He has tried to make the best of his situation. He underwent surgery to remove the tumor and also had radiation therapy and chemotherapy, but none of the treatments was totally effective. He has never achieved remission and his pain has increased. Because of his mother's absence, the health care providers have discussed Andy's treatment options with him, although they actually have made most of the day-to-day decisions.

A significant turning point in Andy's illness occurred when his mother refused to move from her walk-up apartment into an available ground-floor apartment. His deterioration has made it impossible for him to negotiate the stairs, and his mother's resistance to relocating means that he can never return home. Because he is in the final stage of his illness, his doctors have asked Andy to consider whether he wants to continue chemotherapy and he has declined further treatment.

Should Andy's refusal to continue treatment be honored? Is he capable of making this decision? What responsibilities do Andy's care providers have to him as his disease worsens?

The journey from childhood to adulthood is filled with the potential for growth, achievement, and self-fulfillment. It is also fraught with confusion, uncertainty, and risk. Fortunately, most young people have the security of at least one caring and responsible adult to help them navigate the distance. Some are not so lucky.

A special category of minors is the adolescent alone. These young people are actually or functionally alone because they do not have a supportive relationship with an adult in a birth, foster, adoptive, or chosen family. No trusted adult is consistently available to guide and monitor their passage to adulthood or help them evaluate and make appropriate decisions about medical options.

The number of adolescents alone has increased, causing clinicians, researchers, other service providers, and policy analysts to focus on the special challenges they present. Some of these young people have been orphaned because their caregiving parent died of AIDS or other diseases, substance abuse, or violence. Some are functionally alone because their parent, grandparent, or other nominal caregiver is mentally ill, addicted to drugs or alcohol, or simply overwhelmed by poverty or other pressures. Some gay and lesbian youth have been ostracized by their families. Some adolescents have run away from homes where adults physically or sexually abused them. Some in foster care may feel that, although they have both biological and foster parents, they have no one to trust with private information and concerns. Some have parents or other adults who drift in and out of their lives, leaving them without the security of a stable relationship.

The adolescent alone occupies an ambiguous legal status, which can present particularly difficult problems regarding consent and confidentiality in health care. A variety of legal mechanisms may justify the provision of care to the adolescent alone based on his own consent in specific circumstances. These include the emancipated minor and mature minor doctrines, as well as state-specific medical consent laws, discussed above. These doctrines are not accepted in all jurisdictions, however, and consent provisions vary from state to state. For this reason, health care professionals are advised to familiarize themselves with the relevant laws in the states where they practice, particularly those that might provide the basis for the adolescent's legally valid consent. In addition, because clinicians and administrators may interpret the doctrines inconsistently, care may be provided differently to these adolescents within the same state or even within the same institution. Finally, even when the laws are consistently understood and interpreted, they do not adequately address the range of ethical issues presented by the care of the adolescent alone.

Many of the ethical principles that apply to adolescents with adult supports also apply to adolescents alone, including principles that govern capacity and informed consent and those related to the right to refuse and demand care. Thus, health care providers should assess any adolescent's capacity to consent in light of the specific decision at issue and its implications, as well as the young person's developmental characteristics, life situation, and medical history. Heightened concern about the adolescent's capacity is appropriate whenever the decision involves long-term negative health or life consequences. When recommended treatment is refused, health care providers should initiate an extensive discussion with the teen and explore mutually acceptable alternatives. As is true in the adult setting, refusal of treatment is not the end, but only the beginning of discussion with the adolescent patient. Likewise, the same assessment and serious discussion should be initiated by health care providers when the adolescent requests treatment that providers judge to be inappropriate or dangerous.

The obligation to protect patient privacy and confidentiality is as important for the adolescent alone as it is for other adolescents. Breaches of confidentiality may carry particular risks and be especially counterproductive for these vulnerable minors. The result can be their return to the abusive homes from which they fled and the exacerbation of problems that led them to their current difficult situations. At the outset of the clinical relationship, therefore, health care professionals should assure adolescents that confidentiality will be protected except in specific limited circumstances, which should be clearly defined.

Finally, when treating an adolescent alone, the natural inclination of many caregivers is to expand their role to meet many of the youth's unmet nonmedical needs. Although clinicians may feel as if they are acting like family, it should be clear to them and to the adolescent that they are professionals with the skills and the limits of professionals. Far from rejecting the adolescent alone, establishing and reinforcing the boundaries of the therapeutic relationship creates a stable atmosphere of dependability and trust that is so badly needed in their lives.

The special needs and vulnerability of this population make it likely that, if an adolescent alone is receiving care in your institution, the case will come to the attention of your ethics committee. Your familiarity with the ethical and legal issues will enhance the quality of your deliberations and the usefulness of your recommendations to the team caring for the patient.

REFERENCES

Alderman EM, Fleischman AR. 1993. Should adolescents make their own health-care choices? *Contemporary Pediatrics* 10:65–82.
American Academy of Pediatrics. 1994. Guidelines on forgoing life-sustaining medical treatment. *Pediatrics* 93(3):532–36.

American Academy of Pediatrics, Committee on Adolescence. 1996. The adolescent's right to confidential care when considering abortion. *Pediatrics* 97(5):746–51.

American Academy of Pediatrics, Committee on Bioethics. 1995. Informed consent, parental permission, and assent in pediatric practice. *Pediatrics* 95(2):314–17.

Beauchamp TL. 1997. Informed consent. In Veatch RM, ed. *Medical Ethics.* 2nd ed. Sudbury, MA: Jones and Bartlett Publishers, pp. 185–208.

Becker S. 2003. Consent to medical treatment for minors §19.06. In *Health Care Law: A Practical Guide.* San Francisco: Matthew Bender & Co.

Biggs H. 2009. Competent minors and health-care research: Autonomy does not rule, okay? *Clinical Ethics* 4:176–80.

Blustein J. 1982. *Parents and Children.* New York: Oxford University Press.

Blustein J. 1996. Confidentiality and the adolescent: An ethical analysis. In Cassidy R, Fleischman A, eds. *Pediatric Ethics: From Principles to Practice.* Amsterdam, The Netherlands: Harwood Academic Publishers, pp. 83–96.

Blustein J, Levine C, Dubler NN, eds. 1999. *The Adolescent Alone.* New York: Cambridge University Press.

Blustein J, Moreno J. 1999. Valid consent to treatment and the unsupervised adolescent. In Blustein J, Levine C, Dubler NN, eds. *The Adolescent Alone.* New York: Cambridge University Press, pp. 100–110.

Brock D. 1993. Informed consent. In *Life and Death: Philosophical Essays in Biomedical Ethics.* New York: Cambridge University Press, pp. 21–54.

Brock DW. 1996. Children's competence for health care decisionmaking. In Ladd RE. *Children's Rights Re-Visioned: Philosophical Readings.* Belmont, CA: Wadsworth Publishing Co., pp. 184–200.

DeRenzo EG, Panzarella P, Selinger S, Schwartz J. 2005. Emancipation, capacity, and the difference between law and ethics. *Journal of Clinical Ethics* 16(2):144–50.

Dubler NN, Stern G. 1991. *Illusions of Immortality: The Confrontation of Adolescence and AIDS.* A Report to the New York State AIDS Advisory Council from the Ad Hoc Committee on Adolescents and HIV.

English A. 1999. Health care for the adolescent alone: A legal landscape. In Blustein J, Levine C, Dubler NN, eds. *The Adolescent Alone.* New York: Cambridge University Press, pp. 78–99.

English A, et al. 1995. *State Minor Consent Statutes: A Summary.* Cincinnati: Center for Continuing Education in Adolescent Health.

Fleischman AR. 1994. Ethical issues in neonatology. In Oski FA, DeAngelis CD, Feigin RD, Washburn J, eds. *Principles and Practice of Pediatrics.* Philadelphia: Lippincott Williams & Wilkins, pp. 339–42.

Furrow BR, Johnson SH, Jost TS, Schwartz RL. 1991. *Health Law: Cases, Materials and Problems.* 2nd ed. St. Paul, MN: West Publishing Co., pp. 1183–92.

Hastings Center Research Project on the Care of Imperiled Newborns. 1987. Imperiled newborns. *Hastings Center Report* 17:5–32.

In re Sampson, 47 N.Y.2d 648 (1979).

In re Seiforth, 309 N.Y. 80 (1955).

Kopelman LM. 2004. Adolescents as doubly-vulnerable research subjects. *American Journal of Bioethics* 4(1):50–52.

Kuther TL. 2003. Medical decision-making and minors: Issues of consent and assent. *Adolescence* 38(150):343–58.

Lantos JD, Meadow WL. 2006. *Neonatal Bioethics: The Moral Challenges of Medical Innovation.* Baltimore: Johns Hopkins University Press.

Menikoff J. 2001. *Law and Bioethics: An Introduction.* Washington, DC: Georgetown University Press, pp. 298–99.

Mlyniec WJ. 1996. A judge's ethical dilemma: Assessing a child's capacity to choose. *Fordham Law Review* 64:1873–1915.

Paradise E, Horowitz RM. 1994. *Runaway and Homeless Youth: A Survey of State Law.* Washington, DC: American Bar Association Center on Children and the Law.

Quinn MM, Dubler NN. 1997. The health care provider's role in adolescent medical decision-making. *Adolescent Medicine* 8(3):415–25.

Rosato JL. 1996. The ultimate test of autonomy: Should minors have a right to make decisions regarding life-sustaining treatment? *Rutgers Law Review* 49(1):1–103.

Ross LF. 1997. Health care decisionmaking: Is it in their best interest? *Hastings Center Report* 27(6):41–45.

Schneider CE. 1998. *The Practice of Autonomy: Patients, Doctors, and Medical Decisions.* New York: Oxford University Press.

Weir RF, Peters C. 1997. Affirming the decisions adolescents make about life and death. *Hastings Center Report* 27(6):29–40.

Wolfe J, Klar N, Grier HE, Duncan J, Salem-Schatz S, Emanuel EJ, Weeks JC. 2000. Understanding of prognosis among parents of children who died of cancer: Impact on treatment goals and integration of palliative care. *Journal of the American Medical Association* 284(19):2469–75.

CHAPTER 6

Ethical Issues in Reproduction

The ethics and politics of reproductive choice
Assisted reproductive technologies
Surrogacy and gestational carriers
Termination of pregnancy
Maternal-fetal issues
Prenatal/newborn genetic testing and genomic newborn screening

THE ETHICS AND POLITICS OF REPRODUCTIVE CHOICE

To no one's surprise, most of the pressing ethical issues that arise in the clinical setting concern the beginning and the end of life. What may be surprising is that, as we have become more knowledgeable, more skilled, and more technologically savvy, we have also become less rather than more certain about when and how life begins and ends. Solving those mysteries is certainly beyond the scope of this book but this chapter and chapter 9 present ethical issues that your committee may be asked to address.

Reproductive liberty, the freedom to have children, to determine how many to have, and when and with whom to have them is one of the most highly valued liberties in our society. Because reproductive decisions are thought to be among the most personal and deeply meaningful ones that men and women make in their lives, interference with reproductive choice cannot be taken lightly. Because reproductive choice is a fundamental liberty, governmental interference with it can only be morally justified for compelling state reasons and, even then, the interference must impose the least restriction on reproductive choice, consistent with the aims of the intervention.

Given the intimate nature of reproductive issues, one might reasonably think that decisions about them would be confined to the individuals, their partners, and their physicians. One would be wrong. Paradoxically, these most personal issues are also those on which others—family, friends, legislators, religious leaders, politicians, special interest groups, and other complete strangers—feel not only the right but also the obligation to intervene or at least comment. Moreover, their opinions and interventions are highly variable, including those based on proven science and medical evidence, those rooted in theology or law, those intended to further a particular ideological agenda, and those informed by personal religious or philosophical convictions.

When these matters come to the attention of your ethics committee, it is important to be mindful of their polarizing potential and the need to approach discussions with respect and restraint. Patients, families, and caregivers all bring with them their values, beliefs, and personal histories. Your role is to provide the ethics lens through which the parties can view the medical issues and clinical decisions before them, and to keep the focus on those issues. Your concerns are promoting the right of the capable patient to make autonomous, informed, and voluntary decisions; protecting the right of caregivers to decline participation in any activity that violates their religious or philosophical convictions; and preserving the privacy and dignity of the deliberations. Mediating these delicate issues requires interpersonal skill, cultural sensitivity, and focus, and this is precisely what the institutional ethics voice can do most effectively.

While reproductive liberty is greatly valued, there is controversy concerning its ethical contours. New technologies expand reproductive options for men and women, but they also raise questions about their proper use. Should in vitro fertilization (IVF) be used to assist post-menopausal women to become pregnant? Should pre-implantation genetic diagnosis be used for the purpose of sex selection? Should gestational surrogates be paid? Should there be a market in sperm and eggs? Reproductive choice, after all, does not just involve the rights and interests of the woman who is contemplating becoming pregnant. They also concern the medical professionals who assist her, if she seeks or needs assistance; the man, woman, and sometimes additional individuals who donate gametes to make the pregnancy possible; the future child; and society at large, whose norms regarding reproduction may be adversely affected by the reproductive choices that are permitted within it. There are ethical issues in relation to each of these parties, and how they are addressed determines what the right to reproductive choice is actually a right to do.

Reproductive liberty is not, of course, the entire story about the ethics of reproduction. There is also an ethics of reproductive responsibility, and arguments for limiting reproductive liberty often come from this quarter. Having children knowing that one cannot adequately care for them; having a child with a known high risk of a serious genetic disease; or exposing the fetus to alcohol, drugs, or other harms raises the question of whether parents are acting responsibly in how or whether they reproduce.

Parents may be charged with acting irresponsibly if they knowingly bring a child into the world who will suffer from a serious disease or disabling medical condition. Against this, some philosophers have argued that this child is not harmed by being born in this condition since he is not made worse off than he would otherwise have been; he otherwise would not have been at all (Parfit 1984). Others have proposed that, even if this child is not harmed by being born, he is born in a harmed condition, and parents may have a duty to prevent the resulting suffering (Brock 1995).

Concerns about reproductive responsibility can be taken too far when, for example, a woman's reproductive freedom is constrained in the misguided belief that she is not fit to be a parent. To be sure, parental fitness is a legitimate concern but one that is properly based on a person's behavior that has been *demonstrated* to constitute child abuse or neglect. It is certainly not within the scope of practice for health care professionals to *predict* parental fitness and unilaterally restrict the reproductive liberty of those they find wanting. The early twentieth-century witnessed a shameful period when people who were considered socially undesirable—mainly women, people of color, and those who were or had been in prison or psychiatric asylums—were involuntarily sterilized for the good of society. Egregious cases, such as *Buck v. Bell*, discussed in part IV, resulted in strict standards and safeguards to prevent actions justified by the notion that the right to reproductive choice should be balanced against social norms and interests (Suter 2011).

Reproduction is also not just an ethical issue in our society, it is a deeply and an inextricably political one, as well. Differences of opinion about the extent of women's legitimate reproductive freedom are intimately tied up with differing views about the proper role of women and the nature of the family, and they derive much of their intensity from this connection. The right to abortion is still vehemently debated and contested, serving as a political litmus test for politicians on different ends of the political spectrum and continuing to divide opinion more than 40 years after it was legalized in *Roe v. Wade*. States pass restrictive abortion laws and punish women for endangering the health and lives of the children they intend to bear. Religious institutions refuse to provide contraceptive health coverage for their employees and refuse to adhere to government mandates requiring them to do so. There is no set of issues in the field of bioethics that is as heavily and passionately politicized as reproduction.

The polarizing debate about reproductive choice, especially abortion, has very direct and practical implications for health care providers. In an increasing number of states, the effort to overturn *Roe v. Wade* has been supplemented with statutes that require or prohibit what health care providers discuss with women who ask for information about pregnancy termination. These statutory maneuvers are described further in the discussion of abortion below. The same state intrusion into the provider-patient dynamic prohibits discussion of certain other topics as well, such as the ownership, storage, and safe use of firearms. Regardless of one's position on controversial issues, such as abortion or gun control, it should be a matter of concern to health care providers and ethics committees when states legislatively control what practitioners discuss with their patients as part of their health care.

ASSISTED REPRODUCTIVE TECHNOLOGIES

Henrietta Perkins is a 55-year-old divorced high school teacher who recently married John Franklin, 48, a man she met through an online dating service. Henrietta is close to her two grown children from her first marriage, but she is eager for another with her new partner. She and John have talked about the possibility of having a child of their own and both of them feel that this would enhance their marriage. Henrietta is post-menopausal, however, and to conceive she would need both donor eggs and reproductive assistance through IVF. Henrietta's two grown children are not entirely on board with her plan because they are not sure where the donor eggs would come from and they worry about whether their mother would be able to manage child care as she and the child age. The fertility clinic that Henrietta and John visit has the same concerns and is unsure whether it is ethically and medically appropriate to facilitate their plan. The clinic seeks the advice of the reproductive technologies ethics committee to which it frequently brings difficult cases.

Whose interests should count here and in what priority? What risks are associated with the use of IVF in this case, and how should they be weighted? What role does reproductive freedom play here? Would it be ethically responsible for a physician to assist Henrietta in having a child?

In Vitro Fertilization

According to a 1995 survey conducted by the National Center for Health Statistics, an estimated 2.1 million or 7.1% of married couples with a wife of childbearing age are currently infertile. Infertility is defined in the medical literature as difficulty achieving conception after a specified period of time, usually 12 months, despite unprotected intercourse (National Center for Health Statistics 2011). For many couples, infertility is a source of great frustration, pain, and disappointment. Fortunately, with the advent of techniques of assisted reproductive technologies (ARTs), chiefly IVF and its offshoots, such as intracytoplasmic sperm injection and gamete and zygote intrafallopian transfer, infertile couples who want children may be enabled to conceive and complete a pregnancy.

While IVF is not a panacea for infertility, notable improvements have been made since its first documented use in 1978. A single attempt at IVF costs anywhere from $5,000 to $12,000, and it is not uncommon for couples to attempt more than one cycle since the initial cycle is often unsuccessful. According to statistics from the Centers for Disease Control (2012), a woman who uses donor eggs or non-frozen embryos has a 56% chance of having a live birth and a 37% chance of a singleton live birth, increased from 2002, when even the most successful clinics working with the healthiest couples reported success rates only in the mid-30% range. The use of IVF has expanded beyond infertile heterosexual couples in which the women are of childbearing age and now includes men and women without partners, gay and lesbian couples, and post-menopausal women.

Despite improvements in the rate of successful pregnancies, assisted reproduction still raises health concerns. There is a greater chance of multiple births with IVF (and also with fertility drugs) when, as is often the case, multiple embryos are implanted to increase the probability of achieving a pregnancy. Multiple births often lead to prematurity and its attendant, often serious, medical problems for both mother and babies. Miscarriage and premature delivery are common complications of multiple pregnancy, the risk rising exponentially with the number of fetuses (Dickens and Cook 2008). Reports of high-order multiple pregnancies, such as the case of the woman delivering eight babies in her second IVF-created multiple pregnancy (Saul 2009) have increased public awareness of these issues. Heightened scrutiny of the risks posed by multiple pregnancies has raised the question of whether physicians performing IVF should be required to limit the number of embryos implanted, a practice already in place in other countries (Saul 2009).

In addition to health concerns, ARTs pose several ethical questions. In the simple case of IVF, eggs are taken from the woman and sperm from the man since there is either male or female infertility or both; the eggs are fertilized in a laboratory dish and implanted in the woman's uterus 48 to 72 hours after fertilization.

Like abortion, tubal ligation, and vasectomy, ARTs have religious implications. For example, these techniques conflict with the tenets of Catholic doctrine, which forbids any intervention that inhibits conception or substitutes for the conjugal act. Thus, IVF as described in the scenario above, as well as virtually every ART, including artificial insemination by the husband, is opposed by the Catholic Church (Congregation for the Doctrine of the Faith 1987; *Ethical and Religious Directives for Catholic Health Care* 2009). Absent a blanket prohibition on the use of ARTs, a number of ethical issues must be addressed, including respect for the autonomy and religious convictions of patients, partners, and health care providers, and the obligations of providers to promote the well-being of patients, enhance the likelihood of a healthy pregnancy and successful birth, and avoid actions likely to cause harm to mother or fetus.

Variations on the simple case raise additional problems. A couple may undergo IVF with their own gametes and the resultant embryo is then placed in the uterus of another woman, known as a gestational carrier. Critics of such arrangements worry that they are exploitative of the carrier, who may be susceptible to financial pressures, and that they commodify gestation, making the child into an object of monetary value. Further, a woman may receive donor eggs from a variety of sources, including her sister or daughter. These sorts of possibilities have led to worries that IVF can create novel forms of familial arrangement and unsettle the future child's sense of identity, which has traditionally been grounded in biologically unambiguous relationships to others in the family. The general concern here is that IVF forces us to rethink notions of parenting and family that most people have simply taken for granted. With IVF, it becomes possible to assign different parenting roles to different individuals: one individual can serve as the gestational parent, others as the genetic parents, and still others as the social or rearing parents. The close bond linking these different functions could become undone and that, by itself, may be unsettling to some.

Other important ethical questions concern who should have access to assisted reproduction and who should make that determination. Access to IVF and other forms of ART is arguably part of the right to reproductive liberty and, given the fundamental importance of this liberty, there are grounds for claiming that it is unjust to bar or limit access simply because the woman or couple lacks the financial means to pay for it. This, however, is what Medicaid, the public insurance program for the poor, does because it views IVF as an elective procedure that it will not cover. Further, whatever rights flow from reproductive freedom are not absolute; they must be balanced against considerations of reproductive responsibility. As with traditional reproduction, the way ART is utilized is not always considered responsible and, for this reason, unrestricted access to ART may not always be ethically defensible. Consider, for example, a case in which an HIV-positive woman seeks reproductive assistance, but refuses to take any measures to lower the risk of transmission to her offspring.

An additional moral issue that does not arise with traditional reproduction is the rights and responsibilities of the medical professionals who are enlisted to assist individuals and couples to become parents. In addition to the medical factors considered in assessing people requesting IVF, practitioners' attitudes about same-sex unions, racial or ethnic background, and, most recently, gender identity of potential parents may test their ability to make clinical assessments uninfluenced by personal bias (Richards 2014). The medical professional is an independent moral agent who must make her own moral judgments about the appropriateness of providing ART, based on her best understanding of the professional and ethical norms that apply to the case at hand, and these may diverge from those of her patients. Your ethics committee may be asked to weigh in on these matters in consultation or policy review, and your familiarity with these complex matters and their ethical implications will be important.

There are other concerns of a policy nature related to IVF. Currently, the infertility industry in the United States, unlike that in several European countries, is largely unregulated, leaving individual clinics free to charge whatever they want for their services, implant as many embryos in their patients as they see fit, set how much they will pay for donor eggs, and determine what will happen to frozen embryos that are not used by the couple for whom they were created. Weighty and controversial ethical issues, such as whether gametes should be treated as a commodity or whether there should be any constraints on the disposition of unused embryos, are raised by these practices, and it is unsound public policy to leave them entirely up to individual clinics. They argue for greater public deliberation about the merits of these different practices and, informed by this deliberation, a stronger role for the state in regulating them.

The case of Henrietta and John raises a number of concerns, all of which cluster around the issue of the age of the mother. Pregnancy over the age of 50 is associated with a higher risk of medical complications, including hypertension, gestational diabetes, and preeclampsia. There is also an increased risk of genetic defects in the fetus. An additional concern is the respective ages of mother and child; as Henrietta ages, she may have difficulty taking care of an active adolescent when the child is 15 and she is 70. Yet, while the well-established clinical and genetic risks of pregnancy may be within the clinical purview of the benefit-burden-risk assessment and, when the risks are unacceptably high, may justify refusing to perform assisted reproduction, predicting and assessing parental fitness as the woman ages is a more difficult and controversial matter. Finally, there are the important factors related to egg donation, including the identity of the donor and how donation was solicited and reimbursed, discussed below.

As a member of the ethics committee, you should point out that, although it may be "unusual" or "nontraditional" for post-menopausal women to bear children, that is not the same as "unnatural" or "unethical." Instead, your ethical analysis should focus on the rights and health risks of the mother, the medical and psychological welfare of the future child, and the circumstances under which donor eggs are obtained.

Pre-Implantation Genetic Diagnosis

Sybil and Graham Wray, both in their early thirties, are the proud parents of a little girl, Jill, age 5, who suffers from a deadly genetic disease that causes bone marrow failure, eventually resulting in leukemia. Her best chance for survival is a bone marrow transplant from a perfectly matched sibling donor. Sybil and Graham had considered having another child, but decided against it because of a one-in-four chance the child would have the same disease as Jill. But then they heard about pre-implantation genetic diagnosis (PGD), a technique that would enable them to screen out embryos affected with the genetic disease before implantation. Because this technology holds out the prospect of life-saving treatment for Jill, as well as the opportunity to give her a sibling who will not develop the same lethal disease, Sybil and Graham have decided to try PGD.

Whose interests are being served here? Is one person being created to be "used" without his consent to promote the interests of another? Do parents have the right to do what the Wrays are proposing?

Pre-implantation genetic diagnosis has been available since 1990 in conjunction with IVF. One cell (blastomere) is removed from a cleaving embryo ex utero and tested for a particular genetic or chromosomal abnormality. Embryos with these abnormalities can then be discarded, avoiding the birth of a child with a disabling condition, and the embryos without the chromosomal or genetic defect can be transferred to the woman's uterus. New uses of PGD include detecting mutations for susceptibility to cancer and for late-onset disorders, such as Alzheimer's disease (Robertson 2003).

Some uses of PGD are relatively ethically uncontroversial, such as detecting lethal or serious genetic conditions, including Tay-Sachs disease or autosomal recessive polycystic kidney disease (ARPKD), which will profoundly afflict the child from birth. Some commentators have even argued that, in these cases, potential parents have, not just the right, but also an ethical duty, to use PGD to prevent such conditions (Malek and Daar 2012). Somewhat more controversial is using PGD to detect genetic mutations, such as BRCA1&2 genes, which signal significantly heightened risks of cancer and other late-onset disorders, such as Huntington or Alzheimer's diseases. The concerns are that, while early detection of the BRCA genes enables either a decision about terminating the pregnancy or alertness to the need for close monitoring and possible prophylactic intervention for the affected child, detection of susceptibility to Huntington or Alzheimer's risks preventing the birth of a child who may have a healthy and problem-free life for many years.

More controversial still is PGD for the purpose of sex selection. The use of PGD to select the sex of one's offspring is susceptible to the charge of sexism, which is a compelling reason to oppose it. However, parents may also desire to use PGD for sex selection in order to achieve gender balance in their family, which may not be sexist. Nevertheless, the question remains whether achieving family balance is a strong enough moral reason to discard embryos (Ethics Committee of the American Society of Reproductive Medicine 1999).

More speculatively, PGD might be used to select embryos with certain desirable qualities and nonmedical traits, such as perfect pitch or superior intelligence, and to discard those that fall short. These nonmedical uses of PGD, often referred to as creating "designer babies," are especially worrisome because they invoke the reasoning of the early twentieth-century eugenics movement and permit a significantly increased degree of arbitrary reproductive control that may be detrimental to the resulting offspring and, ultimately, to society.

To return to the case of Sybil and Graham Wray, they want to have another child who, in addition to completing their desired two-children family, can serve as a bone marrow donor for Jill, and they want to use PGD for this purpose. Some may find this morally objectionable because it smacks of using a person as a mere means to serve the interests of others. But the case is more complicated than that, or at least it would be, if the Wrays do not consider the second child as a "mere" means. There is, after all, no indication that the Wrays would not love their second child as much as they love Jill or that they would neglect her once she has served her purpose of aiding Jill. As a member of the ethics committee, you could helpfully point out that individuals often have children to serve a variety of purposes of their own, some legitimate and some not, and you could help clarify the differences between those cases in which this is morally acceptable and those in which it is not.

Gamete Donation

Contributing to worries about the commodification of childbearing is the current practice of buying and selling donor eggs on the open market (Daniels and Heidt-Forsythe 2012). Egg donation has become a significant part of the multi-billion-dollar-a year infertility industry. Men who donate sperm receive a small payment; the going rate for eggs is much higher. It is common knowledge at colleges and universities that young female students sometimes decide to donate eggs, assuming the associated medical risks, as a source of income. Infertile couples now offer large sums of money for donor eggs from women who meet certain specifications, such as educational attainment and athletic ability. Payment of some sort for donor eggs seems acceptable and only fair since the process of donating eggs is both burdensome and potentially dangerous. However, if payment is too high, needy donors may be led to discount the risks of donation, making their decision to sell their eggs less than fully voluntary. In addition, infertility clinics may, in their eagerness to obtain high-quality eggs and increase their profits, fail to fully reveal all the risks and possible costs of donation to potential donors, rendering their decision to "donate" less than fully informed. While these issues are or should be addressed during extensive counseling prior to the donation, your ethics committee is encouraged to devote time to their examination.

Posthumous Sperm Retrieval

The chair of your ethics committee has received the following request from the nurse manager in the surgical ICU (SICU): "Okay, I'm in way over my head on this one and I need an ethics consult ASAP. We have a patient who's just been declared brain dead and his wife is asking to retrieve his sperm. Oh, and just to add interest, his parents hate her and they want the sperm."

Mr. O'Reilly, a 34-year-old man, had been admitted with massive brain injury following a head-on motor vehicle accident. After completion of the relevant examinations and tests, the several neurologists agreed that he had lost entire brain function and met the criteria for a declaration of brain death. His immediate and extended family was in attendance and, after careful and detailed explanation, everyone accepted the fact that the patient was now clinically and legally dead. That, however, was where concurrence ended.

Two groups of family members asked to speak privately with the ethics consultant. Mrs. O'Reilly explained that she and her late husband had been trying to start a family and, for the past six months, had been working with an infertility specialist. She tearfully described their shared dreams of parenthood, ending with, "All I have of him now are those dreams and I want so much to make them come true. It's what he would want." Her brother said, "He was so looking forward to being a father." The patient's parents and siblings insisted, "That tramp just wants a kid to inherit his money. She would be a terrible mother. If we can find a nice girl to have his baby, we'll have a grandchild to carry his legacy."

Whose interests are at stake here? What obligations are owed to the late patient, his grieving wife, and his distraught parents? What ethical principles should inform analysis of the situation? What is the appropriate role of the ethics consultant?

Let's begin by clarifying what the purpose of ethics consultation in this case is *not,* which includes determining the validity of Mrs. O'Reilly's claim that she and her late husband wanted to have a child, assessing her character or parental fitness, or mediating family conflicts that predate Mr. O'Reilly's accident and death. The contribution of ethics analysis here is to identify the competing interests and obligations, and ensure that the rights of the now-deceased patient are not violated. It is important at the outset to distinguish this situation from surrogate decision making as discussed in chapter 2. Typically, the surrogate is responsible for making care decisions on behalf of a patient whose welfare is the paramount consideration. Here, the decision will not affect the now-deceased patient's health, only the respect for his prior preferences and the interests of his survivors.

Sperm is commonly procured and preserved in situations in which infertility can be foreseen, such as impending chemotherapy. But retrieval of sperm in cases of unexpected coma or death, while often technically feasible, is ethically extremely problematic. Of major importance here is the deceased man's prior preferences about becoming a parent, specifically whether he consented to retrieval of his sperm for the purpose of fathering a child under the current circumstances. In other words, while Mr. O'Reilly may have ardently desired to become a parent and participated in infertility counseling and ART, those preferences and actions are not evidence of his willingness to *father a child after his death.* For this reason, implied consent is very problematic because of the likelihood that emotionally involved third parties may erroneously assume that consent has or would have been given or that consent would not have been given.

If Mr. O'Reilly had explicitly consented to have his sperm retrieved posthumously for the purpose of reproduction, it would be ethical to proceed under specified conditions. Many hospitals, as well as sperm and egg banks, have policies that require written documentation of the man's prior consent; designation of the intended sperm recipient who will be the child's parent; and prohibition of third parties, such as potential grandparents, having control of the sperm. If the request for sperm retrieval is on behalf of a man who is currently incapacitated, about to begin treatment that is fetotoxic, and expected to regain capacity following treatment, some policies stipulate that a court-appointed guardian assume responsibility for the storage and disposition of the sperm until the man is able to take control or he is permanently incapacitated or has died. But if a man has steadfastly refused to have a child while he was alive, it would be ethically wrong to retrieve his sperm after his death, effectively making him a father against his will (Orr and Siegler 2002). Because any requests for sperm retrieval in your institution will likely generate a clinical ethics consultation, your committee is encouraged to address the matter proactively through discussion and policy development.

SURROGACY AND GESTATIONAL CARRIERS

Baby M was born to Mary Beth Whitehead, conceived with her own oocytes and sperm from William Stern, the husband of Elizabeth Stern, the intended child-rearing parents. The Sterns and Ms. Whitehead entered into a contract according to which Ms. Whitehead would relinquish her parental rights in favor of Mrs. Stern upon the birth of the child. However, she decided to keep the child, so the Sterns sued to be recognized as the child's legal parents. In an important decision by the New Jersey Superior Court, the contract was ruled invalid according to public policy, Ms. Whitehead was recognized as the child's legal mother, and family court was ordered to determine whether Ms. Whitehead, as mother, and Mr. Stern, as father, should have legal custody of the child, according to the traditional "best interests of the child standard." Ultimately, Mr. Stern was awarded custody of Baby M, Mrs. Stern legally adopted her, and Ms. Whitehead was given visitation rights.

Are there legitimate reasons to prevent people from becoming or hiring surrogates or gestational carriers? Is the practice so dangerous, risky, or contrary to the public good that it should be banned? What ethical values are promoted by permitting the practice?

First a word of clarification. A *gestational carrier* is a woman who carries to term a child conceived with the gametes of a couple to whom she relinquishes the child upon delivery. As such, she is a parent only in the gestational, rather than the genetic, sense. A *surrogate*, by contrast, provides her own oocytes, fertilized with sperm from the man in another couple to whom she relinquishes the child upon delivery. Her contribution is both gestational and genetic. Mary Beth Whitehead was a surrogate.

Surrogacy is far more accepted in the United States than in most countries; however, there is no national consensus on how to deal with it even here. As of 2014, 17 states have laws permitting surrogacy, some with restrictions; 6 states prohibit enforcement of surrogacy contracts; and in 21 states, there is neither a law nor a published case regarding surrogacy (Lewin 2014).

The ethical arguments that support allowing women to serve as surrogates or gestational carriers are rooted in several values: autonomy, beneficence, and reproductive freedom. According to the autonomy argument, women should be free to make decisions about their own bodies, including waiving their parental rights before the birth of children they help conceive or carry. The beneficence argument emphasizes the good that surrogates and gestational carriers can provide couples whose desire for a child with all or part of their genetic makeup has been impeded by the woman's infertility or inability to carry a pregnancy to term. Surrogacy also enhances a woman's reproductive freedom to have a child to whom she is genetically related.

Despite these benefits, there are many reasons to be cautious about surrogacy and gestational carrier arrangements. Relinquishing a child whom one has carried to term can be emotionally traumatic for the carrier, as happened in the Baby M case. An additional concern is that women may agree to serve as surrogates because they see this as an opportunity to improve their economic situations and, as a consequence, the inducement of financial compensation is potentially exploitative. According to 2008 statistics, the mean compensation for a gestational carrier in the United States was approximately $20,000 (Brezina and Zhao 2012). Financial compensation for the delivery of a baby also seems to be tantamount to baby selling, which is both immoral and against public policy. These concerns, while worth taking seriously, can be addressed and should not justify complete prohibition of the practice of surrogacy. The concern about the emotional cost to the surrogate or carrier can be addressed to some extent by pre-conception counseling and requiring a waiting period before the surrogate relinquishes her parental rights; exploitation is less a worry if financial compensation is limited to payment for medical expenses associated with or incurred during pregnancy and, because this remuneration is not for the delivery or relinquishing of a baby, it is less likely to be considered baby selling (Steinbock 1988). Nevertheless, because surrogate and gestational carrier arrangements depart so radically from traditional social norms of parenthood, the risks of objectification of women remain (Tieu 2009; Atwood 1986).

Disputes involving surrogates and gestational carriers may sometimes come to the attention of your ethics committee and you may be able to provide useful guidance to the parties involved. The questions that loom large in an ethics analysis are whether the surrogate or gestational carrier is being exploited; what emotional and psychological risks she faces; what the impact of surrogacy on the families of both the surrogate and the receiving parents is likely to be; and whether permitting surrogacy constitutes endorsement of buying and selling babies.

TERMINATION OF PREGNANCY

Marlise Munoz, 33 years old, was 14 weeks pregnant when her husband found her unconscious on the bathroom floor. Rushed to the hospital, she was found to have suffered a massive pulmonary embolism and was declared brain dead. The declaration was final and uncontested by either the hospital or the patient's family. Mr. Munoz requested that, in keeping with what his wife would have wanted, the mechanical supports maintaining her organ function be removed. The hospital responded that state law required that she be kept on "life support"* until sufficient fetal development created a reasonable chance of survival upon delivery, which would require that Mrs. Munoz's body remain connected to mechanical supports for at least an additional eight weeks. Mr. Munoz insisted that, in deference to his late wife's

---

* *Life support* in this context is misleading, since it suggests that Mrs. Munoz's life was being maintained by technological assistance, whereas, in fact, she was legally and medically dead. The importance of language, especially in discussing life and death, is addressed further in chapter 9.

wishes, the hospital disconnect the mechanical supports immediately, even though he recognized that this would prevent the development and delivery of a viable baby (Ecker 2014).

What rights do the mother and the father have in this situation? What steps should be taken to preserve and support the fetus? Should the mother's body be kept on mechanical supports solely to allow a live birth?

The Legal Landscape

Roe v. Wade is the landmark 1973 U.S. Supreme Court case that legalized abortion and one of the most important legal cases in the field of bioethics. The ruling established that a right to privacy under the due process clause of the Fourteenth Amendment of the U.S. Constitution extends to a woman's decision to terminate a pregnancy. But the ruling also balanced this right against two legitimate state interests in its regulation: protecting the potentiality of life and protecting the health of the mother. The Court held that these interests become stronger over the course of the pregnancy, and it employed a trimester approach to make this more precise: for the first two trimesters, the decision is substantially that of the pregnant woman and her doctor; in the third trimester, the state may proscribe abortion in order to protect nascent human life. In a 1992 case, *Planned Parenthood of Southern Pennsylvania v. Casey*, the Court reaffirmed the essential holding of *Roe* but replaced the trimester framework with the "undue burden" standard intended to protect women from unreasonable barriers to abortion. A fuller discussion of the leading Supreme Court cases related to abortion appears in part IV.

Roe v. Wade prompted a national debate on the legality and morality of abortion that continues to this day, dividing the country into so-called pro-choice and pro-life camps. Whether *Roe v. Wade* will survive the many challenges to its constitutionality remains uncertain in light of the conservative bent of the current Supreme Court.

Meanwhile, however, a number of states, as well as the U.S. Congress, have attempted to make the exercise of the right to abortion more difficult for pregnant women. As of this writing, Oklahoma, Texas, and North Carolina require that pregnant women undergo and view fetal ultrasounds, along with graphic explanations of their significance (Rocha 2012). In South Dakota, providers are required to provide information about the gestational age and development of the fetus, show them a fetal sonogram, and say that, if the woman terminates the pregnancy, she will be "ending the life of a separate human being with whom [she has] an enduring relationship." In West Virginia, women considering abortion are required to undergo a vaginal sonogram, even in cases of rape. Some states require that women be told that the list of risks to the procedure includes depression, suicide, and infertility. In 2003, a Republican-controlled Congress passed the controversial Partial Birth Abortion Ban Act, which the pro-life camp defended as protecting the rights of the unborn and the pro-choice camp rejected on the ground that it constituted an unjustified infringement of the woman's right to abortion. The act was ruled constitutional by the Supreme Court in 2007 in *Gonzalez v. Carhart*. A fuller discussion of this case appears in part IV.

Ethical Issues

More has been written about abortion than any other bioethical issue and, despite the vast literature, it is a matter that continues to generate passionate and polarizing debate. Beginning in 1971 with the landmark article, "A Defense of Abortion," by the philosopher Judith Jarvis Thomson and continuing without interruption until today, articles and books have exhaustively explored every facet of the issue. The most general way of stating the ethical problem of abortion is by asking what makes it right or wrong to voluntarily terminate a pregnancy. This divides into two subquestions: (1) what is the moral status of the fetus? and (2) why does a pregnant woman have the right to terminate her pregnancy? The issue of moral status is important because those who have moral status deserve the protection of moral norms, that is, principles and rules that state obligations and rights. Determining the moral status of a fetus or embryo does not settle the question of what may ethically be done to it, for moral status can come in degrees, but even beings with comparatively little moral status deserve moral consideration.

Several answers to when the embryo or fetus acquires moral status have been proposed. One suggestion is that moral status is acquired at conception, even before an embryo, technically speaking, has developed. Another is that the fetus acquires moral status when pathways develop to transfer pain signals from pain sensors to the brain, around 26 weeks or 6 months. Various other developmental milestones have been proposed as marking the advent of moral status, but these are not straightforward empirical determinations. Each suggested milestone has to be defended on moral grounds. To no one's surprise, consensus remains and likely will remain elusive.

Commonly accepted justifiable grounds for abortion, on which there is wide but not universal agreement, are rape, incest, and threat to the life of the mother. More controversial reasons include the mother's maturity, threat to the mother's psychological health, conflict with the mother's other life goals, and lack of support system and financial resources. Selective reduction, in which one or more embryos in a multiple pregnancy are aborted to enhance the likelihood that the remaining embryo(s) will thrive, is problematic because of the painful and difficult selection it requires. Selective abortion of fetuses with disabling conditions has generated particular controversy. According to the disability rights critique, prenatal diagnosis followed by abortion of fetuses with disabling conditions is morally problematic for a number of reasons: it expresses negative or discriminatory attitudes not only about the disabling traits themselves, but about those who have them; it also signals intolerance of diversity in both the family and society at large (Parens and Asch 2000), ultimately altering for the worse what it means to be a parent.

The pregnancy termination case of Marlise Munoz no doubt generates conflicting opinions among individuals depending on their views regarding the ethical permissibility of abortion and the reasons that might legitimate it. Questions to be asked when doing an ethics analysis include the following: What moral significance does the preservation of fetal life have? Is it one factor among others or is it the overriding consideration? What is the fetal prognosis if the pregnancy is maintained for another eight weeks and delivered? Would the mother want her body to be supported mechanically so that her baby could be delivered? What rights does the father have? Should the hospital attempt to override the father's decision to terminate mechanical supports? The goal of your ethics committee deliberations should be to draw attention to these various moral considerations and to try to come to some conclusions about their respective weights.

MATERNAL-FETAL ISSUES

Janet Jones was 32 weeks pregnant when clinical signs began to indicate that all was not right with her pregnancy. Fetal monitoring revealed a decrease in fetal heart rate that could indicate inadequate blood flow through the placenta. She was followed closely by her obstetrician during this time and, when the fetus's decelerations worsened, her doctor recommended delivering the baby by caesarean section before things got worse. Janet, however, refused. She did not believe her fetus was in serious difficulty and, in any case, she had spent her entire pregnancy preparing for natural childbirth and wanted to deliver her baby that way. Her obstetrician, Dr. DiSalvo, and other members of the obstetrical staff tried to convince her of the need for a C-section, but she continued to refuse and, as fetal condition worsened, they became increasingly worried. They felt a responsibility to do whatever they could to deliver her baby alive before it suffered irreversible brain damage. Finally Dr. DiSalvo warned Janet that if she continued to reject his advice, he would have no choice but to get a court order to perform a C-section over her objection. The rest of the obstetrical staff, though bothered by this threat, supported his stand.

According to *Roe v. Wade*, pregnant women in the United States have a constitutional right to terminate an unwanted pregnancy at least during the first two trimesters, which is not inconsistent with their moral obligation to do whatever is necessary to ensure the success of a desired pregnancy. Women who intend to carry their pregnancy to term are advised to take care of their own health for their sake and for the sake of their future child. But, the ethics and legality of abortion are separate matters from the moral responsibilities of women who choose to carry a pregnancy to term and deliver a child. These are obligations that pregnant women have *now* to the *child-who-will-be-born*. Thus, pregnant women are advised not to drink or smoke, not to take illicit drugs, and to avoid exposing themselves to environments that present a risk to the health of the developing fetus.

Women are also expected to agree to medical interventions, such as caesarean section, that their doctors believe are in the best interests of their to-be-born child. The important distinction between a moral and a legal obligation is that, while these intuitively obvious measures can be seen as *moral* obligations, it is a further question whether they should be translated into *legal* obligations (Post 1997). As a general matter, a woman's right to privacy and self-determination cannot be legally conditioned on the well-being of her future child, but neither should she be relieved of the moral obligations to the child she intends to bring into the world.

Yet, restrictions on a pregnant woman's right of self-determination have taken several forms. Women have been ordered by courts to undergo emergency cesarean sections; incarcerated until delivery if they have taken illegal drugs while pregnant; and punished after delivery for engaging in behaviors during pregnancy that, in the opinion of doctors and courts, endangered the fetus. These actions have been justified by states modifying their child abuse and neglect laws to define a "child" as any being from conception on, thereby expanding their *parens patriae* authority to include fetal protection. These measures depart significantly from the customary legal position that personhood within the meaning of the Fourteenth Amendment occurs when a live birth takes place. Only at that point may the state, under its protective powers, intervene on behalf of the neonate, who now has independent and legally protectable rights (Post 1997). The seriousness of these responses to alleged maternal irresponsibility, as well as their punitive, coercive, and, often, arbitrary nature, shows how much rides on others' assessments of maternal conduct and how important it is to proceed cautiously in making them.

There are reasons to be wary of such interventions. First, obstetricians, like all physicians, are not infallible. Many of their past convictions about diet, ideal weight gain, and exercise during pregnancy are now considered obsolete. Moreover, doctors may disagree with their colleagues, as well as with their patients, about what promotes maternal and fetal health. Second, even granting the soundness of the medical advice, as noted above there is a difference between a moral obligation to do or avoid doing something and an obligation that is legally enforceable. Additional arguments, over and above the existence of the moral obligation itself, are needed to justify the use of state authority to curtail a pregnant woman's autonomy and infringe on her liberty.

Especially important in relation to maternal-fetal issues, there are pragmatic as well as moral reasons not to resort to the heavy-handed strategies described above. First, punitive and coercive responses to alleged maternal misconduct threaten to drive pregnant women away from prenatal care, with potentially worse results for the future child than if non-punitive approaches were adopted. Second, there is no bright line that demarcates punishable from non-punishable conduct. If the goal is to discourage irresponsible maternal behavior, why stop at smoking, alcohol, and illicit drugs? What about failure to have regular prenatal check-ups or take prenatal vitamins? If nothing else, this slide along the continuum of undesirable behaviors is increasingly unenforceable. From the standpoint of the future child's well-being, it is generally better to treat the pregnant woman and her fetus not as two separate entities in conflict with each other, but as a single biological and social unit with common interests (Post 1997; Rothman 1986).

There are cases, however, in which a pregnant woman's right against non-consensual bodily invasion may be limited by the overwhelming likelihood of significant and preventable harm to the future child (Chervenak and McCullough 1991). The most common example is refusal of a cesarean section where the harm to the fetus from refusing the surgery is clear-cut, imminent, and potentially devastating. What makes these cases especially difficult for caregivers is that, with surgery, this almost-baby can be saved. The case of Janet Jones may be an example of this type. In some cases, court orders have been obtained to authorize the contested intervention and, as an example, *In re A.C.* is discussed in part IV.

Given the well-settled right of capable patients to refuse unwanted treatment, discussed in chapter 3, this radical departure from legal and ethical precedent has ominous implications. It may have the counterproductive effect of discouraging pregnant women from seeking prenatal care out of fear that they might be forced to undergo unwanted surgery for the sake of their fetus. As noted in chapter 2, refusal of recommended treatment does not, by itself, confirm decisional incapacity. Yet, in these situations, surgery over the patient's objection is sometimes justified by the presumption of incapacity, the logic being that no rational woman would deliberately put her future child at risk. As "A Defense of Abortion" so brilliantly illustrates, it is hard to imagine analogous actions of non-consensual bodily invasion, especially for the sake of another, occurring in any other patient population or clinical setting. An obstetric case that raises the possibility of court-ordered caesarian section might come to the attention of your ethics committee and your careful analysis of the relevant rights, interests, and obligations will be crucial to its resolution.

PRENATAL/NEWBORN GENETIC TESTING AND GENOMIC NEWBORN SCREENING

The increasing ability to detect actual or potential medical problems enables parents and care professionals to intervene in ways that have profound health benefits. To appreciate the ethical implications, however, it is necessary to distinguish two types of assessment: *testing* and *screening*. Prenatal genetic testing is offered to individual prospective parents, generally on the basis of family history, to identify a specific genetic variant or mutation in their offspring. Genetic testing of newborns may be offered on the same familial basis or because suggestive symptoms have already appeared. Currently, this testing is undertaken only for identifiable *early-onset* conditions, the early diagnosis of which can lead to interventions that have therapeutic value. Newborn testing for *late-onset* conditions or for medical conditions for which there is no cure or other type of medical benefit is ethically problematic and may be objectionable because the child may be able to live a normal life for many years before the onset of disease. Also problematic is prenatal genetic testing for the purpose of identifying fetuses with disabilities or minor medical conditions, although this might be defended as an exercise of reproductive freedom. In a more speculative and ethically contentious vein because of its eugenic overtones, there is the use of prenatal genetic testing to create so-called designer babies by identifying genes that are not associated with medical conditions but with desirable traits, such as superior intelligence and memory.

The aim of newborn screening is different. As currently practiced, screening is intended to identify newborns from a particular population who could be helped if their heightened risk of a specific disease were recognized. Parents could then be offered follow-up genetic testing or some type of therapeutic recommendation.

In contrast, whole genome screening (WGS) of newborns, which examines the entire genome, raises ethical and social issues that targeted newborn genetic testing does not. It is now technically feasible to analyze a newborn's entire genome to reveal her genetic variations. One concern, however, is cost: WGS is currently prohibitively expensive for general use. More important, the clinical utility of newborn genomic screening is questionable, given the current state of scientific knowledge. Unlike the relationship between genetic variation and monogenetic diseases, the relationship between genetic variation and polygenetic disorders, which comprise the majority of human genetic diseases, is still not well understood, making it difficult to interpret and, therefore, make diagnostic, prognostic, or therapeutic use of this information.

As to ethical issues, although there is some overlap between those raised by newborn testing and screening programs and genomic newborn screening, the latter raises distinct problems because of the wide net it casts. WGS can provide information on many genetic variants whose significance is not understood and that may not be linked to disease or significant impairment. Or they may be linked to late-onset conditions, such as Alzheimer's disease, or to conditions, such as Huntington disease, for which there is no cure or ameliorative intervention. The danger is that parents anticipating medical problems in their basically healthy children might subject them to interventions that are unnecessary, burdensome, and even damaging. In addition, the psychological impact of this information on young people could be extremely traumatic and disruptive to their lives.

To be sure, genetic testing of newborns raises some of the same ethical issues. There are questions about what the consent process should be and who should be able to provide consent, the impact of the test results on children and families, safeguarding the privacy of the genetic information revealed, and preventing discriminatory repercussions in employment or insurability. But genomic newborn screening magnifies the double-edged implications, potentially providing vast amounts of useful or unnecessary information to health professionals and families, as well as the risk of creating a "medicalized society" (Almond 2006). On the positive side, newborn genomic screening could offer important diagnostic, prognostic, and therapeutic tools, potentially leading to disease prevention, early intervention, and the development of more effective medicines that are tailor-made to a child's specific medical condition.

An additional concern is the effect that the availability of WGS may have on notions of good parenting and parents' procreative decision making. Given the widely advertised possible benefits genomic information might provide, parents may be susceptible to the notion that they have a duty as good and responsible parents to take advantage of this type of screening (Donley, Hull, and Berkman 2012). The corresponding duty is that of the genetics professionals who, in addition to providing accurate information, also provide explanation, interpretation, and counseling. From an ethics perspective, analysis should focus on the potential benefit-burden-harm ratio; the interests and vulnerabilities of the child and the parents; and the obligations of health care professionals to provide information, support, and guidance in making decisions with profound and lasting implications.

REFERENCES

Almond B. 2006. Genetic profiling of newborns: Ethical and social issues. *Nature Reviews/Genetics* 7:67–71.

Atwood M. 1986. *The Handmaid's Tale*. Boston: Houghton Mifflin Company.

Baily MA, Murray T. 2008. Ethics, evidence, and cost in newborn screening. *Hastings Center Report* 30(3):23–31.

Brezina PR, Zhao Y. 2012. The ethical, legal, and social issues impacted by modern assisted reproductive technologies. *Obstetrics and Gynecology International*: 1–7.

Brock D. 1995. The non-identity problem and genetic harms: The case of wrongful handicaps. *Bioethics* 9(2):269–76.

Centers for Disease Control. 2012. Assisted Reproductive Technology National Summary Report, www.cdc.gov/art/ART2012/NationalSummary_index.htm (accessed August 2014).

Chervenak FA, McCullough LB. 1991. Justified limits on refusing intervention. *Hastings Center Report* 21(2):12–18.

Congregation for the Doctrine of the Faith. 1987. *Instruction on Respect for Human Life in Its Origin and on the Dignity of Procreation: Replies to Certain Questions of the Day.* Rome: Vatican.

Daniels CR, Heidt-Forsythe E. 2012. Gendered eugenics and the problematic of free market reproductive technologies: Sperm and egg donation in the United States. *Signs* 37(3):719–47.

Dickens BM, Cook RJ. 2008. Multiple pregnancy: Legal and ethical issues. *International Journal of Gynecology and Obstetrics* 103:270–74.

Donley G, Hull SC, Berkman BE. 2012. Prenatal whole genome sequencing: Just because we can, should we? *Hastings Center Report* 42(4):28–40.

Ecker JL. 2014. Death in pregnancy: An American tragedy. *New England Journal of Medicine* 370(10):889–91.

Epker JL, de Groot YJ, Kompanje EJO. 2012. Ethical and practical considerations concerning perimortem sperm procurement in a severe neurologically damaged patient and the apparent discrepancy in validation of proxy consent in various postmortem procedures. *Intensive Care Medicine* 38:1069–73.

Ethical and Religious Directives for Catholic Health Care Services. 2009. 5th ed. United States Conference of Catholic Bishops.

Ethics Committee of the American Society of Reproductive Medicine. 1999. *Fertility and Society* 72(4).

Goldenberg AJ, Sharp RR. 2012. The ethical hazards and programmatic challenges of genomic newborn screening. *Journal of the American Medical Association* 307(5):461–62.

Malek J, Daar J. 2012. The case for a parental duty to use preimplantation genetic diagnosis for medical benefit. *American Journal of Bioethics* 12(4):3–11.

Murtagh GM. 2007. Ethical reflection on the harm in reproductive decision-making. *Journal of Medical Ethics* 33(12):717–20.

National Center for Health Statistics. 2011. *Assisted Reproductive Technology (ART): Section 4: ART Cycles Using Donor Eggs,* www.cdc.gov/art/ART2011/section4.htm (accessed February 2015).

Orr RD, Siegler M. 2002. Is posthumous semen retrieval ethically permissible? *Journal of Medical Ethics* 28:299–303.

Parens E, Asch A, eds. 2000. *Prenatal Testing and Disability Rights.* Washington, DC: Georgetown University Press.

Parfit D. 1984. *Reasons and Persons.* Oxford: Oxford University Press.

Post LF. 1997. Bioethical considerations of maternal-fetal issues. *Fordham Urban Law Journal* 24(4):757–75.

Rhoden N. 1987. Cesareans and Samaritans. *Journal of Law, Medicine & Health Care* 15(3):118–25.

Richards SE. 2014. The next frontier in fertility treatment. *The New York Times*, January 12, p. A21.

Robertson J. 2003. Extending preimplantation genetic diagnosis: Medical and non-medical uses. *Journal of Medical Ethics* 29:213–16.

Lewin, T. 2014. Surrogates and couples face a maze of state laws, state by state. *The New York Times*, September 14, p. A1.

Rocha J. 2012. Autonomous abortions: The inhibiting of women's autonomy through legal ultrasound requirements. *Kennedy Institute of Ethics Journal* 22(1):35–58.

Rothman BK. 1986. When a pregnant woman endangers her fetus. *Hastings Center Report* 16(1):24–25.

Saul S. 2009. Birth of octuplets puts focus on fertility clinics. *The New York Times*, February 12.

Steinbock B. 1988. Surrogate motherhood as prenatal adoption. *Journal of Law, Medicine & Health Care* 16(1):44–50.

Suter S. 2011. Bad mothers or struggling mothers? *Rutgers Law Journal* 42:695ff.; 35(3):171–75.

Thomson JJ. 1971. A defense of abortion. *Philosophy and Public Affairs* 1(1):47–66.

Tieu MM. 2009. Altruistic surrogacy: The necessary objectification of surrogate mothers. *Journal of Medical Ethics* 35(3):171–75.

CHAPTER 7

Special Decision-Making Concerns of the Elderly

THE OTHER SIDE OF THE MOUNTAIN

Isabelle described the episode to her brother, Adam: "I came to pick Mama up for our weekly outing. Today, we had planned to go to lunch and then to a new exhibition at the Museum of Modern Art. I let myself into her house and, when she wasn't waiting for me in the kitchen, I went to her bedroom. I found her half dressed, hair uncombed, no makeup, sitting on her unmade bed with her arms wrapped around her, rocking back and forth, moaning, and looking terrified. I said, 'Mama, what's the matter?' She whispered, 'I can't find it. Help me find it.' I sat down next to her and took her hands. 'Mama, look at me. What can't you find?' 'Me,' she wailed. 'I can't find me! What's happened to me?' And we sat there and hugged each other and wept."

Some ethical issues raised in other health care settings assume particular significance in geriatrics and others are unique to care of the elderly. In addition to the inherent vulnerability of people who are sick, uncomfortable, anxious, and lacking information, this population faces special challenges, including diminishing autonomy, physical and mental compromise that will increase their dependence on others, role reversals with the children they raised, diminished goals and expectations, and confrontations with their mortality.

In many ways, this chapter presents the mirror image of chapter 5, the gradual but unrelenting erosion of the physical, mental, and emotional development from birth through childhood, adolescence, adulthood, and middle age. If the growth and development process is about learning skills, accomplishing goals, achieving independence, and looking forward, the elder years are about the inevitability of losing much of the physical and psychological self that has been so carefully nurtured, accepting limitations, and recognizing that, as Simon and Garfunkel sang, "all your dreams are memories."

The notion of pediatrics and geriatrics bookending clinical ethics has been described by the bioethicist Eric Kodish as "the bell-shaped curve of bioethical decision making," with autonomous decision making at the bell's apex and the extremes of as-yet-unrealized and diminished capacities at either end. "On the left side of the curve, you have children, who are completely dependent on us when they are born but eventually develop into autonomous beings. On the right side are geriatric patients, many of whom become completely dependent on us before they die" (Kodish 2013, p. 1). Referencing Shakespeare's *Hamlet*, Dr. Kodish's grandfather described this phenomenon as "once a man and twice a child" (Kodish 2013, p. 1).

DIMINISHING AUTONOMY AND DECISIONAL CAPACITY

The bell-shaped curve analogy should not obscure the very real differences between the incapacities of children and the elderly. While children are presumed to lack decisional capacity, their potential to become autonomous informs efforts to model responsible decision making and ensure "a child's right to an open future" (Feinberg 1992; Feinberg 1980). In contrast, seniors are presumed to have decisional capacity unless and until they demonstrate otherwise and their diminishing capacity signals the projected loss of former decision-making ability with its attendant independence, dignity, and self-respect.

Decision making on behalf of these two incapacitated populations differs in other important respects. Seniors typically have an established profile, including settled values, known goals and preferences, and a history of decision making, all of which inform a substituted judgment, such as, "Even though Mama never spoke about this particular scenario, based on everything we know about her, we think this is what she would want in this situation." What is known about the individual provides a behavioral and attitudinal baseline against which people can say, "Yes, that sounds just like Aunt Betty." Of course, this is precisely the value of prior articulation of health care goals and preferences in an advance directive. In contrast, because children have unformed values, preferences, and decision-making patterns, surrogate decision making cannot reasonably ask, "What would *this person* want in this situation based on what we know of her beliefs and values?" Rather, surrogates invoke the best interest standard, asking, "What do *we* think would be in this patient's best interest?"

"PROMISE THAT YOU WON'T EVER PUT ME IN A NURSING HOME"

Mrs. Gibson and her brother, Mr. Noland, finished the tour of Cedar Grove Nursing Home and met with the executive director, the director of nursing, the medical director, and the director of social work. "This certainly is a beautiful facility," Mr. Noland began. "It seems to provide everything Mama might need." He looked at his sister, who was staring at the handkerchief she was twisting into knots. Finally, as tears ran down her cheeks, she looked up and whispered, "Yes, it provides every-thing except what Mama wanted most—to live in her own home, surrounded by the things she and Dad collected over years, and to be the independent person she was always so proud to be. Can you give her any of that? We promised her that. How can we go back on our word?"

Among the themes that pervade the aging population are the twin fears of be-coming so physically and cognitively incapacitated that relocation to a nursing home becomes necessary. The nightmare is being so diminished, so irrelevant, so much a burden that institutionalization is "for your own good." Spouses and adult chil-dren struggle with this decision, especially when they are tethered to the promise never to allow it to happen. Previously independent, dynamic, successful people may feel betrayed, abandoned, and reduced to little more than aging children. They of-ten resent the paternalism that accompanies illness, frailty, and dependence, the notion that others half their age presume to know what is in their best interest. A lifetime of possessions is distilled into a few personal things in an otherwise im-personal room. Meals, personal hygiene, and recreational activities are scheduled and often supervised by others. Everything seems structured to diminish the au-tonomy that has been the hallmark of adult life.

Against that background, nursing homes are encouraged to reframe the vision of elder living they offer to residents. Among the perspectives that should receive greater attention is relational autonomy, a concept that focuses on a broader range of factors affecting autonomy than the traditional account that conceives of the pa-tient as largely divorced from his social circumstances. Relational autonomy views the individual as a social being and highlights the social and environmental fac-tors that can enhance or diminish the exercise of personal autonomy (Nedelsky 2011). This is particularly useful in the nursing home context, where frail elderly residents are often assumed to lack decisional capacity and institutional needs make it dif-ficult to be responsive to their autonomy interests. Relational autonomy also high-lights the continuum of abilities, recognizing that dependence in some areas of liv-ing does not reflect inability to make some decisions or take responsibility for some activities. Greater choice in everyday activities and flexibility in scheduling are rec-ommended as ways of helping residents retain as much control over their lives as possible (Sherwin 2010).

Ethical problems of the frail and cognitively impaired elderly are not confined to nursing homes, of course. They may become apparent when a family member brings the older person to a clinic for medical care or a day care program for social activities, or when a physician or nurse visits the older person's home. But outside an institutional setting, such as a nursing home, there may be few resources for ad-dressing these problems in a systematic and reliable manner. Ethics committees that can help clinicians and administrators deal with the problems of ambulatory pa-tients, including the elderly, are extremely rare, but ethics committees can become integral to the functioning of nursing homes.

Nursing home ethics committees can play an essential role in working with clin-ical and administrative leadership to create a climate that recognizes the capacities of each resident, promotes the exercise of autonomy, and dignifies the need for assistance. Ethics committees can also collaborate with staff in addressing the concerns of families struggling with the current needs of and the previous promises to loved ones. An ethics committee member participating in a consult can elicit family concerns about betraying or abandoning someone who appears to need the structure and support of nursing home residence. "Tell us about your father. What should we know about him in order to provide the most individualized care?" "Your mother sounds like a very loving person who valued her nurturing role. Do you think that she would recognize her own needs for nurturing now?" "When your sister said that she always wanted to live at home, do you think she pictured a situation in which that would not be safe or provide the kind of stimulation she seems to have loved?" "If your uncle could join this discussion, knowing what we know about his health and having seen what Cedar Grove offers, what do you think he would say?" Recognizing and articulating the tensions between and among the ethical obligations of those who care for and about elders can lay the foundation for resolution that accommodates the needs of residents and the concerns of their families.

INDEPENDENCE, DEPENDENCE, AND ROLE REVERSALS

Mr. Peters is an 85-year-old man with advanced Alzheimer's disease who has been living in the Cedar Grove Nursing Home for almost 2 years. About six months ago, his condition began deteriorating and, when he stopped eating several weeks ago, his longtime primary care physician, Dr. Levine, met with the family to consider placement of a feeding tube to provide artificial nutrition and hydration. While Mr. Peters had often said that he would not want to be "kept alive on machines," Dr. Levine suggested that this might be a temporary intervention to promote nourishment that would increase his strength and vitality. The feeding tube was inserted and Mr. Peters returned to the nursing home briefly but developed uncontrolled diarrhea and apparent abdominal discomfort. Two days ago, the tube fell out and the question has been raised whether to readmit him to the hospital for treatment of the diarrhea and possible replacement of the tube. A clinical ethics consult has been requested to consider the ethical implications of the decision.

Mr. Peters opens his eyes and responds to painful stimuli, but does not interact or appear to recognize family members. He is clearly incapable of participating in discussions or decisions about care and he had not created an advance directive to provide guidance about care planning. He does, however, have close family, including his son and granddaughter, who are visiting from California, and his grandson, Jason, who has been very involved in providing and making decisions about his grandfather's care.

The clinical ethics consultation includes Mr. Peters's family, Dr. Levine, the nursing home's directors of medicine and nursing, two nurses who have consistently cared for Mr. Peters, and three members of the Cedar Grove bioethics committee. Under the leadership of the committee chair, discussion focused on clarifying Mr. Peters's condition and anticipated clinical course with and without the feeding tube, the goals of care, and his likely preferences.

Jason described his grandfather as very active and fiercely independent until age 78, when his dementia became apparent. With his wife, he had raised Jason and, when she died, he continued to raise the boy alone until he left for college. When the dementia worsened, Jason arranged for his grandfather and a team of 24/7 care-givers to move into an apartment next to his. That arrangement continued until Mr. Peters required care that could best be provided in a skilled nursing facility.

When asked, "How much of Mr. Peters's current condition is irreversible?" the treating physicians responded that his neurological functioning is likely to continue deteriorating. All three family members agree that, given Mr. Peters's personality, values, and lifetime behavior pattern, he would not want to be permanently main-tained in his current condition, especially if he were dependent on artificial nutri-tion and hydration. Nevertheless, they express concern about the ethics, legality, and clinical effect of not replacing the feeding tube. They are especially uncomfortable with the notion of "starving Grandpop to death."

The Peters family story captures one of the ethical issues unique to the care of geriatric patients and those who, while not elderly, also suffer accelerated cognitive decline. During the past seven years, Mr. Peters and Jason have gradually traded roles, their relationship evolving so that the protector/caregiver/nurturer has be-come the protected / cared for / nurtured. Perhaps most significant, especially in Western societies that value independence, Mr. Peters has gone from "fiercely in-dependent" in managing all aspects of his life to completely dependent for even the most basic personal needs.

Loss of the ability to be self-governing is especially devastating in Western societies where, as the bioethicist Ira Byock (2010, p. 49) observes, "independence and prowess have become the hallmarks of dignity," making those who are frail and dependent feel undignified. Byock notes that he learned about dignity by watching his parents care for his grandmother following her stroke. He also describes John, "whom no one considered undignified, even though he needed diapers, urinated behind furniture, had fits of rage and required constant attention. John was three years old." Byock asks, "Many decades further on, if John develops dementia and acts in similar ways, will his wife and children consider him undignified? If so, why? We do not consider infants and toddlers undignified because they are at a stage in life in which they need physical care, nurturing and patient, loving attention: why are we less tolerant at the end of life?"

Perhaps the answer to Byock's question is that, typically, we expect the depen-dence and self-centeredness of infants and children to be temporary while they are learning skills, gaining self-control, and becoming independent. In contrast, we see the dependence and neediness of the elderly in terms of the skills they have forgot-ten, the self-control they have lost, and the independence they cherished but will never regain. We are profoundly disturbed by their loss and, even more so, by the reminder of the fate that awaits us all.

Mr. Peters would certainly have been aware of his failing memory, unsteadiness, confusion, and need for help with an increasing number of ordinary activities. Given his fierce independence, his support of Jason's education, and their shared antici-pation of future goal achievement, he would likely have resisted as long as possible becoming a burden to his grandson. Under other circumstances, he might have become isolated, lonely, frightened, and hopeless.

But Mr. Peters had a loving and involved family, people who knew him and understood what was important to him. Years before he moved into the nursing home, Jason arranged for his grandfather to live near him, enhancing their close relationship. As Mr. Peters's abilities decreased and his needs increased, Jason filled in the necessary supports so that his life continued with minimal interruption. When his needs for care and security exceeded what Jason could provide in the community, Mr. Peters moved to a nursing home that evidently gave him excellent care and personal attention, in addition to Jason's continued involvement. The result for Mr. Peters was the perception that, rather than being *taken care of*, he was being *cared for*. Throughout the downward trajectory of his physical and cognitive abilities, everything possible was done to preserve his strengths; supplement his weaknesses; and create a climate of affection, security, and respect, a climate conducive to a feeling of dignity.

Mr. Grant is a 95-year-old man who has been attending the Cedar Grove Adult Day Care (ADC) Program for the past 18 months. He is well groomed and dignified in his appearance. He has an expressive face, ready smile, and pleasant, interactive manner. Although he experiences some mild memory impairment, especially with names and other details, he is alert, gracious, and appreciative of any assistance. His health problems include aortic stenosis, hypertension, and glaucoma. He had surgical repair of a hip fracture three years ago and has a history of depression. He is dependent on staff for all toileting needs and transfers, and requires a walker and a contact guard for ambulation. At home he receives assistance from a home health aide for all his personal hygiene and grooming needs. His son is the primary person responsible for assisting him with all his activities of daily living (ADLs).

Mr. Grant became a widower when his wife died after 63 years of a happy marriage. He had been his wife's primary care provider until her death three months prior to his admission to the ADC Program. He had been very resistant to allowing anyone else to care for his wife and, at one point, an anonymous call had been made to Adult Protective Services (APS), although nothing suggested that her care had been inadequate. Upon admission, he denied feelings of depression, but he has been on Prozac for depression.

Several months ago, Mr. Grant's son, daughter-in-law, and granddaughter moved in with him. He was very happy with their decision because his declining health required more assistance and support, and he was eager to have the company of his family. He loved his son and was very proud of him, and he doted on his only grandchild.

Mr. Grant had been coming to ADC four days per week but, three months ago, his attendance was reduced to two days by his son, who believes that the ADC is financially exploiting his father. Recently, Mr. Grant reluctantly began reporting verbal abuse from his son and daughter-in-law, such as "We can't wait to get rid of you," "This house is no longer yours," "You have no more money and will be out on the street soon," "We will be better off when you die," and, just recently, he reported that his daughter-in-law threatened to "slice my head off." He also said that his daughter-in-law has threatened to hit him and he said that, if she hits him, "I'm afraid I may have to hit her back." When his neighbors had a party on Memorial Day weekend and he said how wonderful it was to see them all celebrating as a happy family, he reported that his daughter-in-law responded, "Oh, we'll be partying like that once you die!" He expresses great fear of his family and has requested to stay at Cedar

Grove as a full-time resident. He insists that he has the resources to pay for long-term care "unless my family has found a way to take it all." Mr. Grant knows that APS is involved, but he worries that not enough is being done to protect him. He expresses sadness, embarrassment, anxiety, and fear. This case has been brought to the Cedar Grove bioethics committee by the ADC staff, citing concern that Mr. Grant is being subjected to verbal, emotional, and, potentially, physical abuse by his family.

This case is appropriate for consideration by a nursing home bioethics committee because it raises issues of immediate and long-range concern. While Mr. Grant is not a full-time resident at Cedar Grove, the nursing home is responsible for his welfare during his regular participation in the ADC Program. Care of the elderly begins with appreciation of the inevitable downward trajectory—whether steep or gradual—in physical, cognitive, and emotional abilities. For precisely this reason, care planning in the geriatric population should take account of both short- and long-term needs and goals.

Here, Mr. Grant is demonstrating marked changes in behavior and mood since his family came to live with him. He reports escalating threats to his safety and feelings of insecurity. His access to ADC, an environment where he feels safe and cared for, is being restricted and he is reaching out for help. Because there is no reason to question his decisional capacity, Cedar Grove's responsibility to act on his behalf derives from its ethical obligations to respect his autonomy, promote his best interest, and protect him from harm. Immediate steps would include soliciting information from Mr. Grant's home health aides about the home situation, contacting APS, and sharing Mr. Grant's reports and the staff's concerns.

Mr. Grant's request to become a full-time resident at Cedar Grove should receive immediate attention, including collaboration and assistance with finances, insurance, and legal matters. He should be counseled about the importance of choosing surrogate decision makers because, absent his specific appointments, decisional authority will default to his family when he is no longer decisionally capable. Accordingly, he should be encouraged to execute an advance directive, appointing a trusted health care agent and an alternate agent to make health care decisions for him when he is no longer able to do so. He should also be encouraged to speak with an attorney about appointing a power of attorney (POA) to manage his financial and other nonmedical affairs, beginning immediately or when he is no longer able to manage these matters. Above all, Mr. Grant should be assured that his safety and well-being are the priority of the nursing home and its staff.

PRIOR WISHES AND CURRENT NEEDS

Mrs. Becker, an 82-year-old woman, has been a resident at Cedar Grove for 6 years. Except for increasing dementia and an irregular heartbeat that requires a pacemaker, she has no medical problems that prevent her from participating in her personal care and enjoying her favorite activities. After two recent episodes of atrial fibrillation, the medical director recommended that the pacemaker be replaced.

Mrs. Becker's significant dementia prevents her from understanding her clinical condition and health care decisions are made for her by her two devoted daughters, who are her health care agent and alternate agent. At a meeting to discuss the proposed hospitalization, the daughters tell the care team that they will not consent to replacing the pacemaker because they are honoring what they believe to be their mother's wishes. "Our mother was an elegant, fastidious, and very private person. She always said that, if she were ever incontinent and had to wear diapers, she would not want to live. We know that, if she could appreciate her situation now, she would be humiliated and would not want to continue this way."

Mrs. Becker, however, does not realize that she is incontinent or that her condition would have been a source of embarrassment. At the nursing home, she greets everyone with a smile, enjoys eating lunch in the garden and listening to opera, and loves visits from her grandchildren, even if she does not remember their names or who they are. Should her previous wishes limit care that would allow her to continue what appears to be a enjoyable quality of life? On the other hand, does her dementia deprive her of the right to determine how she will be remembered?

The notion that an individual's settled convictions, characteristic preferences, and cherished beliefs provide a touchstone for decision making on her behalf even after the loss of capacity is the foundation of surrogate decision making. Making decisions on behalf of an incapacitated person would be arbitrary and inauthentic if they did not reflect the choices and principles that have given her life meaning. Advance directives and other forms of advance care planning would be irrelevant if patients' expressed preferences were disregarded.

In a long-standing and lively debate, the justification for adhering to the preferences and decisions of a previously capable person through reference to advance directives or substituted judgment has been challenged by the notion that patients with dementia may have interests that differ markedly from those they had when they were capable (Dresser 1995; Dworkin 1993; Robertson 1991; Blustein 1999; Post 1995). The argument offered is that individuals with profound dementia are, in effect, different people—the *then person* and the *now person*—for whom decisions should be based on their current needs rather than their prior wishes or instructions based on what they anticipated their future needs and interests would be.

Mrs. Becker's daughters and caregivers are struggling with this very dilemma. Her incontinence, while previously a distressing notion to her, does not threaten her health or interfere with a current quality of life she appears to find pleasant. Given her otherwise good level of comfort and function, it would be hard to justify forgoing a life-sustaining measure at this time. Yet, her daughters feel that they will have betrayed the trust she placed in them if they disregard her previously stated wishes.

One important thing for Mrs. Becker's daughters to clarify is whether they believe that her comments were to be taken literally as instructions or figuratively as an expression of her distaste for the condition of incontinence. In other words, what do they think she would have wanted if she could have envisioned her current, otherwise pleasant, situation? Here, it is useful to consider the distinction between experiential and critical interests (Dworkin 1993). The former are interests in having experiences of certain kinds; the latter are more central and important interests that concern one's long-range goals and the arc of one's life over time. How Mrs. Becker's daughters decide may depend on whether they regard her interest in not being incontinent as so critical to her sense of self that she would not have been able to tolerate her current condition.

The analysis would depend on weighing her confirmed current level of comfort, function, and pleasure against the possible harm that might be caused by her distress if she appreciated her incontinence. If the daughters believe that the current benefits of her life outweigh the theoretical harms, replacing the pacemaker can be ethically justified. Moreover, this calculus should take into account the likely shifting of the balance as Mrs. Becker's dementia deepens, co-morbidities develop, and her quality of life diminishes. When the benefits no longer significantly outweigh the burdens, they may decide not to pursue continued life-supporting measures.

Some bioethicists have questioned the link that is normally assumed between autonomy and the possession of values. They have argued that at least moderately demented people can continue to have values and that these may conflict with the values they had when fully capacitated (Jaworska 1999). On this view, the question whether to honor an advance directive is not only a question about whether critical or experiential interests should take priority over the other. It may also involve asking whether a new set of values should take precedence over an earlier set.

INTIMACY AND SECURITY

Mr. John Morgan is an 83-year-old man who has been a resident of Cedar Grove Nursing Home for 2 years, since shortly after the death of his wife, with whom he had shared a happy 56-year marriage. His only sign of early-onset Alzheimer's disease is the distress of some memory loss; otherwise, his health is quite good and he enjoys daily physical activities. He presents as the upbeat, outgoing person he has always been, eager to share his love of literature, music, and dance. His three adult children visit weekly and are very involved in his life.

Mrs. Mary Daniels is a 79-year-old woman who came to Cedar Grove 1 year ago, after her moderate Alzheimer's disease made it impossible for Joe, her husband of 55 years, to continue caring for her at home. His increasing physical ailments and her increasing forgetfulness had resulted in several episodes of random wandering that were distressing and frightening for both of them. While she remains pleasant and sociable, her memory lapses impair her ability to be independent and even prevent her from recognizing her family, including her husband. He still lives in the home they shared and visits Mrs. Daniels as often as possible, meeting with her care team and advocating for what he believes are her best interests.

Six months ago, Mary and John began spending time together, often dining at the same table and sharing recreational activities. The staff noted that Mary often sought out John's company and appeared more comfortable and less tentative when they were together. They also noted that John seemed to laugh more when he was with Mary.

Recently, a nurse found Mary and John in Mary's bed, naked, cuddled together and fondling each other. The horrified nurse instructed John to return to his room and have no further contact with Mary. A team meeting was called and the case was referred to the bioethics committee with a request for a clinical ethics consult to protect a vulnerable resident from sexual exploitation. The staff's concern was that Mary's dementia rendered her incapable of consenting to having sex and that, therefore, John had coerced her into a sexual relationship. Most of the staff recommended immediately notifying both families and crafting strategies to prevent further encounters between Mary and John.

Predictably, the Morgan and Daniels families regarded their parents' relationship somewhat differently. John's children were supportive of their father's attachment to Mary, in light of the loneliness he had experienced since the death of their mother. Mary's husband, Joe, understandably felt shocked and betrayed. He assumed that, given her history as a devoted and loving wife, she had mistaken John for him. He chastised the staff for insufficiently monitoring Mary and insisted that she be protected from further exploitation. Mary's elder daughter agreed, saying that her mother was acting entirely "out of character" and "would be appalled if she could appreciate her behavior." The younger daughter, however, observed that her mother appeared happier and more secure than she had since developing dementia, and wondered whether she might not have current interpersonal needs that did not devalue her devotion to her husband (adapted from Sokowlowski 2012).

The notion of sexuality and intimacy in the geriatric population triggers strong and varying responses, ranging from disgust to ridicule to prurience to uncertain discomfort. A vast literature demonstrates the human need for physical contact and emotional support at the beginning of life. What has received insufficient attention is the relationship between the deprivation of physical and emotional intimacy and the profound loneliness and suffering experienced by elders who have lost spouses, had serious illness or injury, or have been relocated to an institution. Their sense of isolation, especially as the end of life approaches, is exacerbated by the widely held perception of physical intimacy among the elderly as abnormal or, at least, inappropriate, something to be prevented rather than supported.

Not surprisingly, nursing homes, responsible for the security and welfare of the residents in their care, tend to view as problematic any expression of sexuality or physical intimacy. The underlying assumptions are that sexuality among those who reside in an institution are more likely to be coercive, nonconsensual, and, therefore, harmful than similar relationships among elders who are not institutionalized. The result is that, in an attempt to protect vulnerable residents from harm, many nursing homes actively discourage sexual or intimate behavior and, unintentionally, have created what has been referred to as "iatrogenic loneliness" (Miles and Parker 1999).

Mary and John's relationship and Cedar Grove's response to it raise several ethical issues. Physical and emotional intimacy, especially sexuality, should be grounded in the mutual consent of the individuals, reflecting their appreciation of the potential goods and harms that may ensue. While they are unlikely to view their relationship in terms of benefits and burdens, the inherent unpredictability of intimacy requires acknowledged willing participation. Indeed, it is mutual consent that distinguishes true intimacy from exploitation. Concern about the autonomy necessary to valid consent is amplified in the nursing home setting, where residents vary widely in their capacity to understand and remember, advocate for themselves, and make and communicate choices. Here, John appears to function autonomously, while Mary's moderate dementia makes her vulnerable to coercion. Among the chief concerns in nursing homes is balancing the obligation to respect residents' autonomy and the obligation to protect them from harm. As in all such analyses, John's right to exercise his autonomy is limited by Mary's need to be protected, triggering the nursing home's duty to assess her understanding of the situation and her willingness to engage in intimate behavior.

Of course, Mary and John's actions affect more than just the two of them. The Morgan daughters are relieved that their father's loneliness has been lessened, while the Daniels family is profoundly shocked. Joe is especially devastated by what he can only see as yet another loss of his wife. In addition to the personality and intellect he has loved and her physical presence at home, he now must face her emotional and physical attachment to another man. It will be very difficult for him to continue relating to Mary in the same affectionate and supportive manner. The nursing home has the challenging task of responding to not only this situation, but also to others that raise similar issues. If John and Mary are supported in their relationship, surely other residents will expect equal validation.

Mary's behavior is also an illustration of the *now person* versus the *then person* phenomenon discussed above. Her husband and elder daughter insist that her behavior is "completely out of character," thereby invalidating her actions. Her younger daughter's view, however, suggests the possibility that Mary's *now needs* rather than her *then needs* deserve attention. Adopting that view would require both her family and the nursing home to change the way they perceive and respond to Mary, risking the implicit message to the family that the Mary they have known and loved is either gone or devalued.

The response would seem to be a case-by-case assessment of the individuals' capacities to exercise autonomy, including consent or refusal that will be respected; whether one individual's capacity is so diminished that a power imbalance threatens mutuality; and the likelihood that family responses to the relationship would be helpful or harmful. While the nursing home should not intrude into resident relationships without compelling reason, it does have an obligation to assess vulnerability and protect those who cannot protect themselves. If the risk of harm has been minimized, the significant benefits of intimacy, including sexuality, should receive due consideration. The challenge to nursing homes is expressed in the notion that the greatest fear is dying alone. "Death is the challenge to personal life. Intimacy—a place for solace, privacy, confiding, and telling and retelling one's story—is a lathe upon which the challenge of death can be answered. The possibility of intimacy must be one of the promises that healthcare providers make for those at the end of life" (Miles and Parker 1999, p. 41).

TRANSITION FROM HOSPITAL TO HOME OR NURSING HOME

The health of the frail elderly is typically precarious. Even if they are well enough to live in their own home, a sudden accident, such as a slip or a fall, can send them to a hospital and from there to a rehabilitation facility for a considerable period of time. Their physical, as well as their psychological, capacities may decline as a result and may never recover. This turn of events requires a reassessment of their former living arrangements. Even if they are able to return home, they may need much more nursing and assistive care than they had previously, and their family members may have to be much more closely involved in monitoring their well-being. On the other hand, it may be necessary to discharge them to a nursing home, where reported levels of depressive symptoms are higher than among patients who are discharged to live alone or live with others (Loeher et al. 2004).

The need to alter living arrangements because of deteriorating psychological and physical capacities of the elderly is normally addressed by social workers whose job is discharge planning. There are also ethical issues that require more focused attention. What if an elderly patient wants to return home, even though his safety is at risk there? What if he wants to return home but refuses the help of an aide? What if an elderly patient wants to live with her adult children after discharge, but the children object? What if an elderly patient wants to be discharged to a nursing home, even though she could function quite well at home with assistance? These issues may benefit from ethics committee involvement in the hospital as part of discharge planning.

REFERENCES

Blustein J. 1999. Choosing for others as a continuing life story: The problem of personal identity revisited. *Journal of Law, Medicine & Ethics* 27:20–31.

Braun M, Moye J. 2010. Decisional capacity assessment: Optimizing safety and autonomy for older adults. *Generations* 34(2):102–5.

Byock I. 2010. Dying with dignity. *Hastings Center Report* 40(2):49.

Dresser R. 1995. Dworkin on dementia: Elegant theory, questionable policy. *Hastings Center Report* 25(6):32–38.

Dworkin R. 1993. *Life's Dominion: An Argument About Abortion, Euthanasia, and Individual Freedom.* New York: Alfred A. Knopf.

Feinberg J. 1980. The child's right to an open future. In Aiken W, La Follette H, eds. *Whose Child? Children's Rights, Parental Autonomy and State Power.* Totowa, NJ: Rowman and Littlefield, pp. 124–53.

Feinberg J. 1992. The child's right to an open future. In *Freedom and Fulfillment: Philosophical Essays.* Princeton, NJ: Princeton University Press, pp. 76–97.

Hickman SE, Nelson CA, Perrin NA, Moss AH, Hammes BJ, Tolle SW. 2010. A comparison of methods to communicate treatment preferences in nursing facilities: Traditional practices versus the physician orders for life-sustaining treatment program. *Journal of the American Geriatrics Society* 58:1241–48.

Jaworska A. 1999. Respecting the margins of agency: Alzheimer's patients and the capacity to value. *Philosophy & Public Affairs* 28(2):105–38.

Kennedy GJ. 2000. *Geriatric Mental Health Care.* New York: Guilford Press.

Kodish E. 2013. From pediatrics to geriatrics. *Bioethics Reflections.* Cleveland Clinic Department of Bioethics, pp. 1 and 3.

Loeher KE, Blank AL, MacNeill SE, Lichtenberg PA. 2004. Nursing home transition and depressive symptoms in older medical rehabilitation patients. *Clinical Gerontologist* 27(1/2):59–70.

Miles SH, Parker K. 1999. Sexuality in the nursing home: Iatrogenic loneliness. *Generations*: 36–43.

Muramoto O. 2011. Socially and temporally extended end-of-life decision-making process for dementia patients. *Journal of Medical Ethics* 37(6):339–43.

Nedelsky J. 2011. *Law's Relations: A Relational Theory of Self, Autonomy, and Law.* New York: Oxford University Press.

Nolan K. 1990. Do-not-hospitalize orders: Whose goals? What purpose? *Journal of Family Practice* 30(1):31–32.

Post SG. 1995. Alzheimer disease and the "then" self. *Kennedy Institute of Ethics Journal* 5:307–12.

Reamy AM, Kim K, Zarit SH, Whitlatch CJ. 2011. Understanding discrepancy in perceptions of values: Individuals with mild to moderate dementia and their family caregivers. *The Gerontologist* 5(4):473–83.

Robertson J. 1991. Second thoughts on living wills. *Hastings Center Report* 21:6 9.

Sherwin S, Winsby M. 2010. A relational perspective on autonomy for older adults residing in nursing homes. *Health Expectations* 14:182–90.

Sokolowski M. 2012. Sex, dementia and the nursing home: Ethical issues for reflection. *Journal of Ethics in Mental Health* 7:1–5.

Young Y, Barheydt NR, Broderick S, Collello AD, Hannan EL. 2010. Factors associated with potentially preventable hospitalization in nursing home residents in New York State: A survey of directors of nursing. *Journal of the American Geriatrics Society* 58:901–7.

CHAPTER 8

Ethical Issues in the Care of Disabled Persons

DISABILITY AND ITS PLACE IN BIOETHICS

Until recently, the subject of disability has received scant attention within the mainstream bioethics community. Bioethicists have largely focused on the treatment of the sick and on the duties and rights involved in the relationship between health care professionals, chiefly physicians, and the patients who depend on them for medical guidance and care. Disability occupies a distinct but related area of ethical inquiry.

Persons with disabilities are not necessarily sick, although some disabilities, like the inability to walk, may be associated with certain diseases. A person can be disabled but healthy, whether health is defined in negative terms (the absence of disease) or in positive terms (psychophysical flourishing and vitality). The failure to clearly distinguish disability from disease has led to the neglect of ethical issues related to the health care of persons with disabilities. It has also, perhaps unwittingly, lent support to the view that the presumptively appropriate response to disability is medical rather than environmental or social.

In addition, notably missing from much of the bioethics literature are the voices of persons with disabilities. As is apparent in many bioethical and policy discussions of the experience of disability, most non-disabled persons, including health care professionals, imagine that experience to be far worse than reported by the disabled themselves. This mistaken assumption raises profound ethical issues at the times of greatest life impact, often influencing end-of-life decision making for disabled persons and also informing discussions about the ethics of abortion and prenatal genetic testing. The gap between the disabled and the non-disabled can be explained in part by the limited contact between the two groups, which reinforces damaging misconceptions.

This disconnect has important implications for the therapeutic interaction and for health policy. As an example, Walter J. Peace has written poignantly about his experience as a patient and the impact of thoughtless, albeit well-intended, remarks by a physician who implied that, because of his disability, Mr. Peace might understandably want to end his life (Peace 2012). The implications for health policy were illustrated when, during the debate about Medicaid rationing in Oregon in the early 1990s, non-disabled persons assigned a low priority to treatments that would sustain people with quadriplegia, on the grounds of their presumed poor quality of life. Persons with quadriplegia, however, complained that, because they had not been consulted, their first-person perceptions of their life quality had not been reflected in the ranking process (Menzel 1992). While attempts to create a disability experience for non-disabled persons (navigating a room in the dark, accomplishing tasks using one arm or leg, communicating without sound) are contrived at best, understanding the world from the perspective of the disabled is more than an exercise in being polite or sensitive. Taking seriously the views of disabled people about their disabilities is a critical step toward a better appreciation of the obstacles, challenges, and disadvantages they confront.

DEFINING DISABILITY

Even the definition of disability is extremely contentious. Many different kinds of people with different limitations are described as "disabled." Blindness, paraplegia, autism, epilepsy, depression, and HIV have all been classified as disabilities. The term covers such diverse conditions as congenital absence or traumatic loss of a limb or sensory function; progressive neurological conditions, like multiple sclerosis; chronic diseases, like diabetes or arteriosclerosis; the inability or limited ability to perform certain cognitive functions; and psychiatric disorders, such as schizophrenia and bipolar disorder. It is not immediately apparent what these various conditions have in common. Whatever the wording, the definition of disability somehow captures the notion of limited or impeded ability to do something, typically some function that can be accomplished by those without the disabling condition.

According to the definitions of disability offered by the World Health Organization (WHO), the Americans with Disabilities Act (ADA), and other statutes or guidelines, a disability has the following requisite features: (1) an impairment (or perceived impairment), generally defined as "any loss or abnormality of psychological, physiological, or anatomical structure or function" (World Health Organization 1980); and (2) some significant personal or social limitation associated with the actual or perceived impairment, with limitation defined as either relative to the individual or to some norm or population average. The ADA, for example, defines disability simply and clearly as "a physical or mental impairment that substantially limits one or more of the major life activities of such an individual." Of interest is that the ADA and similar statutes do not attempt to define "impairment." They merely note that impairments can be physical or mental abnormalities that range from conditions generally regarded as disabilities, such as blindness, to conditions generally described as diseases, such as cancer.

Despite the lack of definitional consensus, all attempts to define disability are normative in the sense that they presuppose some standard against which the disabled person's functioning is assessed. There is considerable controversy, however, about how the two elements of the definition of disability—impairment and significant limitation—are related to each other. In some views, biological factors are the sole causes of limitation; others attribute the limitation to features of societal organization that impose barriers or impediments to independent functioning. In between are views claiming that both biological impairment and social environment contribute to limitation. This more inclusive view is predominant in current law and commentary on disability and the best known example is the WHO International Classification of Functioning, Disability, and Health, according to which disability is a "dynamic interaction between health conditions and environmental and personal factors" (WHO 2001). The ADA's definition of disability is generally considered to adopt this interactive approach. The importance of the "dynamic interaction" definition is the recognition that, while the biological determinants of disability may not be reversible, the environmental factors that create barriers or challenges to independent functioning may be susceptible to modification (Bickenbach 1993; Altman 2001). From this standpoint, the appropriate response to disability may be a societal one that focuses on eliminating discrimination and socially constructed barriers to inclusion.

THE MEDICAL AND SOCIAL MODELS OF DISABILITY

Implicit in these different definitions are two contrasting models of disability, often referred to as the medical and social models. The medical model perceives disability as a physical or mental impairment of the individual, with personal and societal effects of that impairment. In its extreme form, the medical model holds that the limitations faced by disabled persons are primarily, or exclusively, due to physical or mental defects of the individual. In contrast, the social model views the limitations experienced by disabled persons as socially produced, a result of the societal exclusion of people with certain physical and mental conditions, and the disadvantages that result from such exclusion. The exclusion not only stems from the discriminatory attitudes of non-disabled persons. It is also due to the organization of the constructed environment and the social activity that fails to accommodate atypical functioning (Wendell 1996). In its extreme form, the social model denies the causal relevance of impairment to limitation, attributing limitation entirely to societal factors.

Neither model is usually defended in its extreme form (Bickenbach 1993; Terzi 2004, 2009; Shakespeare 2006). To be sure, the extreme medical model is often adopted unreflectively by health care professionals and bioethicists because of their focus on cure or, failing that, the amelioration of the effects of illness and disease. Even then, this camp recognizes some role for environmental and societal factors, although they are regarded as less significant than biological ones. Defenders of the social model maintain an emphasis on societal or environmental causes, while commonly recognizing a dynamic interaction between social and medical factors in causing disability. The disability rights movement is responsible for installing the social model as the dominant legislative, social science, and humanities paradigm for understanding disability, which naturally highlights societal obligations to remove or modify the socially created or, at least, permitted barriers to more independent functioning.

The different models of disability also favor different responses to disability. Thus, the medical model tends to support correction of the biological condition or some form of compensation when medical correction is impractical. The social model, by contrast, favors changes in the physical and social environment to better accommodate the functioning of disabled persons. Despite their supporters, these models do not always yield straightforward answers to questions about how to respond to the conditions of disabled persons. Consider, for example, passionate debates within and outside the deaf community about the use of cochlear implants, which examine whether the devices are an appropriate medical response to impairment or an objectionable capitulation to discriminatory social norms. A separate issue not addressed by these models is how to understand the relationship between disability and identity, and whether it should be viewed as a contingent feature of the individual or as a defining trait of personal distinctiveness (Solomon 2012).

THE DISABILITY RIGHTS CRITIQUE OF PRENATAL GENETIC TESTING

Melissa, age 30, is 12 weeks pregnant. She is obese and has maternal insulin-dependent diabetes. Because these are known risk factors for spina bifida, she was advised by her doctor to have her fetus tested for this condition. Spina bifida is a neural tube defect in which the spinal column does not close completely, and its effects vary from hydrocephalus (fluid on the brain) to partial or full paralysis, bladder and bowel control difficulties, and learning disabilities. When Melissa told her doctors that she would rather not be tested, they seemed surprised, as if the choice not to be tested were unusual. They asked her whether anyone had met with her to discuss "options," which is often perceived as a code word for "abortion."

As prenatal tests proliferate, many in the medical and lay communities regard their use as an extension of good prenatal care, similar to pregnant women seeing their obstetricians on a regular basis. The reasoning is that prudent parents-to-be would want to have as much information as possible about the health of their future offspring, enabling them to make decisions that will enhance their child's potential. The disability rights movement, however, has criticized the use of these tests to determine whether a child will be born with a disability because of the negative and discriminatory perceptions they perpetuate. Disability scholars claim that prenatal testing for this purpose, which usually results in the decision to terminate the pregnancy if the test is positive for one or more disabling conditions, is morally problematic for several reasons.

Proponents argue that prenatal genetic testing enables parents with family histories of certain inheritable diseases to spare their children and succeeding generations unnecessary suffering. Also, as noted in chapter 6, parents who have a child with an inheritable disease can more confidently pursue family planning if they can identify potential problems prenatally. Critics respond that, practiced on a large scale, prenatal genetic testing recalls the eugenics movement of the early twentieth century and reinforces discriminatory attitudes toward persons with disabilities. They claim it sends a hurtful message that disabled persons' quality of life is so diminished that it would have been better had they not been born at all. Critics also maintain that using prenatal testing to select against fetuses with certain disabilities reflects a flawed conception of parenthood that requires "good" parents to be selective about the children they bear, and warn that its widespread use threatens morally desirable attitudes toward children and parenting. Rather than supporting a welcoming attitude toward one's child, defects and all, prenatal testing reflects an inability or unwillingness to accept anything less than the perfect child. It also encourages parents to measure the value of a child's life by particular (desirable or undesirable) traits that he or she happens to possess. This faulty conception of parenthood perpetuates the tendency to let the part stand in for the whole that underlies the pervasive discrimination experienced by disabled persons (Parens and Asch 2000).

A leading expert on ethical issues in disability, the late Adrienne Asch, forcefully and very influentially argued against the widespread use of prenatal genetic testing, particularly its use for detecting fetal defects. While her position is compatible with a pro-life stance on the question of abortion, this is not the position she embraced. Rather, she supported the legal right to terminate a pregnancy for any reason, including fetal defects. At the same time, she suggested that abortion for fetal defects is much like abortion for sex selection, at least when the defect is not severe enough to cause early death or intractable pain for the future child, and that abortion in both cases is morally questionable. Decisions about pregnancy termination for fetal defects, she claimed, are often ill-informed and reflect social prejudices against the disabled and negative stereotypes about what life is like raising a disabled child (Asch 1986). Asch also argued that the medical model of disability, which drives prenatal testing, reflects a profound misunderstanding of the nature and effects of disability and that, rather than focus on testing to prevent the birth of children with disabilities, efforts should be directed toward changing societal conditions so that all children, including those with disabilities, can reach their full potential (Asch 1999).

These criticisms of prenatal testing are the basis of a number of recommendations for health care providers. Disability rights critics argue that it is important to distinguish tests that professionals should routinely offer, those that should be offered selectively based on family history, and those that should not be offered at all. These critiques accept that some conditions may be serious enough to justify abortion to spare the future child an early death or a life of unremitting suffering. But, in general, they are wary of drawing a line between serious and minor disabling traits because they fear the heightened potential for abuse in a society characterized by its focus on superior appearance and achievement, which perpetuates widespread discrimination against persons with disabilities. Disability rights critics also advocate that genetic counselors make available to prospective parents full and accurate information about life with a disabled child and what to expect, so that they can correct prevailing stereotypes and misunderstandings. To do this, counselors must themselves receive good information about what disability is really like for children and their families, and come to terms with their own misperceptions and biases. On these latter points, critics as well as supporters of prenatal testing find common ground.

Many bioethicists find serious problems with the disability critique of prenatal testing. Some argue that there is a significant moral and practical difference between aborting a fetus with a serious disabling condition and disvaluing the lives of those already living with a disability. They argue that permitting the former does not entail sanctioning the latter. Others have found fault with the claim that a woman should be open to accepting any child she gets and have argued instead that some selectivity in this regard can be compatible with praiseworthy parenting. Despite these controversies, however, there is widespread agreement on all sides that informed consent to prenatal testing is morally imperative and that, in order to make informed decisions, parents must be given information about life with a disabled child that is not distorted by misconceptions about and biases against persons with disabilities.

The case of Melissa brings to the fore an issue about which both proponents and opponents of prenatal genetic testing for disability can find common ground. Melissa was not merely given information about the availability of a test for spina bifida: she was none too subtly pressured to agree to it. She was made to feel inadequate as a parent if she did not have the test done. She was not given information about what life with a spina bifida child would be like and what its effects might be. She was not told that the effects of spina bifida are different for every person and that not all children experience the most serious form of the birth defect. In these ways, she was not given the opportunity to make an informed and uncoerced decision about testing her fetus.

While this case initially appears to focus on decisions related to endocrinology, genetics, and high-risk pregnancy, the ethical issues require careful analysis and the input of the ethics committee or consultation service. Of special concern are Melissa's decisional capacity, the quality and balance of the information recommendations she was provided, her understanding of the information and how she used it to make decisions, the voluntariness of her decision, and the guidance and support she received. An ad hoc meeting of your ethics committee or consult team to consider this case would usefully include representation from genetics, obstetrics, neonatology, and, if indicated, pastoral care. Developing a coordinated interdisciplinary approach to helping Melissa navigate this difficult set of prenatal and postnatal decisions is a task your ethics committee should be well equipped to manage.

SPECIAL CHALLENGES IN THE CARE OF PERSONS WITH SEVERE COGNITIVE IMPAIRMENT

Mr. Frankenheim, 89 years old, has been an orthodox Jew his entire life and has always subscribed to its central tenet, the sacredness of life and the imperative to preserve it above all else. In the past year, however, he experienced two serious blows: he lost his wife of 60 years and was diagnosed with Alzheimer's disease. The disease has progressed to the point of significant dementia. Now that he is hospitalized with pneumonia, Mr. Frankenheim's doctors are disturbed by a request that he has been making with increasing frequency. He tells them he has nothing left to live for and that he wants to die. When his doctors explain to him that he needs antibiotics to treat his pneumonia, he answers, "I don't care. I have had enough. I don't want any medicine." His doctors do not know whether they should honor his request. After all, it signifies a rejection of his previous values, and they question whether he is capable of making rational decisions in his condition. Unfortunately, Mr. and Mrs. Frankenheim lived alone and never had any children, so there is no family to turn to for additional guidance.

Persons with substantial cognitive impairments present physicians and other health professionals with special medical and ethical challenges. Physicians have obligations both to promote the good of their patients and to respect their autonomous choices. Persons with significant cognitive impairments, however, either lack or have limited ability to make autonomous choices and may not have developed or articulated goals, values, or preferences. They are thus often unable to advocate or advocate effectively on their own behalf, and so are vulnerable to receiving inappropriate treatment or being denied treatment they need. In this regard, they are similar to children whose best interests must be determined by others who assume responsibility for acting on their behalf.

Persons with cognitive impairments, however, do not necessarily lack all capacity for self-determination or the expression of preferences and values. In her work on people with Alzheimer's disease, Agnieszka Jaworska (1999) has argued that the capacity to value and exercise autonomy in at least a rudimentary form is not necessarily lost with the onset of major cognitive impairment. What is essential to valuing, in her view, is not that the individual have a conception of what is good for his life as a whole, but that he possess convictions about what is good for him. Depending on the degree of impairment, this conception of personal good is possible for many cognitively impaired persons. Disability scholars have also argued that personal assistants or personal support agents can help these persons exercise their capacities for self-determination, much as assistants of various sorts can help persons with standard cognition carry out their wishes and express their preferences. As long as the assistance of others reinforces rather than substitutes for the impaired person's own preferences and values, they extend the person's cognitive functions and enable him to exercise the autonomy of which he is capable.

It remains controversial, however, whether and to what extent persons with significant cognitive impairment have or retain the capacity to exercise autonomous choice and to determine, even if only with the aid of a personal assistant, the direction of their care. Loving family members and close friends may be in a better position to determine this than health care professionals whose contact with the impaired person is transient and sporadic. Moreover, physicians and other health care professionals have duties not only to respect the autonomy of their patients but also to safeguard and promote their well-being. Because these are distinct duties to some extent, significantly cognitively impaired persons are vulnerable to mistreatment even if their autonomy is not being violated.

The case of Mr. Frankenheim raises a number of questions to which there are no easy answers. How advanced is his dementia? Is he capable of autonomous decision making? Does his request to die reflect a new set of values or merely the rejection of his former values? Should his former religious values take precedence, so that his doctors are justified in refusing to honor his request to die? Though in some important respects Alzheimer's patients like Mr. Frankenheim who are not in the final stages of the disease retain their former capacities, there is also a moral imperative to protect them from the consequences of choices that may be harmful to their well-being.

Here, again, ethics input can be very useful. In addition to exploring issues of capacity, informed consent, and surrogate decision making, your committee may have a role in advocating for a person who has no family or other support system. A meeting of Mr. Frankenheim's care team should also include his rabbi and other members of the religious community that has been so central to his life. Not only can these individuals provide the necessary lens of Jewish doctrine in considering Mr. Frankenheim's situation, their very presence would likely be comforting and supportive to him during this difficult time.

MEDICAL DECISION MAKING AND THE DISABLED

Frances Becker, age 26, suffers from advanced cerebral palsy and severe degenerative arthritis. She recently checked herself into the psychiatric ward of her local general hospital, claiming that she wants to kill herself. After a month, she announced that she was looking for an attorney who would help her force the hospital to keep her comfortable while she starved herself to death. As she said, "If I really could, I would go out there and kill myself. But I can't. I physically can't." Though assisting her to end her life would not be legal without statutory cover or court intervention, a number of physicians caring for her expressed sympathy with her wish to die, saying, "Her quality of life is so poor I'm not surprised she wants to die," "If I were in her place, I would want to die too," "Life as a disabled person is a fate worse than death."*

Concerns about whether disabled persons are capable of making autonomous decisions are not confined to those who are cognitively impaired. Questions have also been raised about how to evaluate the autonomy of people immediately following traumatic injury or the diagnosis of a disease that will lead to increasing disability and, even among disability scholars, there is sharp division. Some claim that the principle of respect for autonomy requires that the clear and consistent decisions of a recently paralyzed individual or an individual recently diagnosed with Parkinson's disease or multiple sclerosis be honored, even if the decision is to forgo life-sustaining treatment. Others argue that the trauma of a major disability upends one's sense of identity, and so renders suspect decisions made in its immediate aftermath. Persons with new physical impairments may make decisions that run counter to their long-term interests, commitments, goals, and values, and, it is argued, paternalism in such cases is justified to protect the recently disabled person from impulsive and irreversible decisions (Powell and Lowenstein 1996). This

---

*This vignette is based on the legal case of Elizabeth Bouvia (1983), which is discussed further in part IV.

argument recalls that, during the early years of the AIDS epidemic, persons who were diagnosed with HIV often identified milestones of debility ("When I lose my hair," "When I'm no longer able to work," "When I'm so weak I can no longer take care of myself") that would signal when life would no longer be worth living. Yet, when those milestones arrived, many infected persons moved the goal posts because they had accommodated to what they had previously thought would be intolerable.

The famous case of Dax Cowart, the victim of a horrific explosion who refused treatment and begged to end his life rather than endure the pain, disfigurement, and disability caused by massive burns, generated and still generates intense debate within the bioethics community about what respect for autonomy requires in the aftermath of a traumatic injury. Dax, long after he had recovered, claimed that, while he was glad to be alive, his autonomy had been unjustifiably violated. Many commentators, however, supported his caregivers, arguing that it takes time to understand what a major disability may imply, or to discover how many roles, activities, and relationships can survive and adjust to the "new normal." Until the individual has had the opportunity to live with his new limitations, the demand for withdrawal of life-sustaining treatment is not truly informed (Cowart and Burt 1998).

This approach raises the ethical question of how long is long enough and who makes that determination. Waiting too long, and one violates the individual's autonomy; not waiting long enough, and one respects a less than adequately informed decision. Perhaps, with time and experience, the disabled person will shift from seeking death to embracing life. But, it may reasonably be asked, why we should suppose that anyone has the right to make this intensely personal decision for another individual. One strategy sometimes used is negotiation: "I understand that at this time you cannot imagine yourself living in this condition and you want to exercise your legal right to refuse further life-sustaining measures. I respect your right and I want to support your decision as long as I am convinced that it is informed and well settled. This is very new right now and your decision is irrevocable, so let's make a deal. Continue as you are for a year [or whatever time seems reasonable]. One year from today, if you still believe that your life is intolerable, I will do whatever is necessary to honor your decision." This enables the patient to retain ultimate control over his life, while giving him the opportunity to make an informed and voluntary decision.

Another obstacle to making autonomous decisions faced by persons with serious disabilities is the social position they occupy. Stigma, discrimination, and the common belief that disability is devastating all combine to create an atmosphere in which persons lacking psychological resilience, social connections, and political consciousness may feel that it would be best if they did not pursue treatment for a treatable medical condition, even if the treatment could save or prolong their lives. They may internalize the attitudes, stereotypes, and expectations of able-bodied persons in a societal context where the prevailing understanding of serious disability is that it significantly diminishes the quality of one's life. Even among disabled persons with social connections and many psychological strengths, there may be a feeling that the deck is stacked against them, generating an exaggerated sense of pessimism about their life prospects. As one disabled person commenting on proposals to legalize physician-assisted dying put it, "My problem, ultimately, is this: I've lived so close to death for so long that I know how thin and porous the border between coercion and free choice is, how it is for someone to inadvertently influence you to feel devalued and hopeless—to pressure you ever so slightly but decidedly into being 'reasonable,' to unburdening others, to 'letting go'" (Mattlin 2012, p. A31). On the other hand, to deny disabled persons the right to end their lives in the belief that they are not exercising truly free or autonomous choice because of societal and familial pressures is also misguided. It presumes that persons with serious disabilities are, by virtue of that fact alone, unable to resist these pressures, and this amounts to an endorsement of the very paternalism that both bioethics and the disability rights movement reject.

The case of Frances Becker illustrates the ease with which health care providers and persons without disabilities assume that a life with a serious disability is not a life worth living. This may even be a view shared by disabled persons themselves, as a result of the relentless obstacles, hardships, and discrimination they experience in our society. Whether Frances has the moral right to end her life, and whether the hospital has an obligation to assist her, are only two of the ethical issues her case raises. In addition, there is the very real concern that discriminatory attitudes toward disabled persons, absorbed by caregivers from the larger society, can interfere with providing or even offering medical care that is in their best interest. Discussion of these issues continues in chapter 9.

Your ethics committee can provide an invaluable service by highlighting these usually unintended, sometimes unconscious misperceptions and biases. Consider using ethics grand rounds to present a series of vignettes, illustrating language and behaviors that either promote or undercut the functioning and dignity of patients or colleagues with disabilities.

REFERENCES

Altman B. 2001. Disability definitions, model, classification schemes, and applications. In Albrecht GL, Seelman KD, and Bury M, eds. *Handbook of Disability Studies*. Thousand Oaks, CA: Sage Publications, pp. 97–122.

Asch A. 1986. Real moral dilemmas. *Christianity and Crisis*, July 14.

Asch A. 1999. Prenatal diagnosis and selective abortion: A challenge to practice and policy. *American Journal of Public Health* 89(11):1649–57.

Bickenbach J. 1993. *Physical Disability and Social Policy*. Toronto: University of Toronto Press.

Cowart D, Burt R. 1998. Confronting death: Who controls? A dialogue between D. Cowart and R. Burt. *Hastings Center Report* 28(1):14–24.

Jaworska A. 1999. Respecting the margins of agency: Alzheimer's patients and the capacity to value. *Philosophy and Public Affairs* 28(2):105–38.

Malek J, Daar J. 2012. The case for a parental duty to use preimplantation genetic diagnosis for medical benefit. *American Journal of Bioethics* 12(4):3–11.

Mattlin B. 2012. Suicide by choice: Not so fast. *The New York Times*, October 31, p. A31.

Menzel P. 1992. Oregon's denial: Disabilities and quality of life. *Hastings Center Report* 22(6):21–25.

Parens E, Asch A, eds. 2000. *Prenatal Testing and Disability Rights*. Washington, DC: Georgetown University Press.

Peace WJ. 2012. Comfort care as denial of personhood. *Hastings Center Report* 42(4):14–17.

Powell T, Lowenstein B. 1996. Refusing life-sustaining treatment after catastrophic injury: Ethical implications. *Journal of Law, Medicine & Ethics* 24(1):54–61.

Shakespeare T. 2006. *The Sexual Politics of Disability.* London: Cassell.

Solomon A. 2012. *Far From the Tree: Parents, Children, and the Search for Identity.* New York: Simon and Schuster.

Terzi L. 2004. The social model of disability: A philosophical critique. *Journal of Applied Philosophy* 21(2):141ff.

Terzi L. 2009. Vagaries of the natural lottery? Human diversity, disability, and justice: A capability perspective. In Brownless K, Cureton A, eds. *Disability and Disadvantage.* New York: Oxford University Press, pp. 86–111.

Wasserman D, Asch A, Blustein J, Putnam D. Disability: Definitions, models, experience. *Stanford Encyclopedia of Philosophy,* http://plato.stanford.edu/entries/disability/ (accessed August 2014).

Wendell S. 1996. The social construction of disability. In *The Rejected Body.* New York: Routledge, pp. 35–56.

World Health Organization. 1980. *International Classification of Functioning, Disability and Health (ICF),* http://whqlibdoc.who.int/publications/1980/9241541261_eng.pdf (accessed August 2014).

CHAPTER 9

End-of-Life Issues

Decision making at the end of life

Defining death

Organ donation: Donation after cardiac death and elective ventilation

Advance health care planning

Honoring patients' end-of-life decisions

Goals of care at the end of life

Forgoing life-sustaining treatment

Protecting patients from treatment

Rejection of recommended treatment and requests to "do everything"

Medical futility

Mr. Tofer is a 77-year-old man admitted for resection of a squamous cell carcinoma of the tongue. The surgery was successful but, on the following day, he experienced respiratory distress that required intubation. Because he was not able to be weaned from the ventilator after three weeks, a tracheostomy was performed to place the ventilator tube directly into his trachea, which would be safer and more comfortable than continuing to pass the endotracheal tube down his throat. He has had two subsequent episodes of low blood pressure and is experiencing progressive renal failure. His mental status has deteriorated during the four weeks he has been in the ICU and he is responsive only to painful stimuli, such as suctioning of his tracheostomy.

Mr. Tofer's only family is his nephew, Lawrence. Although they have not had a close relationship, they have maintained contact over the years and Lawrence appears concerned about his uncle. Lawrence is not Mr. Tofer's appointed health care agent and they have never had discussions about care at the end of life.

The renal team met with Lawrence to discuss the plan of care. Dr. Cooper, the renal attending, said that, although dialysis might improve Mr. Tofer's mental status, it would not change his overall grave prognosis. The consensus of the renal team is that the patient is a poor candidate for dialysis and has less than a 1% chance of surviving this hospitalization. Given the considerable risk and the slight benefit, the team would consider dialysis only if the family insisted. Dr. Cooper also recommended a do-not-resuscitate (DNR) order so that, if Mr. Tofer experienced a cardiopulmonary arrest, resuscitation would not be attempted.

What should Lawrence consider in making decisions about his uncle's care? What are the team's responsibilities?

DECISION MAKING AT THE END OF LIFE

If you were wondering when we would get to the really tough issues, the ones that make up the bulk of your ethics committee agenda and clinical consults, this is it. Some of the most difficult health care choices take place at the beginning and the end of life, and this chapter is the other bookend with chapter 6. Like much in bioethics, the issues related to dying and death are relatively new and would not have been raised a few generations ago when the health care focus was on attempting to cure or control disease or, at least, promote survival, and when life-sustaining technologies and medical interventions were not available. The response to illness and injury was to try all available measures and hope that something would be effective. Questions about whether the patient was receiving too much treatment or whether life was being unnecessarily prolonged would not have been asked.

Since then, we have managed to greatly expand both our treatment options and our ethical dilemmas. We have witnessed the development of medical and surgical interventions that can often return critically ill patients to health; they can also prevent death, even when improvement is not feasible. Decisions about end-of-life care now require greater scrutiny of the likely outcomes of therapy, including the important distinction between physiologic effectiveness (will the treatment work?) and therapeutic benefit (will the patient be better off because of the treatment?). Recognizing that cure-oriented and life-sustaining measures are not always medically appropriate for or even wanted by patients, bioethics works to facilitate decisions about when to deliver the patient from death and when to let death deliver the patient from us.

Sometimes, dying patients are capable of making or at least contributing to decisions about their care. More often, end-of-life decisions are made when the patient is no longer able to participate in deliberations. As a result, they typically involve efforts by others to determine the care plan that would most effectively meet his clinical needs and promote his well-being. As discussed in chapter 2, any decision making on behalf of an incapacitated patient requires that professionals, families, and other surrogates try to identify what his care wishes were or would be or determine what would be in his best interest. You already know from your experience in the clinical setting and on the ethics committee that these decisions become infinitely more difficult when the stakes are life and death.

Faced with the need for substitute decision making at the end of life, clinicians routinely turn to family members, who are presumed by tradition, and often by law, to know and act in the patient's best interest. As a rule, both medicine and law are more comfortable providing than withholding treatment, and considerable authority is customarily granted to family in *consenting* to treatment. Decisions about *limiting* treatment are far more problematic, however, and some states restrict the ability of non-appointed surrogates, even next of kin, to authorize the withholding or withdrawing of life-sustaining treatment.

The profound consequences of the choices, uncertainty about decision-making authority, lack of clarity about patient wishes, and lack of consensus on goals of care make end-of-life decisions among the most challenging in the clinical setting. For this reason, ethics committee consultations are frequently requested as death approaches.

DEFINING DEATH

Gary, a 9-year-old, was admitted to the hospital after infection from an abscessed tooth spread to his sinuses and eventually to his brain. Despite aggressive treatment, his brain swelled in response to the infection, causing increased intracranial pressure. Ultimately, clinical examinations and tests revealed that he met the criteria for brain death. The attending pediatrician and the pediatric neurologist met with Gary's parents to tell them that the massive infection had destroyed his brain and that the condition was irreversible. In an extended discussion, the doctors explained that, because their son's brain had completely stopped functioning, he was no longer alive. His devastated parents refused to accept the determination of death. His mother cried, "Look at him. His eyes are closed and he doesn't answer us, but he's still breathing and his heart is still beating. He just needs more time to get better. You can't take away the machines that are keeping him alive."

What are the obligations of care professionals in planning for and managing care at the end of life? How can the care team help families accept irreversible deterioration, dying, and death?

Although some things should be relatively straightforward, like knowing when a person is dead, this is not always the case. When medical science and technology were less advanced, death was generally agreed to have occurred when the heart and lungs ceased functioning. By the late 1960s, advances in resuscitative techniques and artificial respirators enabled cardiopulmonary function to be maintained even after the brain had stopped working. Ultimately, the traditional definition of death—irreversible cessation of cardiopulmonary function—was supplemented by a definition that accounted for cessation of entire brain function.

The first well-accepted definition of brain death was the product of the Ad Hoc Committee of the Harvard Medical School to Examine the Definition of Brain Death. The committee defined brain death as irreversible loss of total brain function, including "unreceptivity and unresponsivity . . . no movements or breathing . . no reflexes . . . [and] . . . flat electroencephalogram" (Ad Hoc Committee 1968, pp. 85–86). By the time the committee published its report in 1968, the sophisticated medical technology that permitted measurement of brain waves also enabled organ retrieval and transplantation. The generally recognized motivation for developing brain death criteria was the ability to perfuse organs, the only way to keep them viable for transplantation. Thus, the advances in medical and surgical techniques, the need for transplantable organs, and the unacceptability of taking them from a still-living person prompted a new definition of death.

The Uniform Determination of Death Act (UDDA), adopted in 1980 by the National Conference of Commissioners on Uniform State Laws, expanded the definition of death to include both cessation of circulatory and respiratory function *and* brain death. That dual standard was endorsed in 1981 by the President's Commission for the Study of Ethical Problems in Medicine and Biomedical and Behavioral Research in its report, *Defining Death*, which encouraged all states to adopt the UDDA.

While the brain death definition may have clarified and simplified some clinical determinations, it has also created a category of potential confusion. Terminology is critical and, especially in dealing with families, clinicians should clearly distinguish brain death and other conditions in which the patient is unresponsive.

Brain death is the irreversible cessation of the *entire* brain's ability to function, including the upper brain, which controls the higher functions of cognition and memory, and the brainstem, which controls the body's automatic functions, such as breathing and heartbeat. Because the brain's regulation of vital functions has shut down, the person is considered both clinically and legally dead, although the notion of brain death still generates controversy (see, e.g., Nair-Collins 2010, 2013; Sade 2011; Khushf 2010; Evans 2005). While the family comes to terms with the death and considers possible organ donation, mechanical supports may temporarily continue to perfuse the organs and maintain cardiac and respiratory function. It is, however, counterintuitive for grieving families to accept that death has occurred when looking at a body that is warm and healthy-colored, has a heart beat, and appears to be breathing, although this is only because the cardiopulmonary system is being mechanically supported.

In contrast to brain death, the patient in a *vegetative state* has suffered profound *upper* brain damage and has lost cognitive function; yet she retains the *lower* (brainstem) function that controls the systems essential to life, although if her brain stem function is weak, she may need assistance to support respiration. The vegetative state has been further defined as *persistent* or *permanent* (PVS), depending on its duration and irreversibility. "When a vegetative state continues beyond thirty days, it is described as 'persistent.' A vegetative state is generally considered permanent three months after anoxic injury and twelve months after trauma" (Fins 2005, p. 22). The patient has no awareness of herself or her surroundings and no ability to think or interact, but she is alive and might not be dependent on machines to maintain life. Indeed, as the case of Terri Schiavo, which lasted from 1990 to 2005, demonstrated, if nutrition and hydration are maintained and no additional illness or injury intervenes, patients can live for years in PVS.

The *minimally conscious state* (MCS) has been described as a condition in which people who have been in a vegetative state for less than a year occasionally progress to demonstrate "unequivocal, but fluctuating evidence of awareness of self and the environment" (Fins 2005, p. 22). Finally, *coma* is a label used for temporary or permanent unresponsiveness that may result from a variety of conditions, including illness, injury, or chemically induced unconsciousness.

Because these conditions have such different courses and outcomes, clearly distinguishing among them with careful language is essential to helping families adjust their expectations to the clinical realities. For example, describing a patient in PVS as being "comatose" or "in MCS" may unfairly encourage the belief that responsiveness will return. Likewise, it is extremely unhelpful to tell a family, "Your loved one is brain dead, but we are keeping him alive on machines." Saying this is confusing and hinders acceptance of the patient's death. The term *life support* is also counterproductive in this context because it implies that machines are supporting life. It is more honest and compassionate to explain, "Although your husband is no longer alive, these machines are temporarily perfusing his organs and supporting his heartbeat and respirations. Now that death has been confirmed, these mechanical supports are no longer necessary because they are no longer sustaining his life, and they should be discontinued so that his body can rest." Even the term *brain death* may be counterproductive if it is perceived to refer to some special kind of death from which patients might recover. It may be more helpful to explain, "Your brother has died. We know this because his brain has completely stopped functioning. Once that happens, we know that death has occurred. In other cases, we know that death has occurred because the heart stops and cannot be started again. Both situations are irreversible because the patients have died and nothing we do can change that."

Although families often have difficulty accepting the death of their loved ones, some families have specific moral or religious objections to cessation of brain function as a determination of death and may insist that mechanical supports not be discontinued. Brain death regulations are state-specific and New Jersey and New York are the only states with legislative opt-out provisions that allow families to reject the neurological criteria for determination of death in favor of the cardiopulmonary definition of death (Appel 2005). If a family without specific moral or religious objections to the brain death determination is still unable to accept the death, reasonable accommodations may be appropriate for a specified time. These accommodations (e.g., continuing ventilation, nutrition and hydration, or medications) should take place in a quiet private room, if possible not in the Emergency Department (ED) or the critical care unit, which would be counterproductive to the family's acceptance of the death and an unwise use of resources. The clinical staff should emphasize that the accommodations are for the benefit of the *family*, not the now-deceased patient. Efforts to help the family come to terms with the loss may include bioethics consultation, social service intervention, psychiatric counseling, and pastoral care.

ORGAN DONATION: DONATION AFTER CARDIAC DEATH AND ELECTIVE VENTILATION

Clinical organ transplantation, which began in 1954, required a seeming paradox: "the need for both a living body and a dead donor" (Sade 2011, p. 146). In an effort to resolve this paradox, the definition of death was expanded to include neurological criteria, enabling the retrieval for donation of organs and tissues from patients who had suffered whole brain but not cardiac death. Central to the ethical and legal legitimacy of the organ procurement program is the Dead Donor Rule (DDR), which reflects the widely held prohibition against killing one person by removing vital organs in order to save the life of another person. This ethical norm is codified in the DDR's requirement that an organ donor must be dead before vital organs are removed.

As medical science, surgical techniques, and pharmacological innovations developed and the shortage of transplantable organs grew, however, that seemingly bright line has become the subject of scrutiny and debate. Patients with devastating brain injuries that fall short of the brain death criteria may still be organ donors under Donation After Cardiac Death (DCD) or Non-Heart Beating Donor (NHBD) protocols. Ethical justification rests on the strict separation of two well-settled rights of capable patients or the surrogates of patients without capacity: the right to refuse unwanted life-sustaining treatment (LST) and the right to consent to posthumous retrieval and donation of organs. Safeguards protecting against undue pressure and conflict of interest include not raising the subject of organ donation until after the decision is made to withdraw LST; having the patient brought to the operating room, where LST is withdrawn and the patient is pronounced dead by the treating team, which then departs the scene; and having the organ retrieval team assume control only after the patient has been pronounced dead and a short interval of time, usually three to five minutes, has passed.

If DCD enables the deliberate *discontinuation* of LST to enable organ retrieval, elective ventilation (EV) or elective intensive care (EIC) is the deliberate *continuation* of non-therapeutic supportive measures to maintain organs for possible donation. Controversy relates to the notion of providing intensive measures, including ventilator support, pressors, and even CPR that have no prospect of benefiting the patient but may benefit potential organ recipients. EV has been proposed for two types of patients:

- patients definitely evolving toward brain death
- patients who may be suitable as non-heart beating organ donors (NHBD) for whom mechanical ventilation and life-supporting therapies have been assessed as futile (incapable of providing benefit to the patient) (Baumann et al. 2013, p. 139)

EV seems counterintuitive and causes clinicians, as well as ethicists, understandable unease because it seems to violate several fundamental ethical norms by disrespecting the patient's dignity; exploiting the vulnerable patient; using one person as a means to benefit another; putting the patient at risk of evolving toward PVS; creating conflicts of interest for care professionals; and shifting the focus of care from traditional patient-centered values to a utilitarian, technological ethic. Concern was so great that, despite initially increasing the supply of organs by 50% in the United Kingdom, the practice was declared illegal there between 1994 and 2009, when it was again permitted in that jurisdiction. Renewed interest in EV, including in the United States, finds support in the notion that continuing intensive care until the patient's wishes about organ donation can be confirmed and honored demonstrates respect for the patient and benefits the grieving family, as well as society in general (Baumann et al. 2013).

If you are beginning to get the feeling that the notion of "dead" is being twisted into unnatural shapes, you are not alone. Commentators have argued that brain death is a convenient fiction established and accepted for the sole purpose of increasing the supply of transplantable organs and that both moral integrity and the availability of transplantable organs are advanced by rejecting the whole brain criterion and the Dead Donor Rule (Sade 2011; Miller, Truog, and Brock 2010; Truog 1997, 2007; Nair-Collins 2010). Some have gone further and suggested changing the consent process to facilitate organ conscription, and even organ donation euthanasia (Wilkinson and Savulescu 2012).

Concern about the dissonance between established clinical practices and prevailing ethical norms is captured in the intriguing and provocative work that examines moral fictions, tools that permit endorsing a fictitious justification for accepted practices that would otherwise be prohibited. "The moral fictions relating to end-of-life decisions are motivated to make morally challenging medical practices, such as withdrawing life-sustaining treatment and providing pain-relieving medication at the risk of hastening death, consistent with the norm that doctors must not kill, or assist in killing, patients. . . . the underlying fault that the moral fictions conceal lies not in accepted practices, which are justified, but in established norms that cannot withstand critical scrutiny" (Miller, Truog, and Brock 2010). The notion of moral fictions, especially as it relates to end-of-life care and decision making, would be a relevant and thought-provoking topic for an ethics committee meeting or ethics grand rounds.

When life ends, as when it begins, is a matter of profound scientific, moral, legal, religious, and cultural importance that is not likely to be resolved any time soon. And yet, public policy, legal and regulatory frameworks, professional standards of care, and institutional policy imperatives demand consistency and clarity. Your ethics committee will inevitably be asked to weigh in on these matters. Your task will not be to provide definitive resolution to these conundrums, but to engage clinicians and administrators in considering them through the lens of ethical analysis, focusing on the implications and consequences for those in positions of vulnerability and responsibility.

ADVANCE HEALTH CARE PLANNING
Advance Directives

The 1976 case of Karen Ann Quinlan raised what came to be known as the "right to die"—actually, the right to refuse treatment—and brought to national attention the risks to a patient whose treatment wishes are unknown in a high-tech, aggressive, cure-oriented health care environment. Although physicians determined that the 21-year-old was in a persistent vegetative state (PVS) and would not recover, they were reluctant to agree to her family's wishes and discontinue life-support measures. In a unanimous landmark decision, the New Jersey Supreme Court held that if there were "no reasonable possibility" that she would ever return to a "cognitive, sapient state," her ventilator could be removed without fear of criminal or civil liability. The *Quinlan* case highlighted the potential for incapacitated patients to be subjected to unwanted treatment, providing the impetus for the development of advance directives that could guide care according to patient wishes.

Subsequent cases, most notably the 1990 case of Nancy Cruzan, sharpened the focus on determining the prior wishes of the incapacitated patient as the guide to making authentic health care decisions. After the 25-year-old woman had been in PVS for 7 years, her parents petitioned for an order to discontinue artificial nutrition and hydration. The U.S. Supreme Court, in its only such decision, recognized the protected interest of a capable individual in refusing unwanted treatment, including measures necessary to maintain life. The Court also held that, when life-sustaining treatment is refused on behalf of an incapacitated patient, states may but are not required to insist that these decisions be based on clear and convincing evidence of what the *patient* wanted, not what others want *for* her.

Between 1990 and 2005, these issues were revisited in countless decisions about end-of-life care, most publicly as the fate of Terri Schiavo, a 27-year-old when she suffered a cardiac arrest that ultimately left her in PVS, captured national and international attention. Her husband claimed that, as her next-of-kin and authorized surrogate, he was responsible for honoring Terri's wishes to not be maintained on artificial nutrition and hydration. Her parents argued that Terri would want continued life-sustaining measures because she was not in PVS and, therefore, would recover. Adding to the family's stress and grief was the very public involvement of strangers with religious, political, and special interest agendas.

The cases of Karen Ann Quinlan, Nancy Cruzan, and Terri Schiavo, discussed at greater length in part IV, captured such widespread attention for two reasons. First, these were young women in devastating conditions from which they would not recover. Second, and perhaps more significant, decisions about their care were not automatically considered to be the responsibility of those closest to them. In addition to sympathy, these stories prompted many people to say, "Hey, wait a minute. This could happen to me or someone I love. What if no one knows what I would want? What if these decisions are made by doctors or courts or other strangers?"

The answer seemed to be some method of prospectively documenting care instructions to provide clarity and legal authorization for later decision making. Advance directives were developed to provide for treatment preferences, values, and directions to be articulated by a capable person so that they could be communicated and implemented after decisional capacity has lapsed. As discussed in chapter 2, the most common types of directives are instruction directives (living wills) and appointment directives (health care proxies or powers of attorney for health care).

Mr. Jennings is a 24-year-old man who has just been brought to the ED after a traffic accident. Since his initial diagnosis of HIV three years ago, he has been scrupulously taking his antiretroviral medications and receiving regular care in the HIV clinic and, with a CD4 count of 460, his HIV is under good control. He is physically active and was on his way home from playing basketball when his bike was struck by a car. He is unconscious and suffering from a dislocated shoulder and a collapsed right lung.

As the ED team is preparing to intubate Mr. Jennings, his mother and sister arrive with his living will, which says, "If I am ever unresponsive and in respiratory failure, I do not want to be maintained on life support, including ventilatory support." His sister insists, "That may be what he wrote, but it's not what he meant. He's not ready to die. You must do everything to save his life, even putting him on a respirator."

The care team knows that short-term ventilatory support will permit the resolution of the pneumothorax and that Mr. Jennings's chances are excellent for full recovery from his injuries and return to baseline function. The team is concerned that a living will is a legal expression of the patient's wishes and that respecting his autonomy requires that it be honored, even though his clinical condition would benefit from intubation.

And you thought that an advance directive was the answer to uncertainty about patient wishes. As discussed in chapter 2, a living will is a list of instructions reflecting the individual's wishes about the treatments he would or would not want, usually at the end of life. A health care proxy appointment enables a capable person to appoint an agent to make health care decisions whenever capacity has been lost, either temporarily or permanently. The features of both types of advance directive are often combined in one document that provides for the appointment of a primary agent and an alternate agent, as well as the optional articulation of specific treatment wishes. A related type of prospective care planning for patients with life-limiting illnesses is the Practitioner/Physician Orders for Life-Sustaining Treatment (POLST) or Medical Orders for Life-Sustaining Treatment (MOLST), consolidated sets of medical orders (Bomba 2011; Fromme et al. 2012). While advance directives, especially health care proxies, may be used to guide care at any time the patient has lost capacity, they figure prominently in planning care at the end of life. As discussed in this chapter and chapter 10, the approach of death prompts consideration of life-sustaining treatment, palliation, futility, and quality-of-life judgments. Because these issues are most often addressed when the patient is least able to participate, decisions with lasting consequences must be made on his behalf by others based largely on what they believe he would want or need. Advance directives can provide surrogate deciders with the insight and confidence to act in ways that are consistent with the patient's preferences or best interest.

What could be simpler or clearer? As you well know, clinical ethics consultations are often requested to help the care team, families, and health care agents interpret and implement advance directives. Confusion usually concerns the authority of the directives and the meaning of their provisions. Several points should be emphasized. First, both living wills and health care proxies take effect only when the patient has been determined to have lost decisional capacity. The existence of an advance directive, therefore, does not alter the capable patient's decision-making rights; its authority lies dormant until the patient is deemed unable to make health care decisions.

Second, even when decisional capacity has been lost, treatment instructions are implemented only if the patient meets the criteria specified in the directive. Take, for example, a living will that states, "If I am ever terminally ill, permanently unconscious, or unable to recognize or interact with my family, I do not want to be maintained on ventilatory support, dialysis, or artificial nutrition or hydration." Before even considering withholding or withdrawing these life-sustaining measures, a clinical determination would have to be made that the patient is in one of the specified medical conditions.

Dr. Abrams has called to request a clinical ethics consult. His patient, Mrs. Bennett, is a 61-year-old woman admitted with severe leg pain and altered mental status. Her past medical history includes end-stage renal disease, diabetes, and congestive heart failure (CHF). She is found to have necrotic skin ulcers on her legs and a likely explanation is toxicity caused by the Coumadin she takes for her CHF. She refuses dressing changes and screams in pain whenever she is touched. Dr. Abrams says that the recommended treatment would be a two-week chemically induced coma, during which the necrotic areas can be aggressively debrided and treated without subjecting Mrs. Bennett to the trauma of repeated painful treatments. His concern is that Mrs. Bennett's advance directive explicitly rejects specified life-sustaining interventions, including the intubation and ventilatory support that will be necessary during the two-week treatment. The advance directive also appoints her daughter, Elizabeth, as her health care agent and Elizabeth is requesting the proposed treatment.

Dr. Abrams asks, "If we do this, aren't we disregarding the instructions the patient put into a legal document? Does Elizabeth have the authority to do that?"

Third, inconsistencies between the provisions of an instruction directive, such as a living will, and the decisions of a health care agent should be assessed in terms of the patient's current and projected clinical status, and the relationship between the patient and the agent. Because advance directives are executed before the medical condition that will trigger their use, they try to anticipate what the patient would want under circumstances that have not yet occurred. The impossibility of predicting every medical contingency significantly limits the utility of the instruction directive.

In contrast, the appointment directive, such as a health care proxy, is recommended because it employs the agent's knowledge of the patient and her authority to interact with the care team and respond to changing clinical conditions in real time. She is able to consider unanticipated or evolving situations, as well as the clinical judgment of the professionals. Precisely because the agent has the advantage of assessing current medical information in light of the patient's values and wishes, her decisions may exceed or even depart from the living will. Even though the living will may be silent about a specific choice, even though the patient may never have discussed her present medical situation, substituted judgment allows the agent to say, "If the patient knew what we know about her condition and prognosis, this is what she likely would decide."

This means that the spirit, as well as the letter, of the directive should be considered in interpreting the instructions and determining whether they apply to the current circumstances. Mr. Jennings's living will, for example, specifies that he would not want ventilatory support if he were "unresponsive and in respiratory failure." Given his HIV status and his reference to being "maintained on life support," it is very likely that he was anticipating an end-of-life scenario, including permanent unconsciousness, rather than an acute event that would respond to a short course of ventilatory support. This assessment is supported by his mother and sister, whose knowledge of his values and preferences is an important resource. Thus, the patient's prior wishes as expressed in a living will must be considered in light of the current clinical realities, the expected outcomes, and additional insights about what matters to him.

Likewise, Mrs. Bennett's advance directive says that she would not want certain life-sustaining treatments only "if I am ever in an incurable or irreversible mental or physical condition with no reasonable expectation of recovery." She is not currently in one of those specified conditions. Indeed, the reason the chemically induced coma is being recommended is the care team's conviction that the necrosis, if treated aggressively, is reversible. In addition, Elizabeth is able to say with certainty that, if her mother were aware of her condition and the available treatment, she would consent to the proposed plan.

Several important caveats are in order. Despite early enthusiasm for advance directives, the percentage of people implementing them remains low and, when they are used, their effectiveness in the clinical setting is less than optimal. A large and growing literature suggests that a fundamental weakness is the notion that prospective decision making can provide reliable information that will be useful in planning and implementation care when it is needed. The theory that previously articulated preferences about hypothetical clinical situations should determine specific decisions about current, rapidly changing and possibly unanticipated, medical circumstances risks premature and incompletely informed choices. One suggestion is a redefinition of advance care planning to prepare patients and their surrogates to consider advance directives as one valuable piece of information to be used in collaboration with the care team to make optimal "in-the-moment" decisions about current medical conditions (Sudore and Fried 2010).

Another problem appears to be the unfortunate link between advance directives and dying. While advance directives are often very helpful in end-of-life decision making, the emphasis should be that they can guide care *whenever* the patient is unable to make his own decisions. Indeed, it is recommended that, when advance directives are discussed with patients, they *not* be presented as end-of-life planning, which may discourage their use. In a perfect world, care professionals would raise the issue as a routine part of the clinical interaction, saying, "I have this discussion with all my patients because I believe that advance directives are an important part of total health care planning. This is not a matter of how old you are or how sick you are; this is a matter of being responsible for how and by whom your health care decisions are made." Uncoupling advance directives from end-of-life considerations is likely to make them less threatening, more accessible, and ultimately more useful.

The second barrier to the effective use of advance directives is the lack of understanding about them displayed by patients, families, and care professionals. People often mistakenly assume that, by itself, a detailed list of treatments they do or do not want or the appointment of a proxy agent will get the job done. In fact, what they believe to be informed prospective decisions are likely to be counterproductive if they do not discuss their care preferences with their doctors, families, or agents. People frequently refuse treatments in advance without understanding what they are or how they work. They leave instructions that do not apply to the medical situations in which they ultimately find themselves. They authorize agents who have no idea of their authority, the types of decisions they may have to make, or how to interpret patient preferences. In some instances, agents do not even know that they have been appointed until they are called by the ED and it is too late to ask the patient about her preferences.

Lack of communication and coordination has also been shown to interfere with advance directives accurately influencing care. Even when directives have been executed, they often do not make their way to the acute care hospitals when patients are admitted. Professionals are uncertain how to interpret advance directives and when their provisions are applicable. Physicians are sometimes unable to accurately predict patient treatment preferences and are often unaware that their patients even have advance directives. Research reveals the need for earlier, more frequent, and better doctor-patient communication, focusing on the goals of care rather than specific interventions (Berger 2008; Torke et al. 2008; Teno et al. 1998; Fisher et al. 1998; Prendergast 2001; The SUPPORT Principal Investigators 1995; Morrison et al. 1995).

Even a carefully executed advance directive is not sufficient if the patient's values and wishes are unknown or unexplained to those who will base decisions on them. People need to talk with their families, caregivers, and trusted others about what is important to them, allowing their values, rather than their scant knowledge of medical interventions, to be the guide. For example, knowing that Mama would agree to temporary treatment but would not want to be permanently dependent on mechanical supports is more useful than a statement about "no dialysis." Understanding that Dad's notion of an acceptable quality of life is being able to interact with others is more helpful than a statement about "no heroic measures."

More often, the explicit authorization and guidance of an advance directive is lacking and treatment decisions require inferences based on recalled comments or behaviors. Unfortunately, these conversations typically take place in the least opportune circumstances—in the acute care setting at the time of a critical event when the unresponsive patient is in multi-organ system failure, the family is under enormous stress, and professionals seek direction in care planning.

A third barrier is the misperception that the provisions of an advance directive are activated as soon as the document is received by the care team. If patients or families believe that all treatment will be discontinued when the document is entered in the medical record, it is no wonder they often "forget" to mention Mama's advance directive or "neglect" to bring it to the hospital. Encourage the care teams in your hospital to be proactive in reassuring patients and surrogates that the provisions of advance directives are triggered only when the patient is unable to make decisions and when the specified medical conditions have been confirmed.

As noted in chapter 2, the designation "power of attorney (POA)" also can create considerable confusion. When someone shows up claiming decision-making authority based on a POA appointment, it is essential that someone on the care team reads the document before putting it in the patient's medical record. Unless the words "health care" or "medical treatment" appear somewhere in the text, the document should be returned to the individual with the message, "Clearly, the patient trusted you to be responsible for these matters, but the authority does not extend to decisions about health care." Absent specific appointment of a health care agent or a POA for health care, surrogate decision making becomes the responsibility of the individual(s) in order on the hierarchy approved in most states, which typically lists people in descending order, beginning with those most intimately connected to the patient and moving to those less closely related.

POLST/MOLST

A more recent form of advance care planning for a specific patient population is POLST (Practitioner/Physician Orders for Life-Sustaining Treatment) or MOLST (Medical Orders for Life-Sustaining Treatment). These are consolidated sets of *medical orders* that are the product of discussion between patients with life-limiting conditions and their physicians or other specified practitioner about resuscitation, intubation, dialysis, artificial nutrition and hydration, and other life-extending interventions. POLST and MOLST have three important features that distinguish them from advance directives:

- *Advance directives are statements of patient intention*, which physicians (and, in some states, advance practice nurses, or APNs) translate into medical orders under appropriate clinical circumstances. For example, an advance directive that says, "If I am ever permanently unconscious or terminally ill,

I do not want cardiopulmonary resuscitation (CPR)" is not a medical order. Physicians (and APNs) must determine that a patient is in the specified state and that CPR would be clinically inappropriate before entering a DNR order in the medical record to preclude CPR. In contrast, *POLST/MOLST are medical orders*, which are immediately operational.

- *Advance directives are appropriate whenever a person is temporarily or permanently unable to make health care decisions* and, in a perfect world, everyone age 18 and older would have one. In contrast, *POLST/MOLST are intended only for patients with life-limiting illnesses*, typically those expected to live one year or less.

- Advance directives become *operational only when a patient has been determined to have lost decisional capacity*. In contrast, POLST/MOLST are *operational as soon as they are signed, even if the patient is still decisionally capable*.

These consolidated order sets are approved at the state level and, while a growing number of states have authorized some version of POLST or MOLST, not every state has done so. If this type of resource is available in your state, your ethics committee can provide clinicians with valuable information about how it fits into care planning.

Do-Not-Resuscitate (DNR) Orders

Mrs. Marcus is a 72-year-old woman with multiple medical problems, who was admitted from a nursing home after being found unresponsive and hypotensive. This is the second time in recent weeks that Mrs. Marcus has been admitted. She was hospitalized for 18 days with pneumonia and a massive stroke. During that hospitalization, a feeding tube was placed. She was discharged to the nursing home and now readmitted 17 days later with aspiration pneumonia. She was intubated in the ED and successfully extubated several days later.

Mrs. Marcus's daughter, Deborah, is her health care proxy agent. A living will, executed on the same date as the proxy appointment, stipulates that if Mrs. Marcus's "brain has ceased to function," she would not want a variety of potentially life-sustaining interventions, including respiratory support, artificial nutrition and hydration, and antibiotics. Although Mrs. Marcus responds only to deep pain and her physicians do not expect her condition to change, Deborah is in favor of continued aggressive treatment, which she hopes will result in her mother's improvement. The attending believes that, if Mrs. Marcus suffers a cardiopulmonary arrest, she could survive a resuscitation attempt but would almost certainly be left in a much worse condition. For that reason, the care team has recommended a do-not-resuscitate (DNR) order to spare Mrs. Marcus an intervention that would increase her suffering without providing benefit.

Deborah refuses to consent to a DNR order because the wording of the living will does not clarify what is meant by the "brain has ceased to function," and she does not think that forgoing resuscitation reflects her mother's wishes. She says that the living will is clear that her mother would not want to linger in a coma. Because she is not yet in that condition, however, Deborah is unwilling to consent to a DNR order or consider less-than-aggressive cure-oriented treatment at this time.

Another type of prospective decision making is the do-not-resuscitate (DNR) order. A DNR order means that cardiopulmonary resuscitation (CPR), including mouth-to-mouth resuscitation, external cardiac massage, intubation, and stimulants, will not be attempted if the patient suffers a cardiopulmonary arrest. Consent to a DNR order can be given either by a capacitated patient or by someone authorized to consent on the incapacitated patient's behalf.

The ethical dilemma is that CPR's ability to prevent death can greatly benefit some patients and greatly burden others. In a young or otherwise healthy person, if cardiopulmonary function can be restarted within approximately four minutes, avoiding irreversible damage to brain and other organs, CPR can give back a life. In an elderly, demented, terminally ill person, one who has multiple serious health problems or has suffered severe and permanent damage, CPR can deprive the individual of a peaceful death.

Unfortunately, reports of successful resuscitations and dramatic television and film depictions of heroic rescue have played into popular belief in CPR's life-saving certainty. In fact, the brutal procedure is rarely effective on frail, debilitated, or terminally ill patients and may simply impose suffering and prolong dying. The critical distinction between attempting and successfully achieving resuscitation accounts for widespread efforts to change the term from DNR to the more accurate DNAR (do not *attempt* resuscitation). Because of its profound implications, consent to forgo CPR is explicit and limited, not inferred or automatically transferred from one setting to another. Thus, DNRs must be renewed periodically, a specific discussion is necessary to suspend a DNR order during the perioperative period, a new DNR order must be entered upon admission to another care facility, and a nonhospital or community DNR must be written if the patient is returning home or to another residential situation.

Even experienced physicians know that advising patients or, more often, families that CPR is not recommended is among the most difficult discussions in the clinical setting. No matter how sensitively it is presented, suggesting that life-saving efforts not be undertaken is distressing and frightening, an index of just how hopeless the patient's condition has become. Unfortunately, a common misperception is that DNR means do not treat, signaling a collective resignation to impending death and a scaling back of all treatment. Indeed, patients and families are often resistant to considering a DNR order because of the fear that the patient will receive less attentive care. A crucial task is clarifying for patients, families, and clinical staff that DNR forgoes only one intervention—cardiopulmonary resuscitation—and does not alter the rest of the care plan or the team's commitment to the patient. These discussions require all the judgment, skill, and compassion that practitioners can muster, and ethics consultations are often requested to assist in the process.

Rather than an isolated conversation, the DNR discussion should be part of the overall review of the patient's changing clinical condition. Just as other interventions are evaluated in terms of whether they promote the patient's well-being, resuscitation should be subjected to a benefit-burden analysis. Patients, families, and staff should clearly understand that it is the physiologically futile or clinically inappropriate *attempt* rather than successful resuscitation that will be withheld. Discussions with Deborah should balance the benefits and burdens of resuscitation to help her view a DNR order as a way to *protect* her mother from a painful and violent but, ultimately, ineffective intervention, rather than *deprive* her of potentially beneficial treatment.

It is unfair to ask families to take full responsibility for the difficult and painful decision to forgo resuscitation. Asking "If Mama's heart stops, do you want us to start it again?" is mean, as well as unethical. First, the question implies that the intervention would be successful, but if that is not anticipated it is wrong to suggest that outcome. Second, the question puts the entire burden on the family to say, "No, don't save my mother," a burden that will haunt the family long after the patient's death. At every Thanksgiving dinner, someone will say, "If we had just insisted on resuscitation, Mama would be sitting right there." If CPR is not clinically indicated because it is not expected to improve the patient's condition, the physician's clear recommendation, rationale, and support should be central to the discussion. "Let me tell you why we believe that, if your mother's heart were to stop, attempting to restart it would not benefit her" sends an entirely different message, one of collaboration and concern for both the patient and the family. Once the decision has been made, it is often the consent document that may be most distressing, as if putting pen to paper is the act that seals the patient's fate. The most common expression is, "I feel like I'm signing the death warrant." It is far more compassionate to avoid that trauma by obtaining verbal and witnessed consent.

Finally, there are times when, even though the disadvantages of attempting resuscitation have been explained, families cannot or will not authorize a DNR. However well intended, repeated efforts to obtain consent begin to feel like harassment. The issue risks becoming the focus of the clinical interaction and the signed consent perceived as a trophy. In these circumstances, ethics committee involvement may be helpful to redirect attention to other care goals that are more important and achievable.

Attempted and Assisted Suicide

Chapter 10 addresses the critical distinction between and among actions by clinicians that permit, promote, or hasten death, including aid in dying (AID), formerly known as assisted suicide. As discussed later, the more neutral and accurate AID reflects the fundamental differences in intent, deliberation, and rationale between the decision of a terminally ill person and a person who is not terminally ill to end their lives. To maintain this distinction, two situations involving attempted suicide are presented here. When patients who appear to have attempted suicide are brought to the hospital, caregivers are faced with competing and seemingly irreconcilable ethical obligations of respect for patient autonomy, beneficence, and nonmaleficence. Because these matters implicate moral, religious, and professional values and convictions, your ethics committee is likely to be consulted.

One manifestation of this dilemma is how caregivers should respond to an individual whose suicide attempt is followed by a refusal, either contemporaneously or in an advance directive, of life-saving measures, illustrated by the following case in Great Britain: "Kerrie Wooltorton was a twenty-six-year-old woman with psychiatric problems. She had repeatedly tried to poison herself but each time doctors intervened to save her life. In 2007, she again took poison and called an ambulance. At the hospital, she refused treatment and presented a document saying she had come to the hospital to avoid a painful and lonely death and wanted no lifesaving measures. The hospital staff followed Wooltorton's wishes, and she died the next day." The ensuing inquest supported the hospital staff's decision to withhold life-saving measures (Dresser 2010, p. 10).

Analysis of care professionals' obligations considers the well-settled right of competent individuals to refuse unwanted treatment, including life-sustaining treatment; the well-settled duty of care professionals to intervene in attempted suicides; relevant notions of intent (while the patient's intent was to end her life, the staff's intent was to respect her treatment refusal rather than assist her death), causation (was death caused by the patient's actions or the withholding of medical treatment?), and timing (is treatment refusal several months after a suicide attempt a continuation of suicidal behavior or a separate assertion of her right to refuse unwanted treatment?) (Dresser 2010, p. 10).

A variation on this theme concerns caregivers' response to DNR orders for patients who attempt suicide.

Mr. Herman, an 81-year-old man with a long history of chronic obstructive pulmonary disease (COPD) and depression, was found by his daughters shortly after he had accidentally or deliberately ingested several bottles of opioid analgesics. He was awake but unable to respond. The daughters called 911 and Mr. Herman was taken to the nearest hospital, where he was admitted to the medical intensive care unit (MICU). In discussion about the patient's condition, the critical care attending noted that, given his advanced COPD, Mr. Herman was likely to develop respiratory failure, leading to a cardiac arrest that would require resuscitation to prevent death. The daughters replied that their father's clear and consistent wish had been to avoid resuscitation and he had insisted that, under these circumstances, he wanted a DNR order. The critical care resident explained that, even if a DNR order had been written or requested, standard clinical practice called for resuscitation if respiratory failure or cardiac arrest were precipitated by a suicide attempt (Geppert 2011).

As discussed in chapter 1, ethical dilemmas arise when two or more moral principles or obligations are in conflict and cannot be honored simultaneously. Here, the ethical dilemma is the collision between the ethical principles of autonomy (patient right to refuse treatment) and beneficence (professional obligation to promote patient best interest and protect patients from harm) or nonmaleficence (professional obligation to avoid actions likely to cause harm). The literature reveals that arguments for overriding an existing or, as in this case, a requested DNR order in this situation would rest on the one or more of the following assumptions:

- attempting suicide is the act of a person suffering from treatable mental illness who, therefore, cannot be considered capable of an autonomous refusal of life-sustaining treatment;
- patients who have requested DNR orders often do not fully understand what they are refusing and/or cannot anticipate the specific situations in which the need for resuscitation might arise; and
- the DNR order should be considered part of the suicide attempt and honoring it would constitute assisting a suicide, exposing caregivers to legal liability

In contrast, justifications for honoring existing or requested DNR orders in the setting of attempted suicide include recognition that

- the suicide attempt and the refusal of CPR are not necessarily related, especially if the wish not to be resuscitated was longstanding and consistently articulated;
- physician concerns about responsibility for maleficence and legal liability often lead to overestimating the potential for a good outcome and underestimating the harm from attempted resuscitation;
- lack of physician knowledge about patients' values and goals often obscures the importance of refusing unwanted interventions; and
- even if the suicide attempt were the impulsive act of depression or mental impairment, the wish to avoid resuscitation is typically rational and well settled.

Your ethics committee is likely to be consulted when a patient believed to have attempted suicide has or has requested a DNR. The literature (e.g., Geppert 2011; Loertscher et al. 2010; Cook et al. 2010) discusses this matter in greater detail than is possible here and you are encouraged to become familiar with the issues and arguments. The takeaway message here is the importance of considering the specifics of each case through the ethical lens of competing principles and obligations, and focusing on the timing and intent of the separate elements. Unless the validity of the DNR order is suspect or it is clear that the order is an integral part of the suicide attempt, a DNR order should be viewed as an independent expression of patient autonomy and honored as such.

HONORING PATIENTS' END-OF-LIFE DECISIONS

Mr. Gonzalez is a 61-year-old man with recently diagnosed pancreatic cancer. His condition is rapidly deteriorating and he understands that he is dying. Mrs. Gonzalez, his wife of 38 years, however, cannot bring herself to accept the gravity and irreversibility of his condition. She comes to the hospital every day and sits at the bedside, anticipating that her husband will improve. She insists that he does not need pain medication because "it makes him sleepy and he wants to be awake when I come" and, on two occasions, she has disconnected the patient-controlled analgesia (PCA).

Mr. Gonzalez has had several long discussions with the palliative care team and, when he consented to a DNR order, he told the attending physician, "I know that my wife will never agree to this." Three days later, he arrested and when the rapid response team (RRT) arrived, Mrs. Gonzalez hysterically threw herself at the feet of the team and cried, "Do something! You must save my husband!" Mr. Gonzalez was resuscitated, intubated, and transferred to the ICU and his code status was changed to "full code," the reasoning being, "When the patient is unable to make decisions, we always turn to the family."

What's wrong with this picture? Too often, the keening of the grieving family is allowed to divert attention from the wishes of the now-silent patient. One of your most important committee functions is to emphasize that the decisions of capable patients survive the loss of capacity. When a patient with decisional capacity makes an informed and voluntary decision to forgo CPR, the care team makes an implicit promise: "When you are at your most vulnerable and cannot advocate for yourself, we will advocate for you." Patients depend on that promise and, unless we expect them to sit up in the middle of a code and remind us that they have a DNR order, we have an obligation to honor the commitment we have made.

It is, however, difficult to face the grieving family of an arresting patient with the explanation that we are honoring the dying patient's wishes. In addition to the instinctive urge to fix the situation and make the patient better, there is always the concern about angry families responding to what appears to be a deliberate failure to save the patient's life. Your committee can help focus attention on the following:

- Health care professionals are not legally liable when they honor the instructions of capable patients, but they may be liable when they do not. Imposing treatment over the patient's explicit objections may be considered battery, which is actionable.
- When patients engage in discussion about resuscitation and provide informed and voluntary consent to a DNR order, the next questions should be, "Does your family know that you've made this decision? If not, will you tell them or allow us to tell them?" It is not fair to families when they find out about a DNR order as the patient is arresting and the care team appears not to be responding. It should be emphasized that the intent is not to secure family permission—capable patients do not require family ratification of their decisions. This is about letting families know what to expect. Of course, some patients will explicitly forbid alerting their families about their decisions, often to spare themselves the incessant pressure to rescind their decisions, and this should be respected. But it is worth engaging patients in a discussion of the merits of sharing their plans with their families.
- Experienced care professionals can identify family situations likely to be problematic because of dysfunctional dynamics, poor communication, or lack of consensus on goals of care. While it should be understood that the responsibilities of the care team and your committee do not include family therapy, it is important to recognize and plan for situations likely to be problematic. Mr. Gonzalez and his wife, for example, gave fair warning that his appreciation of his impending death and his wishes about end-of-life care were not shared by his wife. Things might have played out differently if, when he arrested, someone had been ready to put an arm around Mrs. Gonzalez and say, "Come sit with me. I know how hard this is for you but, remember, we talked about this being what your husband wanted. We all have an obligation to respect his wishes and our promise to honor them."

GOALS OF CARE AT THE END OF LIFE

Mrs. Diller is an 86-year-old woman admitted from home after suffering her second stroke. Following her last stroke, she recovered some mobility and could enjoy some of her favorite activities, such as Bingo. The attending physician, Dr. Tanner, has discussed the case with the neurologist, Dr. Moon, who thinks that it is still too early to predict the potential for recovery because, when strokes are this deep, patients may take longer to improve. She recommends tissue plasminogen activator (TPA), a complex and potentially dangerous therapy that should be instituted immediately. Based on his prior experience with Mrs. Diller and familiarity with her priorities, however, Dr. Tanner favors a care plan that focuses on comfort.

On this admission, Mrs. Diller was responsive and, although she had great difficulty speaking, she insisted that she did not want to "be like this again." Since then, her level of consciousness has deteriorated and she is largely unresponsive, although her family insists that she squeezes their hands when asked. Dr. Tanner has observed the patient squeezing a hand placed in hers, but believes that this is reflexive rather than a response to command.

Before her initial stroke, Mrs. Diller had appointed one of her daughters, Lila, as her proxy agent. Additional instructions in the proxy document include her wish not to be resuscitated if she has a cardiac arrest and not to receive artificial nutrition and hydration if she has a terminal condition or is in an irreversible coma.

Her family describes her as a very independent woman who would be distressed by her current significantly compromised condition but disagrees about the appropriate care plan. Although Lila feels obligated to honor her mother's expressed wishes, she does not want the responsibility of forgoing life-sustaining treatment. Another daughter notes that Mrs. Diller improved considerably after her last stroke and insists that the same thing could happen this time. The patient's brother argues for the TPA advocated by Dr. Moon, while one granddaughter insists that she would not want to be "tortured" with tubes and machines and should be allowed to die in peace. Another granddaughter pleads that, as long as her grandmother can squeeze her hand, she should be kept alive as long as possible.

Perhaps the single most important question in clinical decision making and the one that is central to any ethics analysis is, "What are the goals of care for this patient?" or "What do we intend to accomplish with our diagnostic and therapeutic efforts?" Identifying the care goals, especially at the end of life, requires professionals, families, and, when possible, patients to clearly articulate what they understand and expect. While the care team understands that the goals of care change as the patient's condition evolves, the patient and family may not appreciate that process. If they are still relying on the goals established three weeks ago, there will be a disconnect that leaves the team referring to the "demanding family" and the family referring to the "unresponsive team." If recovery or substantial improvement is unrealistic in light of a terminal diagnosis and steady deterioration, the goals and plan of care should be revised. If the aim is to relieve suffering and not prolong the dying process, then interventions aimed at cure are inconsistent and serve only to distract from the primary objective.

Regularly reassessing the goals in response to clinical changes permits the care plan to reflect accurately what is both feasible and desirable, especially as death approaches. Critical considerations during this time include the determination that the patient is dying, the initiation or forgoing of particular interventions, and the involvement of additional resources, such as palliative care. As discussed in chapter 10, the relief of pain and suffering is a moral imperative central to the entire clinical interaction, which becomes more prominent at the end of life.

Focusing on the goals of care guards against the risk of resorting to interventions because they are available rather than clinically indicated. The temptation to use everything in the therapeutic arsenal makes it easy to justify this treatment, which triggers that one and then, of course, the one that follows. Rather than asking, "What is the goal of this particular intervention?" the patient is better served by asking, "Where does this intervention fit into the overall plan of care? If it advances the agreed-upon goals, we may appropriately begin or continue it. If not, it is probably not indicated."

Keeping the goals at the center of care planning also permits a wider range of treatment options, which is especially important at the end of life. Interventions should be evaluated in terms of what they can accomplish for the patient rather than categorized according to conventional labels. For example, surgery, radiation, or antibiotics can be appropriately considered for a dying patient when it is clear that the goal is comfort rather than cure.

Clarifying *whose* goals are being considered is a key element in care planning. A frequent source of ethical tension is the presumption of consensus on care goals when, in fact, the patient, family, and care team may not share the same understanding of the clinical picture or possible outcomes. The patient may want to spare his family the pain of seeing him deteriorate and the emotional and financial burden of his care. His children may want him to continue aggressive therapy in hopes of a cure. His wife may want him to come home with the focus on symptom management so that his remaining time can be spent comfortably finishing his work and interacting with his family. His sister may want to protect him from the knowledge that he is dying. His caregivers may feel that he could benefit from a clinical trial of an experimental protocol.

Mrs. Diller's family and care providers find it hard to agree on a plan of care because of their differing perceptions of her condition, prognosis, and wishes, as well as their own notions of what is in her best interest. Dr. Moon and the patient's brother believe that not pursuing aggressive treatment would be giving up prematurely. Dr. Tanner and one granddaughter urge a focus on comfort measures to protect the patient from treatment that would increase and prolong her suffering. As the health care agent, Lila feels bound to honor her mother's expressed preferences, which appear to be forgoing specific life-sustaining treatments. Finally, while differences between physicians' clinical impressions are not uncommon and can be useful in arriving at accurate prognoses, families often find their lack of agreement frustrating.

How the goals of care are articulated and justified will influence the therapeutic and interpersonal dynamics. Inconsistent expectations inevitably lead to descriptions of the family as "unreasonable" or "demanding," and charges that care professionals have not been clear and candid in their explanations or responsive in their treatment. Insufficient attention to what is really being communicated or avoided permits people to mistakenly believe that what they have said has been heard and understood. Your involvement through clinical ethics consultation can be especially helpful when the parties need to clarify the clinical realities, identify the patient's interests and values, and focus on the goals in developing an appropriate end-of-life care plan.

Mr. Giles is a 58-year-old man who has had AIDS for 14 years, apparently the result of a long history of intravenous drug abuse. He has multiple medical problems, including hypertension, asthma, chronic obstructive pulmonary disease (COPD), panic disorder, colitis, stroke, meningitis, and multiple pneumonias, two episodes of which required ventilation. He has been receiving hemodialysis for one year to treat end-stage renal disease. He was admitted from a long-term nursing facility with seizures and changes in mental status. He is nonverbal and only intermittently responsive.

An MRI revealed a brain tumor. Given Mr. Giles's AIDS status, he faces specific risks. Surgery carries a high risk of hemorrhage, which could leave an immediate, severe, and permanent neurologic deficit, such as hemiplegia (one-sided paralysis). Without surgery, his seizures and cognitive changes can be controlled with anticonvulsant medication, but he faces progressive decline in mental status, as well as a slow evolution of hemiparesis (one-sided weakness). Mr. Giles has no family or others involved in his care. Despite encouragement from the nursing facility, he has not completed an advance directive.

An important consideration in setting end-of-life care goals is the quality of the patient's remaining time. For example, it is not uncommon for an intervention to be recommended because it will "improve the quality of life" or for a prognosis to be described in terms of a "poor quality of life." It is worth noting that assessments of quality of life are not *medical* determinations but *value* judgments with implications for what is or is not worth pursuing medically, and clinicians have no special expertise in defining it. Indeed, defining beneficence and best interest ultimately remains the responsibility of the patient and his surrogates, for whom the requested interventions have the most significance. Clinicians have a critical role to play: they can describe the likely range of comfort and function that the patient will experience and help guide the patient's or family's decision making. However, it can be argued that only the patient or those who know him well can assess how those projections will be perceived in terms of the patient's life quality. When, as in Mr. Giles's case, the patient is without capacity, surrogates, or advance directives, the care team has no insight into his values, wishes, or the quality of life he would consider acceptable. In these circumstances clinicians must rely exclusively on a best interest standard to try to assess what plan might benefit the patient.

Setting therapeutic goals should be a fully collaborative effort by the patient or trusted surrogates and the care team, reflecting not only what is possible but also what is desirable. This balance calls for articulation and periodic review of the meaning of success, recognizing the deeply personal nature of quality-of-life assessments. Despite the superiority of professional medical knowledge and skill, the perspective that matters most is that of the patient who will experience the life and death that are achieved.

FORGOING LIFE-SUSTAINING TREATMENT

Mrs. Lewis is a 72-year-old woman with progressive dementia of unknown etiology, progressive renal failure, and hypertension, admitted with an acute gastrointestinal

(GI) bleed. She has been living at home with her daughter and has received care through the family practice group. She has neither a living will nor a health care proxy.

Prior to admission, Mrs. Lewis could use a walker and a bedside commode. She has not been hospitalized recently and generally manages well at home. While her renal failure has been progressive, her current deterioration may be the result of her acute GI bleed and might be reversible, although the renal attending thinks this is unlikely. Her primary care physician favors a trial of dialysis to see if her renal function improves and her mental status clears, but he doubts the utility of chronic dialysis. Mrs. Lewis's acute bleeding has stopped, but she is not eating and the gastroenterologist has placed a temporary nasogastric tube to provide nutrition. He says that, shortly, a more permanent feeding tube will be necessary for continued nourishment. The chief resident describes Mrs. Lewis as "a little old lady curled up in bed who responds only to noxious stimuli and occasionally utters a single word." He is concerned that dialysis and tube feeding will prolong her dying and increase her suffering.

Her daughter is anxious about making decisions without knowing what her mother would want. In particular, she is concerned about eliminating dialysis from consideration without knowing whether it would be effective.

It's a safe guess that much of your ethics committee agenda and consultation requests concern withholding or withdrawing life-sustaining treatment, especially from patients without capacity. Decisions about deferring or permitting death are difficult for clinicians and administrators; they are painful and often paralyzing for those who act on behalf of their loved ones. If abandoned to make these choices alone, the family or other surrogate is likely to feel solely responsible for the outcome. The lingering regret is likely to be, "If only we had insisted on continued treatment, Papa could have had more time with us." Clinicians can help make the process more bearable by sharing the burden of making these hard decisions.

Whether end-of-life care choices are made by capable individuals or surrogates, using a benefit-burden analysis as a template for decision making can provide structure, consistency, and support for patients, families, and staff. Central to this analysis is the overarching goal of providing only care that benefits the patient without needlessly increasing suffering or prolonging the dying process. When the burdens of an intervention or a course of care are shown to outweigh its benefits, the decision to look for alternatives is more easily and comfortably justified.

One useful strategy is to solicit the family's or other surrogate's agreement to a therapeutic trial. A treatment plan with potential benefits is implemented for a specified period of time, after which its effectiveness is evaluated and it is either continued or discontinued. The key is clearly setting out in advance the proposed length of the trial, as well as the goals, limits, and criteria for success. For example, "Let's try three dialysis treatments during the next seven days. If Mrs. Lewis's renal function and mental status improve, we can consider the benefit of further treatments. If she shows no improvement, we'll know that dialysis is ineffective for her and should not be continued." Consensus on the goals and indices of success encourages the trial of appropriate interventions without the fear that, once begun, they cannot be stopped. Therapeutic trials also provide important reassurance that no potentially beneficial treatments have been left untried.

Productive end-of-life decision making depends on clarity and candor. As discussed in chapter 3, offering false choices when there are no real alternatives frustrates patients and families, and diminishes their exercise of genuine autonomy. Asking, "Should we continue your husband's antibiotics?" or "Do you want us to intubate Mama if she is struggling to breathe?" is not helpful if it is clear that these interventions are not clinically indicated. It is more responsible and compassionate to say, "The antibiotics we tried are no longer fighting your husband's infection. Because they're not helping him and may be creating other problems, they should be discontinued," or "Let me tell you why we believe that, if your mother requires intubation, she is unlikely to ever come off the ventilator." These are not quality-of-life-judgments, but clear indications for patients and families of what is medically achievable.

These discussions are never easy, but they can be made less threatening with careful language and reassurance that the patient will not be abandoned. "Withholding" or "withdrawing" treatment sounds as though something necessary is being snatched away. "Forgoing" treatment conveys the sense that the surrogate has more control in the decision-making process, although with greater control comes the responsibility to exercise that control wisely and ethically. When specific interventions will be eliminated or discontinued, the focus should be on those that will be continued or added. While we may "withdraw treatment," we never "withdraw care." It is critical to emphasize that, while the goals of care may change to reflect a greater priority on comfort than cure, the team's commitment to the patient's well-being remains unaltered.

PROTECTING PATIENTS FROM TREATMENT

Decisions about forgoing life-sustaining measures usually arise when death is imminent and continued intervention will not improve the clinical condition but may only contribute to suffering. How these issues are resolved depends greatly on how they are framed. Forgoing treatment can be seen either as *depriving* the patient of needed care or *protecting* the patient from the burden of ineffective or harmful interventions. It is the latter that should be the message. When continued treatment will only prolong dying or increase suffering, it is appropriate to help the patient's loved ones give themselves permission to make hard choices, within applicable state law, that will be in his best interest.

An example is considering artificial nutrition and hydration (ANH) at the end of life when the burdens of the intervention will outweigh the benefits. Research has shown that patients with advanced dementia typically stop eating as the end of life nears because their bodies are shutting down and no longer need the nutrition. For these patients, continued tube feeding often creates considerable discomfort, including bloating, gas, nausea, cramping, and diarrhea (Huang and Ahronheim 2000; Ahronheim 1996). When the dying process cannot be reversed and an intervention imposes only pain or other distress, it can be argued that discontinuing the treatment—even nutrition and hydration—protects the patient from harm and promotes comfort as death nears. Although some commentators regard ANH as particularly significant because of its symbolic connection to normal feeding and nurturing, the emerging consensus is that it is a life-sustaining intervention similar to mechanical ventilation and dialysis, and that like them, it must be subjected to a benefit-burden analysis.

The frustration and despair of those closest to the dying patient are directly related to their feelings of helplessness as his condition deteriorates. No matter what they do, they cannot prevent the inevitable. But, while they cannot determine *whether* he dies, they can influence *how* he dies. Assessing the care plan according to its relative benefits and burdens, they are able to make decisions that shield their loved one from interventions that create more harm than good. At the end of life, the notion of family as protector can be a powerful and comforting one that can and should be reinforced. Your committee can be influential in supporting the reframing of issues at the end of life so that patients, families, and care professionals share a common vision of patient benefit and best interest.

REJECTION OF RECOMMENDED TREATMENT AND REQUESTS TO "DO EVERYTHING"

Mrs. Abrams is a 70-year-old woman who came into the hospital for surgical closure of her colostomy. She had been living independently at home and, on admission, she was interactive and fully capacitated. Her medical history includes emphysema from years of cigarette smoking. The surgery was successful but, shortly thereafter, Mrs. Abrams developed abdominal fistulas that required another operation. She was so weakened by her multiple surgeries that she required ventilatory support. Despite strong initial resistance to intubation, she reluctantly agreed to it after discussion with her pulmonologist.

The following day in the ICU, Mrs. Abrams lets it be known in no uncertain terms that she wants to be extubated. Her surgeon is playing a marginal role in her care and all important medical decisions are being made by her pulmonologist. Mrs. Abrams's three daughters are deeply troubled by their mother's decision to refuse further intubation. The house staff caring for Mrs. Abrams do not know how to proceed or what is legally and ethically appropriate. They believe that removing the vent would mean almost certain death, which they find personally and professionally very disturbing.

When patient or family decisions conflict with physician recommendations, clinical judgment and skill are tested. Patients often reject proposed interventions likely to be beneficial or even life saving. While respect for patient autonomy requires that capacitated care decisions be honored, the refusal of treatment should be the beginning, not the end, of the discussion. As discussed in chapter 3, the professional obligation is to ensure that all consents and refusals are informed, thoroughly considered, and voluntary. Because of their profound implications, refusals of life-sustaining treatment should receive heightened scrutiny. Special attention should be given to the adequacy of the information presented and the quality of the explanation, possible language or cultural barriers to understanding, the patient's capacity and appreciation of the consequences of forgoing treatment, and the voluntariness of the decision.

In addressing Mrs. Abrams's request for extubation, the care team should clarify the length of time ventilatory support is recommended, the anticipated benefits, and the likely outcomes of premature vent removal. Carefully probing her concerns should reveal fears and misconceptions that can be addressed. For example, she may be afraid that she will be permanently dependent on ventilatory support, when, in fact, her doctors anticipate that she should be weaned from the ventilator within a few weeks.

Although Mrs. Abrams's ability to communicate will be hampered by the endotracheal tube, adequate time and effort should be invested in assessing her capacity, her goals for care, her expectations, and the consistency of her wishes. Throughout the process, which may take several days, she should be reassured that her request is being carefully considered, especially in light of its significant consequences. A clinical ethics consultation, including Mrs. Abrams, her daughters, and the care team, can facilitate a clinically, legally, and ethically acceptable resolution. If the patient remains committed to discontinuing ventilatory support, the care plan should focus on promoting her comfort, including measures to minimize air hunger, anxiety, and other symptoms of respiratory distress.

Physicians may also be faced with patient or family instructions to "do everything," including requests for specific interventions judged to be therapeutically inappropriate or otherwise not indicated. The "do everything" request almost always signals desperation—the family or patient desperately want something, they just do not know what it is. At the end of life, family members often feel the need to be good advocates, to ensure that their loved ones are not neglected and that no potentially beneficial treatment is left untried. Unable to enumerate all the interventions that might be effective, they assume that "do everything" covers the therapeutic landscape. Especially when they do not know what to anticipate or how much confidence to place in the care professionals, they may insist on all available therapies in the hope that one of them will be effective.

Is the customer or, in this case, the patient or family always right? The short answer is, of course not. Because there is no obligation to provide treatment just because it is requested and because physicians must be guided by their clinical judgment and professional ethics, they should not comply with requests that fall outside the standard of care. That position, however, is only the beginning of the ethics analysis. Like treatment refusals, insistence on inappropriate treatment should trigger further discussion and clarification.

These requests should be seen as an important signal that the parties to the interaction may not share the same understanding of the patient's condition and prognosis, goals of care, available treatment options, and expected outcomes of the proposed interventions. The first question should be, "What does 'everything' mean to you, and what do you expect to happen if we do it?" This is an opportunity to help the family unpack the bucket of "everything" and recognize that there is less in it than they thought. The focus should be on identifying unrealistic expectations, clarifying the goals of care, the potential for the proposed treatments to achieve those goals, the obligation to prevent suffering without benefit, and further explanation of the recommended plan of care.

MEDICAL FUTILITY

"He never had time to even catch his breath and already it's come to this." Ari was talking about his father, Dr. Dole, a 54-year-old physician who had diagnosed his own pancreatic cancer just 9 weeks ago. He was found to have significant metastases and his condition has deteriorated very rapidly. Now he is in the ICU, intubated and comatose, and his colleagues are finding it increasingly difficult to keep his organ systems from failing. Even with aggressive management, there is reluctant consensus within the medical team that the therapeutic options are running out and nothing further can be done to stem multi-organ failure.

When the critical care team met this morning to discuss Dr. Dole's care, several suggestions were offered for continued and even accelerated interventions. Finally, Dr. Birch said quietly, "Let's face it. This is medically futile."

Judgments about providing or limiting treatment frequently invoke the notion of medical futility. Despite vast literature and vigorous debate, there is still considerable disagreement on how it should be defined. Its narrowest and most useful definition describes the *physiologic impossibility* of an intervention achieving its therapeutic objective. In that strict sense, physicians are excused—even precluded—from burdening patients with treatment that will be clinically ineffective and, therefore, possibly even harmful.

This narrow and value-neutral definition does not apply, however, to the vast majority of cases in which the notion of futility is raised. Far more often, interventions or care plans are labeled "futile" when they are expected to produce a clinical effect that falls below a specified standard. For example, dialysis may successfully assume the function of failing kidneys, but not contribute to returning the patient to an acceptable overall health status. Depending on the long-range clinical goals, the intervention may be considered futile in achieving the desired objective. In addition to the physiologic definition above, suggested definitions have focused on quantitative criteria (e.g., if the intervention has not been effective in the last 100 cases it can be considered futile); benefit (failure of an intervention to provide a benefit to the patient); normative (impossibility of an intervention achieving one or more value-based goals held by the patient, family, or other surrogate decision maker); and obligation-based (providing the intervention would divert resources better spent elsewhere or would violate the professional's integrity) (Schneiderman 2011; Mosely, Silveira, and Goold 2005; Lo 2005; Schneiderman, Jecker, and Jonsen 1990). As some of these definitions suggest, notions of futility may have more to do with what is perceived to be an acceptable quality of life than with actual clinical effectiveness.

Care providers faced with new and often competing pressures may misuse the notion of futility in the service of what they see as their ethical responsibilities to patients, families, and society. Mindful of their conflicting obligations to promote the best interests of patients by providing only beneficial treatments, not raise unrealistic expectations, and provide cost-effective care, physicians may label questionably effective interventions "futile" as a way of withholding them. Futility can also function as the trump card to discourage families from insisting on treatment that care providers consider inappropriate. While some physicians see futility determination as the ethical way to manage end-of-life care, others see it as a way to take control of decisions from demanding families.

Families and patients sometimes request non-beneficial treatments (Brett and McCullough 2012), but labeling inappropriate interventions as "futile" distorts the meaning of the term and obscures the message that should be communicated. The more accurate and accessible approach might be to explain that, regardless of what is done, the patient is dying and what matters is the quality of that dying. Invoking futility as a kind of discussion stopper for end-of-life issues should be replaced with reality checking—clarifying that the patient is dying, reassessing the goals and expectations of care, defining benefit and burden, and identifying ways to promote physical and emotional comfort.

Seen in this light, further efforts to reverse Dr. Dole's clinical course can be considered medically futile because the interventions are not meeting their physiological objectives and he is dying regardless of treatment. Continued cure-oriented measures would not only be ineffective, they would also be counterproductive and, as discussed in chapter 10, the goals of care are now more appropriately palliative than curative. In other cases, discussion might well reveal that, rather than strict futility, decisions for the dying patient concern quality of life and death.

In an effort to create fair, balanced, transparent, and accessible processes for addressing conflicts about treatment requested by the patient or family and considered medically futile by the care team, professional guidelines, ethical frameworks, and discussion suggestions have been offered (Code of Ethics of the American Medical Association 1999; Winkler, Hiddermann, and Marckmann 2012; Brett and McCullough 2012) In addition, many care-providing institutions are developing consensus-based futility policies. These frameworks provide a step-wise process of corroborating the attending physician's finding of medical futility, including other attending physicians, department chairs, and the chief medical officer; review by the ethics committee and the legal department; and offers to transfer the patient's care to another physician or facility willing to provide the requested interventions. Each step is followed by another attempt to reach consensus with the patient or family. When all the steps have been exhausted without achieving consensus, the futile treatments may be refused or discontinued. Some policies offer the family the option of seeking judicial intervention (Schneiderman 2011; Standley and Liang, 2011; Fine 2001). A sample policy, Managing Requests for Treatment Judged to be Medically Futile or Harmful, appears in chapter 17.

Finally, language matters in the clinical setting, certainly in discussions about medical futility. When the collective opinion of the care professionals is that specific interventions are no longer clinically indicated, words that should never be uttered are "We've done all we can" or "We have nothing left to offer," which are the sound of abandonment. We may not have any more treatments intended to cure the patient's disease or effect improvement, but *we always have something left to offer*—comfort, security, companionship, hope for achievable goals. Specific interventions may be futile; patients are never futile.

REFERENCES

Ad Hoc Committee of the Harvard Medical School to Examine the Definition of Brain Death. 1968. A definition of irreversible coma. *Journal of the American Medical Association* 205(6):85–88.

Ahronheim JC. 1996. Nutrition and hydration in the terminal patient. *Clinics in Geriatric Medicine* 12(2):379–91.

Appel JM. 2005. Defining death: When physicians and families differ. *Journal of Medical Ethics* 31:641–42.

Arnold RM. 2002. A rose by any other name. *Journal of Palliative Medicine* 5(6):807–11.

Baumann A, Audibert G, Lafaye G, Puybasset L, Mertes PM, Claudot F. 2013. Elective non-therapeutic intensive care and the four principles of medical ethics. *Journal of Medical Ethics* 39:139–42.

Berger JT. 2008. Surrogate decision making: Ethical theory and clinical practice. *Annals of Internal Medicine* 149:48–53.

Blustein J. 1999. Choosing for others as continuing a life story: The problem of personal identity revisited. *Journal of Law, Medicine & Ethics* 27(1):20–31.

Bomba P. 2011. Landmark legislation in New York affirms benefits of a two-step approach to advance care planning including MOLST: A model of shared, informed medical decision-making and honoring patient preferences for care at the end of life. *Widener Law Review* 17(475):475–500.

Brett AS, McCullough LB. 2012. Addressing requests by patients for nonbeneficial interventions. *Journal of the American Medical Association* 307(2):149–50.

Brock DW. 1991. Surrogate decision making for incompetent adults: An ethical framework. *Mount Sinai Journal of Medicine* 58(5):388–92.

Brock DW. 1997. Death and dying. In Veatch RM, ed. *Medical Ethics*. 2nd ed. Sudbury, MA: Jones and Barlett Publishers, pp. 363–94.

Brody H, Campbell ML, Faber-Langendoen K, Ogle KS. 1997. Withdrawing intensive life-sustaining treatment—recommendations for compassionate clinical management. *New England Journal of Medicine* 336(9):652–57.

Byock I. 1997. *Dying Well: Peace and Possibilities at the End of Life*. New York: Riverhead Books.

Christakis NA, Iwashyna TJ. 1998. Attitude and self-reported practice regarding prognostication in a national sample of internists. *Archives of Internal Medicine* 158(21):2389–95.

Code of Ethics of the American Medical Association, 2.037 Medical Futility in End-of-Life Care. 1999. *Journal of the American Medical Association* 281:937–41.

Cook R, Pan P, Silverman R, Soltys SM. 2010. Do-not-resuscitate orders in suicidal patients: Clinical, ethical, and legal dilemmas. *Psychosomatics* 51(4):277–82.

Cranford RE. 1995. The persistent vegetative state: The medical reality (getting the facts straight). In Arras JD, Steinbock B, eds. *Ethical Issues in Modern Medicine*. 4th ed. Mountain View, CA: Mayfield Publishing Co., pp. 172–77.

Cruzan v. Director, Missouri Department of Health, 497 U.S. 261 (1990).

Davis JK. 2008. Futility, conscientious refusal, and who gets to decide. *Journal of Medicine and Philosophy* 33:356–73.

Dresser R. 2010. Suicide attempts and treatment refusals. *Hastings Center Report* 40(3):10–11.

Dresser RS, Robertson JA. 1989. Quality of life and non-treatment decisions for incompetent patients: A critique of the orthodox approach. *Journal of Law, Medicine & Health Care* 17(3):234–44.

Dubler NN, Post LF, Barnes B. 1999. Making health care decisions for others: A guide to being a health care proxy or surrogate. New York: Montefiore Medical Center.

Dworkin R. 1993. *Life's Dominion: An Argument About Abortion, Euthanasia, and Individual Freedom.* New York: Alfred A. Knopf.

Evans HM. 2005. Reply to: Defining death: When physicians and families differ. *Journal of Medical Ethics* 31:642–44.

Fine RL. 2001. The Texas Advance Directives Act of 1999: Politics and reality. *HEC Forum* 13(1):59–81.

Fins JJ. 2005. Rethinking disorders of consciousness: New research and its implications. *Hastings Center Report* 35(2):22–24.

Fins JJ, Miller FG, Acres CA, Bacchetta MF, Huzzard LL, Rapkin BD. 1999. End-of-life decision-making in the hospital: Current practice and future prospects. *Journal of Pain and Symptom Management* 17(1):6–15.

Fisher GS, Tulsky JA, Rose MR, Siminoff LA, Arnold RM. 1998. Patient knowledge and physician predictions of treatment preferences after discussion of advance directives. *Journal of General Internal Medicine* 13(7):447–54.

Fromme EK, Zive D, Schmidt TA, Olszewski E, Toll SW. 2012. POLST Registry, do-not-resuscitate orders and other patient treatment preferences. *Journal of the American Medical Association* 307(1):34–35.

Geppert C. 2011. Saving life or respecting autonomy: The ethical dilemma of DNR orders in patients who attempt suicide. *Internet Journal of Law, Healthcare and Ethics* 7(1), http://ispub.com/IJLHE/7/1/11437 (accessed August 2014).

Gillick MR. 2000. Rethinking the role of tube feeding in patients with advanced dementia. *New England Journal of Medicine* 342(3):206–10.

Harrington SE, Smith TJ. 2008. The role of chemotherapy at the end of life: "When is enough, enough?" *Journal of the American Medical Association* 299(22):2667–78.

Helft PR, Siegler M, Lantos J. 2000. The rise and fall of the futility movement. *New England Journal of Medicine* 343(4):293–96.

Huang ZB, Ahronheim JC. 2000. Nutrition and hydration in terminally ill patients: An update. *Clinics in Geriatric Medicine* 16(2):313–25.

In re Quinlan, 355 A.2d 647 (N.J. 1976).

Kagawa-Singer M, Blackhall LJ. 2001. Negotiating cross-cultural issues at the end of life: "You've got to go where he lives." *Journal of the American Medical Association* 286(23):2992–3001.

Kalkut G, Dubler NN. 2005. The line between life and death. *The New York Times*, May 10, p. A17.

Khushf G. 2010. A matter of respect: A defense of the dead donor rule and of a "whole-brain" criterion for determination of death. *Journal of Medicine and Philosophy* 35:330–64.

Lo B. 2005. Palliative sedation in dying patients: "We turn to it when everything else hasn't worked." *Journal of the American Medical Association* 294(14):1810–16.

Loertscher L, Reed DA, Bannon MP, Mueller PS. 2010. Cardiopulmonary resuscitation and do-not-resuscitate orders: A guide for clinicians. *American Journal of Medicine* 123(1):4–9.

Loewy EH. 1998. Ethical considerations in executing and implementing advance directives. *Archives of Internal Medicine* 158(4):321–24.

Luce JM. 1995. Physicians do not have a responsibility to provide futile or unreasonable care if a patient or family insists. *Critical Care Medicine* 23(4):760–66.

Lynn J, Teno J, Dresser R, Brock D, Nelson HL, Nelson JL, Kielstein R, Fukuchi Y, Lu D, Itakura H. 1999. Dementia and advance-care planning: Perspectives from three countries on ethics and epidemiology. *Journal of Clinical Ethics* 10(4):271–85.

Meisel A, Snyder L, Quill T. 2000. Seven legal barriers to end-of-life care: Myths, realities, and grains of truth. *Journal of the American Medical Association* 284(19): 2495–501.

Mezey MD, Cassel CK, Bottrell MM, Hyer K, Howe JL, Fulmer TT, eds. 2002. *Ethical Patient Care: A Casebook for Geriatric Health Care Teams*. Baltimore: Johns Hopkins University Press.

Mezey M, Dubler NN, Mitty E, Brody ΛΛ. 2002. What impact do setting and transitions have on the quality of life at the end of life and the quality of the dying process? *The Gerontologist* 42(Special issue III):54–67.

Miller FG, Truog RD, Brock DW. 2010. Moral fictions and medical ethics. *Bioethics* 24(9):453–60.

Morrison RS, Olson E, Mertz KR, Meier DE. 1995. The inaccessibility of advance directives on transfer from ambulatory to acute care settings. *Journal of the American Medical Association* 274(6):478–82.

Moseley KL, Silveira MJ, Goold SD. 2005. Futility in evolution. *Clinics in Geriatric Medicine* 21:211–22.

Nair-Collins M. 2010. Death, brain death, and the limits of science: Why the whole-brain concept of death is flawed public policy. *Journal of Law, Medicine & Ethics* 38(3):667–83.

Nair-Collins M. 2013. Brain death, paternalism, and the language of "death." *Kennedy Institute of Ethics Journal* 23(1):53–104.

Orentlicher D. 2001. *Matters of Life and Death: Making Moral Theory Work in Medical Ethics and the Law*. Princeton, NJ: Princeton University Press.

Post LF. 1999. Decisions to permit death: Whose interests should determine the outcome? *Geriatric Care Management Journal* 9(4):16–23.

Post LF. 2006. Living wills and durable powers of attorney. In Schulz R, Noelker LS, Rockwood K, Sprott RL, eds. *The Encyclopedia of Aging*. 4th ed. New York: Springer Publishing Company, vol. 2:668–71.

Post LF, Blustein J, Dubler NN. 1999. The doctor-proxy relationship: An untapped resource. *Journal of Law, Medicine & Ethics* 27(1):5–12.

Prendergast TJ. 2001. Advance care planning: Pitfalls, progress, promise. *Critical Care Medicine* 29(2) *Supplement* N34–39.

President's Commission for the Study of Ethical Problems in Medicine and Biomedical and Behavioral Research. 1981. *Defining Death: A Report on the Medical, Legal and Ethical Issues in the Determination of Death*. Washington, DC: U.S. Government Printing Office.

Quill TE. 2000. Initiating end-of-life discussions with seriously ill patients: Addressing the elephant in the room. *Journal of the American Medical Association* 284(19):2502–7.

Rhoden NK. 2003. The limits of legal objectivity. In Steinbock B, Arras JD, London AJ, eds. *Ethical Issues in Modern Medicine*. 6th ed. Boston: McGraw-Hill, pp. 368–75.

Sade RM. 2011. Brain death, cardiac death, and the dead donor rule. *Journal of the South Carolina Medical Association* 107(4):146–49.

Schneidermann LJ. 2011. Defining medical futility and improving medical care. *Bioethical Inquiry* 8:123–31.

Schneiderman LJ, Jecker, N, Jonsen A. 1990. Medical futility: Its meaning and ethical implications. *Annals of Internal Medicine* 112:949–54.

Silveira MJ, DiPiero A, Gerrity MS, Feudtner C. 2000. Patients' knowledge of options at the end of life: Ignorance in the face of death. *Journal of the American Medical Association* 284(19):2483–88.

Singer PA, et al. 2001. Hospital policy on appropriate use of life-sustaining treatment. *Critical Care Medicine* 29(1):187–91.

Sprung CL, Eidelman LA, Steinberg A. 1995. Is the physician's duty to the individual patient or to society? *Critical Care Medicine* 23(4):618–20.

Standley C, Liang BA. 2011. Addressing inappropriate care provision at the end-of-life: A policy proposal for hospitals. *Michigan State University Journal of Law and Medicine* 15:137–76.

Steinhauser KE, Christakis NA, Clipp EC, McNeilly M, McIntyre L, Tulsky JA. 2000. Factors considered important at the end of life by patients, family, physicians, and other care providers. *Journal of the American Medical Association* 284(19):2476–82.

Sudore RL, Fried TR. 2010. Redefining the "planning" in advance care planning: Preparing for end-of-life decision making. *Annals of Internal Medicine* 153(4):256–61.

The SUPPORT Principal Investigators. 1995. A controlled trial to improve care for seriously ill hospitalized patients: The Study to Understand Prognoses and Preferences for Outcomes and Risks of Treatments (SUPPORT). *Journal of the American Medical Association* 274(20):1591–98.

Teno JM, Stevens M, Spernak S, Lynn J. 1998. Role of written advance directives in decision making: Insights from qualitative and quantitative data. *Journal of General Internal Medicine* 13(7):439–46.

Terry PB, Vettese M, Song J, Foreman J, Haller KB, Miller DJ, Stallings R, Sulmasy DP. 1999. End-of-life decision making: When patients and surrogates disagree. *Journal of Clinical Ethics* 10(4):286–93.

Torke AM, et al. 2008. Rethinking the ethical framework for surrogate decision making: A qualitative study of physicians. *Journal of Clinical Ethics* 19(2):110–19.

Truog RD. 1997. Is it time to abandon brain death? *Hastings Center Report* 27(1):29–37.

Truog RD. 2007. Brain death—too flawed to endure, too ingrained to abandon. *Journal of Law, Medicine & Ethics* 35(2):273–81.

Truog RD, Frader JE, Brett AS. 1992. The problem with futility. *New England Journal of Medicine* 326(23):1560–64.

Wicclair MR. 2001. Medical futility: A conceptual and ethical analysis. In Mappes TA, DeGrazia D, eds. *Biomedical Ethics*. 5th ed. New York: McGraw-Hill, pp. 340–50.

Wilkinson D, Savulescu J. 2012. Should we allow organ donation euthanasia? Alternatives for maximizing the number and quality of organs for transplantation. *Bioethics* 26(1):32–48.

Winkler EC, Hiddemann W, Marckmann G. 2012. Evaluating a patient's request for life-prolonging treatment: An ethical framework. *Journal of Medical Ethics* 38:647–51.

Wissow LS, Belote A, Kramer W, Compton-Phillips A, Kritzler R, Weiner JP. 2004. Promoting advance directives among elderly primary care patients. *Journal of General Internal Medicine* 19(9):944–51.

Zeleznik J, Post LF, Mulvihill M, Jacobs LG, Burton WB, Dubler NN. 1999. The doctor-proxy relationship: Perception and communication. *Journal of Law, Medicine & Ethics* 27(1):13–19.

CHAPTER 10

Palliation

FROM CARING TO CURING AND BACK AGAIN

Providing comfort, especially at the end of life, is neither a new concept nor a departure from the traditional responsibilities of the caring professions. Until the middle of the twentieth century, the cure of disease and the prevention of death were largely beyond the capability of those who ministered to the sick by trying to relieve their pain. With the development of biotechnology, the obligation to provide *care* became the obligation to provide *cure*, where cure often meant prolonging life, and a focus on comfort was reserved for those times when "nothing more could be done." Rather than an inevitability, death was often perceived as a failure of skill and the very notion of dying made professionals feel uncomfortable, even guilty. Increasingly sophisticated science and technology inflated both professional and lay expectations about the power of medicine. The resulting belief that cure is always possible led to a perceived requirement to "do everything" and a sense of defeat whenever patients did not recover or improve.

Beginning in 1974, palliative care was initially delivered in the United States through community-based hospices. As efforts to promote comfort and relieve suffering came to be seen as coexisting with cure-oriented care rather than being reserved for dying patients, palliative care services for inpatients were added to hospitals during the past decade and are now offered in almost two-thirds of U.S. hospitals. In a 138% increase since 2000, consultative palliative care services are provided in 63% of hospitals with more than 50 beds. Palliative care clinics now offer services for outpatients and, more recently, community-based palliative care (CPC) has been proposed to complete the outreach by providing services to patients at home, in residential care-providing facilities, in rehabilitation centers, and in transition across care settings. Regardless of location, these services span the illness trajectory, including management of acute and chronic symptoms (Kamal et al. 2013).

Palliative care as a discipline has successfully reintroduced the notion that relieving pain and suffering is central to the complete and authentic practice of medicine. Its defining philosophy is that cure and comfort are consistent objectives that may assume greater or lesser prominence, depending on the patient's condition, prognosis, and values. Critical to its full appreciation and optimal application is the recognition that palliative care is not synonymous with end-of-life care or a prelude to hospice, but an essential part of the entire therapeutic continuum. Symptom management is *always* an integral element of care.

The therapeutic enterprise seeks a balance of curative and palliative care that responds to the patient's changing condition. When the potential exists for significant improvement, the plan of care emphasizes aggressive curative interventions, supplemented by comfort measures. As the likelihood of remission fades and the patient approaches the end of life, the goal of care shifts and aggressive palliation becomes the primary focus. Perhaps the clearest explanation is the now-iconic diagram (see figure), which illustrates the coexistence of disease-modifying (curative) treatment and palliative care throughout the entire therapeutic continuum, and the gradual shift in emphasis as the clinical condition evolves and the end of life nears.

This transition, which occurs over time rather than at a given moment, depends on attention to the evolving medical status; the clinical effectiveness of specific interventions; and the wishes and values of the patient, family, and others who are authorized to make decisions on the patient's behalf. Helping patients, families, and professionals to adjust their goals and make decisions in ways that are clinically sound and ethically defensible is an important contribution of the ethics committee.

One effort to clarify the palliative approach suggests changing the terminology from palliative *care* to palliative *treatment* as a way to emphasize its importance and efficacy. "Because an intervention with proven benefit is generally referred to as a treatment, and because there is clear evidence that palliative measures are effective in reducing suffering, these interventions qualify as treatments. Labeling evidence-based, goal-directed interventions that ameliorate suffering as treatment is important so that physicians and patients alike may view such treatment as important, effective, and based on good science" (Kon and Ablin 2010, p. 644).

Reproduced with permission from the EPEC Project. Emanuel LL, von Gunten CF, Ferris FD, Hauser JM, eds. The Education in Palliative and End-of-life Care (EPEC) Curriculum. © EPEC Project, 2003.

Mrs. Heller has been a resident of a long-term care facility for many years, during which her chronic obstructive pulmonary disease, diabetes, and osteoarthritis have become more severe. She is now confined to a wheelchair because of the intense pain in her back and hips, which she often describes as excruciating. The mild analgesics, including Tylenol, that have been prescribed do not bring relief and she has become increasingly immobilized, withdrawn, and depressed.

When her nephew, Dr. Agin, visited recently, he was alarmed by the deterioration he saw in his aunt. The person he remembered as vibrant and active was now saying, "I have no life. All I have is pain." When he asked what she would like to be able to do that the pain prevented, he expected her to talk about missing her hiking, gardening, and painting. Instead, she replied, "Sleep. I don't remember the last time I was able to sleep without being awakened by pain."

Dr. Agin has requested a meeting to discuss his aunt's pain management.

THE EXPERIENCE OF AND RESPONSE TO PAIN
Pain

Despite its subjective quality, the experience of pain is very real and can be consuming. As one writer describes it,

> Pain is dehumanizing. The severer the pain, the more it overshadows the patient's intelligence. All she or he can think about is pain: there is no past pain-free memory, no pain-free future, only the pain-filled present. Pain destroys autonomy: the patient is afraid to make the slightest movement. All choices are focused on either relieving the present pain or preventing greater future pain, and for this, one will sell one's soul. Pain is humiliating: it destroys all sense of self-esteem accompanied by feelings of helplessness in the grip of pain, dependency on drugs, and being a burden to others. In its extreme, pain destroys the soul itself and all will to live. (Lisson 1987, p. 654)

Whatever the clinical setting, medical condition, or technological sophistication, one caregiver mandate remains constant and compelling—the relief of pain. Even when cure is impossible, the duty of care includes palliation. Moreover, this obligation is central to the therapeutic interaction, unquestioned and universal, transcending time and cultural boundaries. Whether the source of the pain is physiological or psychological, its relief is considered a primary moral goal of medicine because of the unique and intimate connection between those who hurt and those who comfort.

Pain and Suffering

A related distinction has been made between pain and suffering. Dr. Eric Cassell (1982) has written about pain as a physiological response of the body and suffering as an existential assault on the person. He describes how one can experience pain without suffering when the goal is a noble or joyous one, using as an example the pain of childbirth. Conversely, a person can suffer without physical pain when he feels the disintegration of his personhood and his sense of control. When pain and suffering *are* closely related, Cassell claims, it is because the patient perceives the pain as overwhelming, uncontrollable, or unending. Emotional isolation may be added by the suggestion that the pain is only imagined. Pain of this kind represents suffering that is a threat, not only to life but also to the integrity of the patient's sense of self.

It is impossible to spend any time in a clinical setting without recognizing this distinction. Patients are often asked to endure pain in the pursuit of a cure or remission. In weighing the benefits and burdens of a proposed treatment, current discomfort for clear and likely future relief seems ethically appropriate. The calculus is different when the intervention will impose pain or suffering with no benefit. Likewise, suffering without pain is evident in the patient with aphasia that prevents him from communicating with his family, the trained athlete who can no longer care for her most basic physical needs, the father who must accept that his infant will never develop, and the artist trying to create faster than her eyesight is failing.

Responses to Pain

Mr. Peters is a 27-year-old African American man with sickle cell anemia, admitted to the ED in sickle cell crisis. He is experiencing severe pain in his thighs, arms, hands, and feet. He is also dehydrated and anemic. An emergency medicine resident orders an injection of Demerol for pain and admits him to the hospital.

Following admission, Mr. Peters continues to complain of pain and asks the nurses repeatedly about the medication that has been ordered for him. During morning rounds the following day, the medical team is impressed by how much he knows about his disease and its management. He reports that, most of the time, he is able to manage his pain with an anti-inflammatory drug, such as Motrin. During a sickle cell crisis, however, the only effective pain relief is achieved with intravenous morphine, and he specifies the dosages and schedules that have been successful. He says that, during past hospitalizations, self-administering the morphine with a patient-controlled analgesia (PCA) pump has allowed him to achieve a constant blood level of medication, with supplementary morphine as needed for breakthrough pain.

The attending tells Mr. Peters that Demerol will be available when he requests it to control his pain. She also asks where and from whom he usually receives care, and Mr. Peters names several hospitals where he has been treated during crises. During post-rounds discussion, several residents express concern about the patient's detailed request for a particular opioid in specific dosages. They suggest that this may be drug-seeking behavior by an addict. One resident recounts a similar case during his internship, concluding, "That patient conned us for two days before we caught on. When we cut off her drugs, she left the hospital."

Nothing should be more self-evident than the clinical and ethical imperative to relieve pain. Yet, pain is a complex phenomenon for both patients and care providers in several important ways. First, pain is solitary, experienced only by the patient. Unlike other indications of illness or injury, clinicians rely heavily on patients' first-person descriptions of their pain, although corroborative objective signs accessible to others may also be present. This reliance on patient assessment of symptoms makes the evaluation and treatment of pain significantly different from other patient-physician interactions.

Second, although universally acknowledged, the experience and understanding of pain is influenced as much by personal values and cultural traditions as by physiological injury and disease. If the perception of and response to pain are to be understood in a useful way, they should be examined in the context of culture, gender, power, morality, and myth. These factors are especially important in the health care setting, where pain becomes an interpersonal encounter between the sufferer and the reliever. How pain is experienced and expressed by the patient and how it is understood and responded to by the provider are influenced by these factors and largely determine how it is valued and, ultimately, how it is treated (Brennan, Carr, and Cousins 2007).

Both patient and clinician attitudes are affected by their respective personal and cultural values. For example, physicians' clinical judgments about and responses to pain are influenced by group-based factors, including age, gender, race, ethnicity, and physical appearance. The balance of power between provider and patient is yet another theme in the pain management interaction. So long as therapeutic control is vested in the caregiver, the patient remains the passive victim of pain, a supplicant in the standard p.r.n. (as circumstances require) regimen that requires the patient to ask for medication each time it is needed (Post et al. 1996).

Third, both patients and their doctors are influenced by their understanding—often misunderstanding—of pain and the agents for its relief. Studies have shown that physicians are inhibited by their inadequate professional education about analgesia, misconceptions about opioids and addiction, and fears about regulatory and legal liability. Similar misconceptions are shared by the lay public, and Americans have been shown to reject what they believe to be effective medicinal pain relief because they fear over-reliance and addiction. Reluctance to provide sufficient pain medication has also been related to clinician fears that use of opioids will "kill patients" by depressing respirations and hastening death. These fears, plus concerns about legal liability and suspicions that patient requests for pain medication are a cover for drug-seeking behavior, are reflected in the stringent laws regulating drug prescription. The unsurprising and unacceptable result is the routine under-medication of even terminally ill patients (e.g., Fine 2007; Furrow 2001; Post et al. 1996).

Mr. Peters's case illustrates several of these issues. He comes to the ED requesting morphine, a potent opioid, and specifying the dosages and intervals that he would prefer. The care team has no prior experience with him and no way of confirming his history of sickle cell or its prior management. Mindful that morphine's effects are euphoric as well as analgesic, and also potentially addictive, the team believes that it must consider the possibility that he is a drug seeker rather than simply a patient in pain. While no explicit mention has been made of his race, it may influence some team members' perception about the likelihood that he abuses drugs. Even if he had not requested an opioid, by specifying dosages and intervals, Mr. Peters may have seemed "demanding" or "bossy" to some caregivers, who prefer to be in control of the clinical interaction. Individually or in combination, these factors may result in his claims of pain and requests for relief to be discounted.

Patients who appear to exhibit drug-seeking behaviors trigger an intense and, usually, counterproductive dynamic. On one level are the care team's explicit efforts to determine what the patient needs and what therapy will be most effective. On another level, caregivers often react to patient requests for pain medication with resistance, disbelief, and anger. The inchoate reaction is, "This guy's looking for drugs and he's trying to scam me. Well, I'm on to him and I'm not going to let him get away with his con on my watch." Left unacknowledged, the result can be an exercise in power playing, disrespect, and erosion of trust. Your ethics committee can help caregivers recognize the implications of their understandable but unhelpful response, and replace it with a more informed and professional approach.

When dealing with patients in pain, especially pain that is chronic or intermittently intense, it is important for caregivers to understand the nature of the discomfort, its effects, and useful ways to respond to it. Assuming that Mr. Peters suffers from periodic sickle cell crises, it is reasonable that he is very familiar with the medications, dosages, and schedules that most effectively treat his pain. Unless and until he demonstrates that his description of symptoms is inaccurate or that he has another motive for his requests, the primary clinical goal should be to relieve his pain as quickly and completely as possible. Collaborating with him in this endeavor has the added benefit of helping him to regain some control over a situation that may well make him feel repeatedly helpless.

Mr. Charles is a 32-year-old man with end-stage AIDS. He is wasted and noncommunicative, but responsive to painful stimuli. His rapid breathing, sweating, and restlessness indicate that he is experiencing considerable discomfort. His attending, Dr. Fellows, has written a standing order for Tylenol to be given every four hours, with Demerol to be given "if the patient appears especially uncomfortable."

When Mr. Charles's sister, a nurse, arrives from another state, she is appalled by her brother's condition. She discusses his pain management with Dr. Fellows and asks why he is not receiving constant intravenous morphine. Dr. Fellows replies, "Morphine will depress his respirations and may speed up his dying. I will not be responsible for contributing to his death. We can keep him comfortable by increasing his other medication." She responds, "He's dying now and nothing will change that! Why should he have to die this horribly?"

A critical distinction supporting adequate palliation, especially at the end of life, is the doctrine of double effect, which responds to the ethical tension between the obligations to promote patient well-being and to avoid inflicting harm. The doctrine holds that a single act having two foreseen effects, one good and one bad, is not morally or legally prohibited *if the harmful effect is not intended*. The doctrine requires that three conditions be met: the act itself is not wrong; the good effect is the direct result of the intentional act, not the result of the bad or harmful effect; and the benefits of the good effect outweigh the foreseen but unintended bad effect. All three conditions are essential to prevent the doctrine from being abused or perverted in an effort to justify actions intended to cause harm.

The doctrine of double effect recognizes that, while the administration of sufficient opioids to manage pain at the end of life risks depressing respirations enough to hasten death—although the risk is generally small with careful management of the administration of pain medication—the clinical and ethical mandate to relieve suffering is paramount. Mr. Charles may not be verbally asking for analgesia, but he gives every clinical indication (rapid shallow breathing, rapid pulse, elevated blood pressure, perspiration, grimacing) that he is in terrible pain. As his sister points out, he is actively and irreversibly dying, so the question is not *whether* he will die, but *how*. His death is not preventable, but dying in pain is. Under these circumstances, the only thing that can be done to benefit him is to relieve his suffering and make his remaining time more bearable. Using the rationale of the doctrine of double effect, the palliative intervention is both justified and protected. Helping physicians appreciate this distinction so that they can confidently and comfortably provide adequate palliation at the end of life is often an important part of ethics committee involvement.

THE MORAL IMPERATIVE TO RELIEVE PAIN

Carla is a 9-year-old girl who was diagnosed several months ago with Ewing's sarcoma. She has received radiation and chemotherapy, and was recently hospitalized for amputation of her entire left leg. Following surgery, Carla's pain was being successfully managed with a continuous IV morphine drip supplemented by patient-controlled IV morphine to be used when she felt she needed additional pain control. On the third postoperative day, one of her physical therapists told her that she should not activate the patient-controlled morphine until the pain became unbearable because, if she overused narcotics, she would become addicted. An intern who overheard this statement corrected the physical therapist, explaining that addiction is not associated with use of opioids in the immediate postoperative period and is rarely the result of even chronic use to control severe pain. He emphasized using the term *opioids* rather than *narcotics*, and reassured Carla, telling her that she should activate the morphine as often as she needed it and that she would not be risking addiction.

Carla's parents, however, became very concerned about the potential danger of addiction and tried to discourage her from using the patient-controlled morphine. When she continued to use the medication, they insisted that her oncologist, Dr. Brader, stop both the continuous IV drip and the patient-controlled morphine. Dr. Brader replaced the morphine with non-opioid analgesia, which was much less effective, and Carla began to experience severe pain. Dr. Brader has recommended restarting the morphine to relieve Carla's pain, but her parents are adamant that she not receive any opioid medication, which they insist on referring to as "narcotics."

Do the obligations of care professionals include the relief of pain? Does pain management require the informed consent of a capable patient or an authorized surrogate? Can the conflict between Carla's doctor and her parents be resolved in a way that prevents her from suffering?

More than a professional obligation, the relief of pain has traditionally been considered a moral imperative. It is also an endeavor that reflects the tension between the two fundamental ethical principles of autonomy and beneficence. As discussed in chapter 3, the notion of autonomy is expressed in the health care setting in the doctrine of informed consent. Under this doctrine, capable, knowledgeable, and voluntary consent, either by or for the patient, is required for legally and ethically valid authorization for most diagnostic and therapeutic interventions.

Yet, the requirement of informed consent is conspicuously absent from the relief of pain. The reason goes to the very core of the caring interaction and invokes the mandate to relieve pain and suffering. This imperative is so powerful that it gives rise to the presumption that, unless patients explicitly object, they would want their pain relieved. In that circumstance, respect for autonomy requires that a capable patient's decision to refuse analgesia—either because she finds the experience of pain meaningful or she does not want to chemically compromise her awareness—must be honored.

As discussed in chapters 2 and 3, however, beneficence is elevated over autonomy in protecting and benefiting patients who are vulnerable because they cannot make decisions or advocate for themselves. Thus, an incapacitated patient who is clearly in pain must not be deprived of relief because she is unable to provide informed consent. While honoring the wishes of a capable individual shows respect for the person, withholding relief from one who cannot decide or communicate would be an indefensible abandonment. It would also be indefensible not to provide pain relief simply because a family member finds it objectionable. Rather, principled and compassionate caring embraces both the respect for and the protection of persons. No explicit informed consent is required precisely because relieving pain is central to the very notion of healing and, for that reason alone, it requires no additional justifications.

Accordingly, adequate relief of Carla's pain may not be impeded by her parents' well-meaning but misguided rejection of morphine, including the repeated use of the term *narcotic* to equate the medication with illicit drug use. Every effort should be made to help them understand the considerable benefits and minimal risks of opioid use in managing her severe pain, and the distinction between increasing tolerance and addiction. Including the palliative care service in this discussion would be helpful in educating and reassuring her parents about the care plan. The care team should be supportive of their desire to be responsible guardians and the focus should be on the shared goal of promoting Carla's best interest and protecting her from harm. Ultimately, however, her parents must know that, with or without their consent, Carla's pain will be managed according to the standard of care and the ethical requirements of professional practice.

Here too, language matters. While *opioids* and *narcotics* are often used interchangeably, their impact is powerful, which is why the terms should be distinguished. Both opioids and narcotics are a class of drugs derived from opium that have potent analgesic and mood-altering effects. *Narcotics*, however, are persistently associated, especially in the lay community, with illicit, recreational, and risky drug use. This negative association has been reported as a barrier to patient and family acceptance of appropriate analgesia. In contrast, the connotation of the term *opioids* is that of therapeutic, safe medication approved by the medical community and included in standard of care. Pain specialists are increasingly encouraging all caregivers, as well as professional journals and lay media, to use the more accurate and neutral term *opioids* when referring to this class of medication (Wallace et al. 2012; Quinn and Miller 2008).

An important contribution of your ethics committee is ensuring that the care team appreciates that symptom management does not require surrogate consent. Rather than requesting permission, the approach should be, "Let me assure you that everything possible will be done to promote Carla's comfort. We will begin with a low dose of medication and increase it only until it is effective."

Mrs. Heller, the nursing home resident with multiple medical problems, is experiencing pain severe and persistent enough to interfere with her activities and her sleep. Despite her best efforts, pain has become the focus of her attention and has profoundly impaired her quality of life. Far from rejecting pain medication, she is clearly asking for relief. Her care team has both a clinical and an ethical mandate to assess her pain carefully; discuss with her the benefits, burdens, and risks of the analgesic options; and provide her with sufficient medication to relieve her suffering. The team should also identify and address the barriers to adequate pain relief that have prevented her symptoms from being recognized and managed appropriately.

If, as appears happened here, the care plan is still not adequately managing Mrs. Heller's pain, additional resources should be involved. The nursing staff should ensure that her primary care physician (PCP) is aware of her continuing discomfort. If the PCP appears reluctant to modify the analgesic regimen, the nursing home medical director should be enlisted to speak with him. In addition, an ethics consultation requested by the care team or, as here, the family, can be critical in highlighting Mrs. Heller's needs and goals, emphasizing the moral and legal imperative of pain relief, and reassuring the care team, including the treating physicians, that the benefits of palliation outweigh any possible risks.

ASSISTED AND PERMITTED DYING

The lab results of Diane's blood tests confirmed Dr. Timothy Quill's worst fears—she did have leukemia. His distress reflected the disappointment common to physicians whose patients contract life-threatening illnesses, as well as the special concern he had for someone who had been his patient for many years and with whom he had developed a close and trusting relationship. In addition, he greatly admired the resilience and determination with which she had overcome significant physical and emotional difficulties. In the process, she had strengthened her relationships with her husband, son, and friends, and reinvigorated her business and artistic work.

Now they faced this devastating news together, going through the confirmatory tests and discussing with her husband the various options, including chemotherapy, followed by radiation and possible bone marrow transplants. Even with the most aggressive treatment regimen, the chances for long-term survival were 25%; the certain outcome of no treatment was death within a few months. After considerable discussion, Diane decided not to undergo chemotherapy because she was convinced that the quality of whatever time she had left was more important than the unlikely benefits of treatment. Despite Dr. Quill's misgivings and her family's attempts to persuade her to change her mind, she remained steadfast in her determination to make the most of her time at home. Ultimately, her family and physician reluctantly supported her decision.

Dr. Quill had known throughout their relationship that, for Diane, regaining and maintaining control of her life was a central value. Now he realized that being in control of her dying was just as important to her as she faced the end of her life. She became preoccupied with deteriorating, lingering, being helpless and in pain. Her anxiety about the prospect of a protracted death became so severe that it threatened to undermine the quality end of life she had as her goal. She asked Dr. Quill to help her avoid the painful, debilitating, and dehumanizing ravages in store by providing drugs that she could take to end her life when she chose. She was convinced that having the ability to control her death would give her the dignity and peace of mind that she needed.

After extensive discussion and psychiatric consultation, Dr. Quill acceded to Diane's unwavering determination, prescribed the barbiturates, and provided the information necessary for her to take her own life. She was able to spend the next several months focusing on the people, relationships, and activities that were most important to her. She received aggressive palliative treatment but, eventually, she determined that the benefits of life no longer outweighed its burdens. Her death was on her own terms, at the time and in the manner of her choosing. Yet, concerns about potential legal liability prevented her from having her family or physician with her at the end, and she died alone. When Dr. Quill writes or speaks about this episode, he invariably says that not being with his patient as she died is his only regret (Quill 1991).

Distinguishing Forgoing Life-Sustaining Treatment, Euthanasia, and Assisted Dying

Discussions about end-of-life issues inevitably refer to behaviors that promote, permit, or hasten death. Because these concepts are highly charged with medical, legal, ethical, and emotional significance, it is critical that we begin by distinguishing their definitions.

- *Aid in dying* (AID) or *assisted dying** is clinician facilitation of a patient's death by providing the means and information (prescription, medication, instructions) that enable the patient to perform an act that results in self-inflicted death. The clinician's actions are taken with the knowledge that the patient

---

* Until recently and in the first edition of *Handbook for Health Care Ethics Committees*, the practice of a terminally ill patient self-administering physician-prescribed medication to achieve a peaceful death was referred to as "physician-assisted suicide (PAS)" or "assisted suicide (AS)." Language matters, however, and the highly charged and pejorative connotations of "suicide" have increasingly been distinguished from and replaced by the more neutral and accurate "dying," based on the following reasoning: "Terminology is evolving because of an understanding in both the mental health field and in the legislation and case law of many states that a mentally competent, terminally ill patient bases a decision to end his or her life for fundamentally different reasons than a clinically depressed person uses to justify suicide" (personal letter from Kathryn L. Tucker, director of Legal Affairs, Compassion & Choices). Accordingly, this edition of the handbook adopts the more accurate terms "aid in dying (AID)" or "assisted dying."

intends to use the provided drugs and information to end her life, but the agent of death is the *patient*. Aid in dying is legal in five states (Oregon, Washington, Montana, Vermont, and New Mexico), which have adopted formal, multi-step protocols with safeguards for its limited use. The legal climate appears to be changing, however, as more states are considering legalizing AID (Orentlicher, Pope, and Rich 2014).

- *Euthanasia* is clinician administration of a lethal agent with the intent of relieving the patient's untreatable suffering or pain. Whether the act is performed at the request of the patient (*voluntary euthanasia*) or without the patient's request (*nonvoluntary or passive euthanasia*), the agent of death is the *clinician*. Euthanasia of either kind is illegal in all 50 states and the District of Columbia and all other countries, except the Netherlands, Belgium, and Luxembourg (Siegel, Sisti, and Caplan 2014; Menzel, Steinbock, and Summer 2013).

- *Forgoing life-sustaining treatment* is the withholding or withdrawing of interventions that maintain one or more organ system functions necessary to keep the patient alive. When these interventions are discontinued, the patient's death is considered to be the result of the *underlying disease(s)*. Patients with decisional capacity, health care proxy agents, and, in some states, other surrogates acting on behalf of patients without capacity have the well-settled legal and moral right to refuse unwanted life-sustaining treatments. Even when that refusal leads to or hastens death, the action is not considered suicide, assisted dying, or euthanasia.

- *Aggressive palliation* is the provision of therapeutic interventions, including opioid medications, to relieve pain and manage other symptoms effectively, throughout the therapeutic continuum and, especially, at the end of life. While these interventions may have two possible effects, one positive (e.g., pain relief) and one negative (e.g., depression of respirations), when the intent is palliation, the action is considered medically, ethically, and legally justified under the doctrine of double effect. Therefore, although aggressive palliation at the end of life may hasten the patient's death, the action is not considered suicide, assisted dying, or euthanasia.

It is worth noting that even the U.S. Supreme Court went out of its way in 1997 to articulate that patients at the end of life have a protected liberty interest in pain relief and are entitled to sufficient analgesia *even if it hastens death*. In June 1997, the Court ruled in two cases, *Washington v. Glucksberg* and *Vacco v. Quill*, which sought to turn the right to refuse treatment into a constitutionally protected right to assisted death. (The cases are discussed in part IV.) These two rulings are more significant for what they say about palliative care than about assisted death. Repeatedly, the Court reaffirms the doctrine of double effect, saying that it is both legally and ethically appropriate to give terminally ill patients as much medication as necessary to relieve pain, recognizes the unintended potential for hastened death, and explicitly distinguishes between forgoing life-sustaining treatment and assisted dying. The critical take-away message is that providing sufficient medication to manage pain effectively at the end of life is a clinical and ethical imperative, not to be confused with assisted death or euthanasia. The importance of these rulings to compassionate end-of-life care cannot be overstated.

Ethical Issues

It is beyond the scope of this handbook to discuss adequately the multiple and complex aspects of aid in dying. For our purposes, it is enough to raise some of the ethical issues, including caregiver obligations, individual autonomy, public policy, and the moral imperative to relieve suffering. Some argue that respecting patient autonomy includes respecting the wish of the terminally ill to control when and how death occurs. Consistent with the principle of nonmaleficence, however, the concept of facilitating patient death is counterintuitive to those who devote themselves to promoting and protecting life. Yet, many have come to see assisting the rational decision of a capable person to effect a peaceful death as the last act in a compassionate continuum of care and forcing the patient to take that final step alone as abandonment. Some suggest that, in vulnerable and disempowered populations, such as the poor and elderly, the right to die may become the obligation to die as a way of relieving family or society of the unwanted burden of their care (e.g., Hardwig 1997). Yet these and similar worries about permitting withdrawal of life-sustaining measures have not been borne out by experience. Moreover, others argue that these same marginalized populations, which often lack access to health care and providers, may be deprived of the opportunity to end their suffering under physician care. Ultimately, there is concern that the individual, morally justified act of aid in dying could become the generalized policy of euthanasia (e.g., Emanuel 2012; Prokopetz and Lehmann 2012; Shalowitz and Emanuel 2004; Bascom and Tolle 2002; Emanuel, Fairclough, and Emanuel 2000; Salem 1999; Thomasma 1996).

While assisted death is not a legal option in 45 states and the District of Columbia, it highlights issues that demand attention in all care settings. Both the public and professionals are troubled by the reality of overtreated disease and undertreated pain, especially at the end of life. Considerable research demonstrates that the medical profession does an inadequate job of pain management and that many people who request assistance in ending their lives are actually asking for the assurance of pain relief. It is a matter of concern when the debate centers on the alleged moral right of terminally ill patients to receive physician assistance in *ending* rather than *easing* their lives.

Among health care's most pressing challenges, then, is introducing and improving palliation along the entire therapeutic continuum, especially as death approaches. Encouraging clinicians to collaborate with palliative care specialists can be a valuable contribution of clinical ethics consultation. In particular, your ethics service can help care teams to distinguish cases that are appropriate for ethics consultation, those that require palliative care expertise, and those that will benefit from involvement of both services. Consider, for example, the following requests for clinical ethics consultation:

- Mr. Cowan, a 78-year-old man, is admitted with altered mental status and delirium, which are considered potentially reversible with psychotropic medication. His son has agreed to the care plan but his daughter has been refusing medications and a recommended peripherally inserted central catheter (PICC) line, and threatening to sign the patient out against medical advice (AMA).

- Mrs. Epstein is an 84-year-old woman admitted with fever, hepatic abscesses, and advanced acute myelogenous leukemia (AML). According to the treating oncologists, she is no longer a candidate for chemotherapy. Her husband and daughter are unable to appreciate the gravity and irreversibility of her condition, and are insisting on continued aggressive, cure-oriented measures that are increasing her suffering.
- Samuel is a neonate, born at 30 weeks' gestation with a rare, lethal syndrome that includes skin blistering, skin absence, and pyloric atresia. Life expectancy for afflicted children is typically five to six months. The parents are struggling with a decision about surgically repairing the intestinal atresia and taking Samuel home for whatever time remains or instituting a comfort care plan and allowing him to die.

The case of Mr. Cowan is appropriate for a clinical ethics consult because it raises ethical issues related to identifying the most appropriate surrogate decision maker and setting boundaries for family members to prevent interference with the delivery of care and protect a vulnerable patient from harm. Mrs. Epstein's case is appropriately referred to the palliative care service because it requires the assessment of medical needs, symptom management, and goals and plan of care. Samuel's case can benefit from both ethics and palliative care consultation to help the parents and care team sort out the medical, surgical, and palliative options, and analyze the ethical imperatives of the options. Although there is often no sharp distinction between when ethics intervention and when palliative care involvement are appropriate, assisting care teams in identifying and requesting consults that will be most effective in each case is one of your ethics service's most valuable contributions.

PEDIATRIC PALLIATIVE CARE

Eric is a 16-year-old boy who has undergone a second bone marrow transplant for sickle cell disease, after rejecting his first transplant. His second post-transplant course has been complicated by septic shock and coding, post-transplant lymphoproliferative disorder (a type of secondary cancer), prolonged intubation requiring tracheostomy and a gastrostomy tube, amputation of several fingers, peripheral neuropathy, pain, and depression/anxiety. On this admission, Eric's pulmonary status is deteriorating, despite aggressive antimicrobials and extensive respiratory support.

These complications, as well as the very poor prognosis, have been discussed at length with Eric's mother. Because the treating doctors concur that, if Eric were intubated, it would not be possible to subsequently extubate him, the decision has been made not to intubate him if he goes into respiratory failure. This difficult decision has not been explained to Eric because of the concern shared by his mother and the treating team that it may exacerbate his anxiety. The goals of the comfort care plan are to manage Eric's pain with continuous opioids, which may also help his breathing and manage the attendant anxiety.

Eric's case illustrates several factors unique to pediatric palliative care. Most adults who receive palliative care have typical and predictable trajectories that allow for more realistic goal setting. In contrast, because of their resilience combined with the rarity of their diseases, children frequently have very unpredictable medical courses. A child may be, literally, "one in a million," leaving care teams and families without similar cases as precedents or FDA-recommended medications known to have been effective. This prognostic uncertainty may be among the most difficult challenges with which practitioners and parents grapple as they try to chart a therapeutic course that neither overlooks potentially effective therapies nor subjects the patient to unnecessary, nonbeneficial treatment in an effort to "do everything" or, at least, "do something." Here, pediatric palliative care can play an invaluable role in guiding parents and, in many cases, patients in focusing on quality of life and revising their goals to those that are achievable.

Children are not small adults. Capable adults are routinely engaged in determining the goals and plan of care, following disclosure of the diagnosis and likely prognosis, the benefits, burdens, and risks of the treatment options, and the alternatives. As a result, patients are accorded not simply the courtesy of involvement, but the basic dignity and control that accompanies self-determination about what happens to one's body and one's future. As noted in chapter 5, children are presumed to lack the capacity to make autonomous decisions because they have not yet developed the maturity, judgment, and ability to take a long view and recognize that the unexpected may still be manageable. With parents/guardians as primary decision makers for minors, care planning is a delicate balance of parental hopes, fears and anticipatory grief, and the wisdom of involving the patient to the extent possible, while considering the effect of decisions on the patient's siblings and extended family.

As discussed in chapter 4, withholding information is an imperfect enterprise at best. Even when families insist that the patient does not know, does not want to know, or would be harmed by the information, there is no guarantee that the information can be successfully withheld. The greater likelihood is that patients sense when things are being kept from them and inevitably imagine something far worse than the actual situation. The erosion of trust, the anxiety, insecurity, and isolation are as true and damaging for children as for adults. "If my parents and caregivers can't even talk to me about whatever's going on, it must be really awful and I have no one to tell how scared I am." While not every minor is eager to or capable of receiving certain information, the ethical imperative is to determine what each patient knows and wants to know. Because minors' cognitive and emotional capacities are so variable, this ongoing assessment is especially important. Whenever possible, children deserve to know what to expect in terms they can handle. Eric, at 16 and having had more than his share of experience with illness, is likely wondering about his future and how his care will be managed. His mother, in collaboration with the pediatric palliative care service, can help him know that he is not alone with his concerns.

Finally, in addition to caring for sick children, pediatric palliative care cares for parents during some of the worst times of their lives. When, because of illness or injury, parents are unable to meet their most central responsibility of protecting their children from harm, it can be unbearable for them and painful for those around them. Their anguish can be lessened by reframing their decision making in terms of protecting their child. Discussions with the parents of a dying child about forgoing curative treatment, especially at the end of life—surely the most counterintuitive interactions imaginable—can be made tolerable by helping parents see themselves as protecting their child from the burden of interventions that cause suffering or prolong dying without compensating benefit. Helping parents regain their role as protectors is among the most important things that pediatric palliative care offers, especially as the end of life nears.

Pediatric palliative care serves to balance many of the core ethical issues—relief of suffering, best interest, quality of life, truth telling and disclosure, parental autonomy and permission, pediatric assent, futility and hope, access to care and resource allocation—in the setting of non-autonomous patients and the people who care for and about them.

PALLIATIVE CARE AND HOSPICE

Mr. Choi is an 82-year-old man with end-stage colon cancer. According to his son and daughter, he had not disclosed his symptoms to avoid being a burden to his family. By the time his illness was recognized, the cancer was widely metastasized and the consulting physicians agreed that he was not a candidate for surgery, radiation, or chemotherapy. After several meetings, during which the son and daughter translated for their Korean-speaking father, the family, the care team, and, presumably, the patient agreed on a care plan that focuses exclusively on comfort. Given Mr. Choi's repeated request to return home, a meeting was scheduled with the hospice coordinator and a Korean interpreter to discuss home hospice.

Just before the meeting began, the patient's children took the coordinator aside to say, "Our father does not know that his cancer is untreatable or that he will be receiving hospice care. He thinks he is going home to get stronger so he can have treatment. All he knows about hospice is that it is for dying people. If he knew he were on hospice, if he even heard the word 'hospice,' he would give up all hope and just stop living. We want to make whatever time he has left comfortable and meaningful, and we need your help to make that happen."

Hospice, either at home or in a dedicated inpatient facility, remains the model for providing palliative services to patients approaching the end of life. While symptom management and palliative care services can and should be integrated into the entire illness trajectory, hospice services are focused exclusively on a subset of terminally ill patients[†] for whom the goal of cure has been replaced with the goal of maximizing comfort, minimizing suffering, and preventing prolongation of the dying process. There is a common misconception that invasive treatments, such as various types of surgery, are precluded by hospice. As long as these procedures are designed to keep patients comfortable and relieve pain and suffering, they promote and do not frustrate the aim of hospice.

Although the moral imperative to provide comfort has always been central to caregiving, a constellation of developments over the past several decades has brought

[†] The criterion most often referenced is the Medicare hospice benefit, which reserves eligibility for terminally ill patients expected to live six months or less "if the disease runs its normal course" (Kamal et al. 2013, p. 255).

to public attention the need for and benefits of high-quality, specialized, inter-disciplinary care for terminally ill patients and their families.[‡] The result is that providers of inpatient or home hospice services have become a ubiquitous and essential health care resource. Yet, for many this is an emotionally charged concept and, often, patients or their families respond to the suggestion of hospice with, "Is it really that hopeless?" Mr. Choi is a good example of a patient whose family wants to protect him by not disclosing the truth about his condition or the care he will be receiving. This well-intended but unsustainable deception is one of the issues that frequently comes before hospice ethics committees.

As noted in chapter 1, hospices often have their own ethics committee or share access to a regional ethics committee. In addition to the issues typically addressed by all health care ethics committees, hospice ethics committees have special strengths and face unique challenges. The strengths include the self-selected membership, which includes clinicians and other members of the interdisciplinary team who are experienced and skilled in the care of dying patients. Likewise, the bedside care-giving team tends to have a more intimate relationship with patients and families than in the acute care setting. Hospice patients are cared for either in their own homes or in an inpatient unit devoted to end-of-life care.

Challenges for hospice ethics committees include geography-related issues for home hospice staff, such as finding a mutually convenient meeting time and place or the awkwardness of asking family to leave the room to protect patient confiden-tiality. The rather brief length of stay for hospice patients (median 18.7 days nation-ally) (National Hospice and Palliative Care Organization 2013) means that ethical issues that might benefit from clinical consultation may not be recognized in time to be addressed. While there is a growing body of literature on hospital ethics com-mittees and the dilemmas they routinely address, there has been far less written on the ethical issues confronting hospice patients, families, and clinicians, and vir-tually nothing specifically for hospice ethics committees. This dearth of material for reference and guidance will begin to be filled by *Hospice Ethics* (Kirk and Jennings 2014), but the field deserves more educational and practice resources (private correspondence with Timothy Kirk, co-chair Visiting Nurse Service of New York Hospice Ethics Committee).

[‡] When she founded St. Christopher's Hospice in London in 1967, Dame Cicely Saunders identified three core elements in end-of-life care—pain and symptom relief, preservation of patient dignity, and attention to psychological and spiritual suffering as death approaches—which remain the bedrock of hospice care. *On Death and Dying*, a ground-breaking book by Dr. Elisabeth Kübler-Ross (1969), described the five emotional stages experienced by dying patients. A series of legislative provisions by the U.S. Congress, especially the creation of the Medicare hospice benefit in 1982, reflected the growing societal consensus that the hospice resource was a necessary part of comprehensive health care. The 1995 SUPPORT (Study to Understand Prognosis and Preferences for Outcomes and Risks of Treatment) concluded that 50% of dying patients had unrelieved severe pain; 20% of family members experienced financial devastation when they left their jobs to care for a dying relative; and 30–40% of fam-ily caregivers lost most of their savings. A 2004 study of end-of-life care in home and institu-tional settings as assessed by bereaved family members revealed a significant deficit of atten-tion to pain management, physician-patient communication, and respect for patients (National Hospice Foundation 2011; Cassin 2007).

Joyce died in her apartment, two months after she voluntarily stopped eating and drinking. She was 31 at the time of her death and had been quadriplegic since breaking her neck in a diving accident 6 years previously. Initially after the accident, Joyce tried to resume her life, continuing her career as a musician by learning to use mouth-operated electronic equipment and advocating for stem cell research and the needs of the paralyzed. She was convinced that her strong will would sustain her until she was cured.

Gradually, however, Joyce began to realize that a cure for her paralysis was not on the horizon and that her increasing physical and psychological suffering was not temporary. She developed decubiti and autonomic dysreflexia, which caused her body to overreact to pain she could not consciously feel. Even more difficult was the loss of independence and privacy, especially the embarrassment of having others manage her personal needs. She spoke of "living in a body that is no longer mine."

Eventually, Joyce began researching her options for legally ending a life she considered intolerable. She consulted attorneys and physicians, read articles in journals and online, and had two psychological evaluations. When she asked the opinion of her home hospice nurse, Geri gently reminded her that assistance in dying was not something that hospice could provide.

Joyce finally decided to stop eating and drinking. Recognizing the extent of her physical and psychological suffering, her mother and her close friends understood and supported her decision (case adapted from Braun 2012). Geri, however, was deeply conflicted about her role. Her empathy for her patient and her obligation to provide comfort seemed to conflict with her obligation to protect her patient and the prohibition against assisted dying. Geri requested a consultation with the hospice ethics committee.

Voluntarily stopping eating and drinking (VSED) is a situation in which "a patient who is otherwise physically capable of taking nourishment makes an active decision to discontinue all oral intake and then is 'allowed to die' gradually, primarily of dehydration or some intervening complication" (Quill, Lo, and Brock 1997, p. 2099). Because this action is considered to fall within the well-settled right of capable patients to refuse any unwanted interventions, including life-sustaining measures, VSED is a legal option in all states and the District of Columbia. The ethics are somewhat more complicated because of the competing moral imperatives. The care professional's obligation to respect the autonomy of a capable patient by honoring decisions based on personal values and preferences is in tension with the obligation to protect the patient from harm. Refusing to provide supportive care to a patient who has decided on VSED, however, would violate a fundamental moral obligation not to abandon a suffering patient.

The hospice ethics committee had addressed these issues one year earlier after learning about a hospice patient in another state who elected to forgo nutrition and hydration. "How would we manage that situation if one of our patients chose that course?" the committee chair asked. "Shouldn't we think this through and have an agreed-to policy and procedure ready?" Over the next several months, the ethics committee deliberated about VSED and the unique role of hospice in caring for patients considering that option. Discussions included patient rights, caregiver responsibilities, determination of patient best interest and harm, the potential abuses inherent in VSED, and the unique role of hospice. The consensus of the committee, reflected in the policy and procedure it drafted, addressed the following:

- The core ethical principle of respect for autonomy that grounds the right of capable patients to accept or refuse any treatment is as central to hospice care as any other health care setting. Accordingly, decision making in hospice defers to the capable patient's assessment of the benefit-risk-burden ratio when considering therapies. When a capable patient has determined that the harm is continued suffering and the benefit is release from suffering through death, VSED is an ethically and legally acceptable option. The only risk is that, if not managed carefully, the dying process may be unnecessarily burdensome if it is protracted and uncomfortable.

- Because VSED is legal, unregulated, and able to be accomplished without the involvement of care professionals, the following potential abuses may go unrecognized: uninformed or coerced decisions to VSED, especially if the patient is concerned about being a continued burden; coercion to continue the process even if the patient requests nourishment and fluid; without professional support, inadequate palliation of symptoms; unrecognized treatable depression; and lack of support if "starving" is considered morally repugnant.
- The mission of hospice is to maximize the quality of life for patients with life-limiting illnesses by maximizing physical and emotional comfort, minimizing suffering by omitting measures that have no palliative value, and enhancing the dignity and self-determination of patients by honoring their preferences whenever possible.

When Geri requested an ethics consultation to address Joyce's decision and her own concerns, the committee was well prepared to consider the issues. The consensus was that, with appropriate safeguards against potential abuses, Joyce's right to refuse nutrition and hydration should be honored and that the moral obligation of hospice to comfort and not abandon a patient justified Geri providing supportive measures during Joyce's dying. The distinction between providing comfort and support, on the one hand, and actively assisting in a patient's death on the other, was crucial in reframing Geri's perspective and helping her to see her services as an extension of the traditional hospice role. A sample hospice policy, Responding to a Patient's Desire to Voluntarily Stop Eating and Drinking, appears in part IV.

PALLIATIVE CARE: GIVING UP OR GIVING PERMISSION

While the shift in goals from cure to comfort is a process rather than a sudden decision, there comes a time when the care team, family, and often the patient need to acknowledge that palliation is now the focus of care. Recognizing and accepting this reality is unlike other care decisions because of the profound implications for everything that follows. For many people, reliance on palliative care is accompanied by a sense of loss and defeat. The expectation of cure, sometimes even the goal of improvement, must be relinquished. Belief in the power of medicine is exchanged for frustration and lingering doubts about whether all possible options have been explored. The common but unfortunate distinction between "aggressive" and "comfort" care reinforces the notion that palliation represents a lesser level of attention and commitment while waiting for death. The unintended but clear message is, "We have given up and you should too."

The perception can and should be reframed, and this can be one of your ethics consultation service's most important contributions. Rather than abandoning hope, the focus on palliative care can be seen as liberating the patient, family, and care team from increasingly counterproductive efforts to reverse the inexorably deteriorating clinical course. With the investment of time and skill, those who care for and about the patient can give themselves permission to focus on an aggressive palliative care plan that will enhance the quality of the life that remains. Indeed, as recognized by many hospice programs, the therapeutic options can be expanded. Precisely because palliation remains on the care continuum after cure is no longer the goal, it may encompass particular comfort measures posing risks to life, including higher doses of more potent medication that might not have been acceptable when cure was still the goal of care. Rather than "Death is approaching and it must be resisted as long as possible," the message becomes "Life is continuing and its quality must be enhanced as much as possible" (Post 2007, p. 221). Hope is never extinguished; rather, the objects of hope can change and revised goals can be achievable. Among the unique skills that characterize palliative care practitioners and the ethics committees that support them is the ability to help patients, families, and clinicians envision a different, more comfortable, more hopeful ending to their story.

REFERENCES

Alpers A, Lo B. 1999. The Supreme Court addresses physician-assisted suicide. *Archives of Family Medicine* 8:200–205.

American Board of Internal Medicine. Committee on Evaluation of Clinical Competence. 1996. *Caring for the Dying: Identification and Promotion of Physician Competency*. Philadelphia: American Board of Internal Medicine.

Bascom PB, Tolle SW. 2002. Responding to requests for physician-assisted suicide: "These are uncharted waters for both of us . . ." *Journal of the American Medical Association* 288(1):91–98.

Blackhall LJ, Frank G, Murphy ST, Michel V, Palmer JM, Azen SP. 1999. Ethnicity and attitudes towards life sustaining technology. *Social Science & Medicine* 48(12):1779–89.

Braun B. 2012. For Freehold woman, paralyzed life became too much to bear. *The Star Ledger*, February 14.

Brennan F, Carr DB, Cousins M. 2007. Pain management: A fundamental human right. *Anesthesia and Analgesia* 105(1):205–21.

Brock DW. 1997. Death and dying. In Veatch RM, ed. *Medical Ethics*. 2nd ed. Sudbury, MA: Jones and Barlett Publishers, pp. 363–94.

Cassel CK, Vladeck BC. 1996. ICD-9 code for palliative or terminal care. *New England Journal of Medicine* 335(16):1232–34.

Cassell EJ. 1982. The nature of suffering and the goals of medicine. *New England Journal of Medicine* 306(11):639–45.

Cassin C. 2007. Hospice care. In Blank AE, O'Mahoney S, and Selwyn A, eds. *Choices in Palliative Care: Issues in Health Care Delivery*. New York: Springer, pp. 45–61.

Davies B, Sehring SA, Partridge JC, Cooper BA, Hughes A, Philp JC, Amidi-Nouri A, Kramer RF. 2008. Barriers to palliative care for children: Perceptions of pediatric health care providers. *Pediatrics* 121(2):282–88.

Dresser R. 2010. Suicide attempts and treatment refusals. *Hastings Center Report* 40(3):10–11.

Dworkin R. 2003. Assisted suicide: The philosophers' brief. In Steinbock B, Arras JD, London AJ, eds. *Ethical Issues in Modern Medicine*. 6th ed. Boston: McGraw-Hill, pp. 382–85.

Dworkin R, Nagel T, Nozick R, Rawls J, Scanlon T, Thomson JJ. 2003. The philosophers' brief. In Steinbock B, Arras JD, London AJ, eds. *Ethical Issues in Modern Medicine*. 6th ed. Boston: McGraw-Hill, pp. 386–94.

Emanuel EJ. 2012. Four myths about doctor-assisted suicide. *The New York Times Opinionator*, October 27.

Emanuel EJ, Fairclough DL, Emanuel LL. 2000. Attitudes and desires related to euthanasia and physician-assisted suicide among terminally ill patients and their caregivers. *Journal of the American Medical Association* 284(19):2460–68.

Emanuel LL. 1998. Facing requests for physician-assisted suicide: Toward a practical and principled clinical skill set. *Journal of the American Medical Association* 280(7):643–47.

Feudtner C, Friebert S, Jewell J. 2013. Policy statement: Pediatric palliative care and hospice care: Commitments, guidelines, and recommendations. *Pediatrics* 132(5):966–72.

Fine RL. 2007. Ethical and practical issues with opioids in life-limiting illness. *Proceedings (Baylor University Medical Center)* 20(1):5–12.

Fischberg D, Meier DE. 2004. Palliative care in hospitals. *Clinics in Geriatric Medicine* 20(4):735–51.

Furrow BR. 2001. Pain management and provider liability: No more excuses. *Journal of Law, Medicine & Ethics* 29(1):28–51.

Hardwig J. 1997. Is there a duty to die? *Hastings Center Report* 27(2):34–42.

Hyman CS. 1996. Pain management and disciplinary action: How state medical boards can remove barriers to effective treatment. *Journal of Law, Medicine & Ethics* 24(4):338–43.

Johnson JA. 2004. Withdrawal of medically administered nutrition and hydration: The role of benefits and burdens, and of parents and ethics committees. *Journal of Clinical Ethics* 15(3):307–11.

Johnson SH. 1996. Disciplinary actions and pain relief: Analysis of the pain relief act. *Journal of Law, Medicine & Ethics* 24(4):319–27.

Joranson DE, Gilson AM. 1996. Improving pain management through policy making and education for *medical* regulators. *Journal of Law, Medicine & Ethics* 24(4):344–47.

Kamal AH, Currow DC, Ritchie CS, Bull J, Abernethy AP. 2013. Community-based palliative care: The natural evolution for palliative care delivery in the US. *Journal of Pain and Symptom Management* 46(2):254–64.

Kirk TW, Jennings B. 2014. *Hospice Ethics*. New York: Oxford University Press.

Kon AA, Ablin AR. 2010. Palliative treatment: Redefining interventions to treat suffering near the end of life. *Journal of Palliative Medicine* 13(6):643–46.

Kübler-Ross E. 1969. *On Death and Dying*. New York: Simon and Schuster.

Lisson EL 1987. Ethical issues related to pain control. *Nursing Clinics of North America* 22:649–59.

Lo B. 2000. *Resolving Ethical Dilemmas: A Guide for Clinicians*. 2nd ed. Philadelphia: Lippincott Williams & Wilkins.

Lopez SR. 1989. Patient variable biases in clinical judgment: Conceptual overview and methodological considerations. *Psychological Bulletin* 106(2):184–203.

Mangione MP, Crowley-Matoka M. 2008. Improving pain management communication: How patients understand the terms "opioid" and "narcotic." *Journal of General Internal Medicine* 23(9):1336–38.

Menzel PT, Steinbock B. 2013. Advance directives, dementia, and physician-assisted death. *Journal of Law, Medicine & Ethics* 41(2):484–500.

Miller FG, Fins JJ, Snyder L. 2000. Assisted suicide compared with refusal of treatment: A valid distinction? *Annals of Internal Medicine* 132:470–75.

Morrison RS, Meier DE, Cassel CK. 1996. When too much is too little. *New England Journal of Medicine* 335(23):1755–59.

National Hospice and Palliative Care Organization. 2013. NHPCO's Facts and Figures: Hospice Care in America, www.nhpco.org/sites/default/files/public/Statistics_Research/2013_Facts_Figures.pdf (accessed August 2014).

National Hospice Foundation. 2011. National Hospice Foundation & FHSSA: 2011 Annual Report, http://nationalhospicefoundation.org/files/public/2011_NHF_Annual_Report.pdf (accessed August 2014).

Orentlicher D, Pope TM, Rich BA. 2014. The changing legal climate for physician aid in dying. *Journal of the American Medical Association* 311(19):1961–62.

Pereira J. 2011. Legalizing euthanasia or assisted suicide: The illusion of safeguards and controls. *Current Oncology* 18(2):e38–e45.

Post LF. 2007. Ethics and the delivery of palliative care. In O'Mahony S, Blank AE, eds. *Choices in Palliative Care.* New York: Kluwer Academic / Plenum Publishers.

Post LF, Blustein J, Gordon E, Dubler NN. 1996. Pain: Ethics, culture and informed consent to relief. *Journal of Law, Medicine & Ethics* 24(4):348–59.

Post LF, Dubler NN. 1997. Palliative care: A bioethical definition, principles and clinical guidelines. *Bioethics Forum* 13(3):17–24.

Prokopetz JJZ, Lehmann LS. 2012. Redefining physicians' role in assisted dying. *New England Journal of Medicine* 367(2):97–99.

Quill TE. 1991. Death and dignity: A case of individualized decision making. *New England Journal of Medicine* 324(10):691–94.

Quill TE, Lo B, Brock DW. 1997. Palliative options of last resort: A comparison of *voluntarily* stopping eating and drinking, terminal sedation, physician-assisted suicide, and voluntary active euthanasia. *Journal of the American Medical Association* 278(23):2099–2104.

Quill TE, Meier DE. 2006. The big chill: Inserting the DEA into end-of-life care. *New England Journal of Medicine* 354(1):1–3.

Quinn TE, Miller K. 2008. Opioid, opiate, narcotic? *Yale Cares: News & Notes on Supportive Care, Symptom Management, and Care at the End of Life* 2(12):1–2, www.yalecancercenter.org/research/education/471_90466_YaleCares_December2008.pdf (accessed August 2014).

Salem T. 1999. Physician-assisted suicide: Promoting autonomy—or medicalizing suicide? *Hastings Center Report* 29(3):30–36.

Shalowitz D, Emanuel E. 2004. Euthanasia and physician-assisted suicide: Implications for physicians. *Journal of Clinical Ethics* 15(3):232–36.

Siegel AM, Sisti DA, Caplan AL. 2014. Pediatric euthanasia in Belgium: Disturbing developments. *Journal of the American Medical Association* 311(19):1963–64.

Steinbock B, Arras JD, London AJ. 2003. Moral reasoning in the medical context. In Steinbock B, Arras JD, London AJ, eds. *Ethical Issues in Modern Medicine.* 6th ed. Boston: McGraw-Hill, pp. 1–41.

The SUPPORT Principal Investigators. 1995. A controlled trial to improve care for seriously ill hospitalized patients. The Study to Understand Prognoses and Preferences for Outcomes and Risks of Treatments (SUPPORT). *Journal of the American Medical Association* 274(20):1591–98.

Thomasma DC. 1996. When physicians choose to participate in the death of their patients: Ethics and physician-assisted suicide. *Journal of Law, Medicine & Ethics* 24(3):183–97.

Vacco v. Quill, 521 U.S. 793 (1997).

Wallace LS, Keenum AJ, AbdurRaqeeb O, Miser WF, Wexlwe RK. 2012. Terminology matters: Patient understanding of "opioids" and "narcotics." *Pain Practice* 69(14):1184–86.

Washington v. Glucksberg, 521 U.S. 702 (1997).

Weissman DE, Block SD, Blank L, Cain J, Cassem N, Danoff D, Foley K, Meier D, Schyve P, Theige D, Wheeler HB. 1999. Recommendations for incorporating palliative care education into the acute care hospital setting. *Academic Medicine* 74(8):871–77.

CHAPTER 11

Justice, Health, and Access to Health Care

Mrs. Gomez is an undocumented person from Colombia. Since coming to this country in 1976, she has been employed as a housekeeper. Because she has no health care coverage, she has received all of her care in the emergency rooms of various local hospitals.

Last week Mrs. Gomez came to General Medical Center quite ill and was admitted to the medical unit, where she was found to be in kidney failure. She was begun on dialysis and remained in the hospital for three days, until she had been dialyzed twice. When she was ready for discharge, the medical resident in charge of her care inquired whether she would be eligible for Medicare support for her future dialysis under the end-stage renal disease program. He was told that, although Mrs. Gomez's inpatient costs might be covered by Medicaid—something that still needed to be determined—she was clearly not eligible for Medicare.

The medical resident, not to be defeated in his pursuit of care for his patient, asked the ER staff what is usually done when a patient in kidney failure who needs dialysis comes to the ER. He was told that, under an arrangement between the ER and the dialysis unit, these patients are transferred directly to the unit for emergency dialysis treatment. The medical resident told Mrs. Gomez to come to the ER three times a week so she could have the dialysis she needs. When this plan was discovered, the director of the ER exploded and said that this could break the budget for his service. He also pointed out that a nearby city hospital with a dialysis unit is designed to take care of poor people with no insurance.

If the topics of this chapter, justice and access to health care, seem abstract and unrelated to your committee's function, you may want to reconsider. As the case of Mrs. Gomez illustrates, clinical decision making and the therapeutic relationship do not exist in a social vacuum. They are affected in myriad ways, directly and indirectly, by the laws and public policies that determine the availability of health care services and access to health care. These laws and policies, on the local, state, and federal levels, provide the context within which health care providers work, influencing and constraining what they can do on behalf of their patients. In a federal system such as that of the United States, it is the laws and policies on the federal level that have the most far-reaching effects on access to care. Though health care providers may not often rub up against issues of social justice in the care of their patients, it is the sometimes visible, sometimes invisible framework that influences their decision making and shapes their practice. Your ethics committee may be called on to consult on cases that raise these issues in a particularly pronounced way, and the purpose of this chapter is to help you address them.

Because of this dependence of medical practice on features of the larger health care system, we have to acknowledge a difficult truth: it is hard, though not impossible, to be an ethical practitioner in a health care system that is in very significant ways unjust. "But wait," you may say. "Even if the nation's health care delivery system needs work, we can't be expected to take on those huge problems. We have enough to worry about right here in our own health care facility." This is true. As the local arbiter of moral reasoning and ethical practice, your committee's responsibilities include monitoring and guiding the way organizational decisions are made and how they affect the delivery of health care in your institution. But the purpose of this chapter is not to get you to take up the cause of changing our health care system, however worthwhile this would be. Rather, it is to make you aware that a complete ethical analysis of issues that arise on the clinical level may sometimes require you to look beyond the bedside encounter or the organizational environment to the societal factors that condition it.

ACCESS TO HEALTH CARE IN THE UNITED STATES

Any discussion of health care entitlement should begin by distinguishing between a *moral* right and a *legal* right: a moral right might exist even if it is not recognized by law. Health care in the United States, with some exceptions, is not a legal right. If, however, it is a moral right, then serious questions must be raised about whether the inequalities in access to care that exist in our society are unjust.

The following overview examines the extent to which there is a *legal* right to health care in the United States. Since World War II, most health insurance in this country has been private, a fringe benefit of employment. Employers provided health insurance, often for the individual employee and his dependents; later, the employee contributed as well. Such a system of providing health insurance is extremely vulnerable to fluctuations in the economy and job market. Those who are not wealthy enough to either purchase outright all the health care they want or buy enough insurance to cover their needs depend on their employers for coverage. In periods of economic downturn, unemployment rises and many employers cut back on the benefits they provide their employees. In addition, people are constrained in their search for career opportunities because their health care insurance is tied to their current employer.

The two main public insurance programs in the United States are Medicaid (a joint federal and state program, mainly for the poor) and Medicare (a federal program, mainly for the elderly, but also for persons with end-stage renal disease and some disabilities). Enormous variation exists in the percentage of poor people covered by state-run Medicaid programs, and states are free to restrict the range of "optional" services and the number of allowable hospital days for Medicaid patients. Moreover, contrary to popular belief, Medicaid is not an entitlement program. Physicians often refuse to treat Medicaid patients because of low reimbursements and hospitals that treat a predominantly Medicaid population are sorely understaffed and undersupplied.

Medicare, by contrast, has been an enormously successful program. It provides universal access to generally high-quality health care for those over 65 and has kept many elderly people from the brink of bankruptcy due the high cost of medical care. Concerns have been raised, however, about the adequacy of coverage. For example, despite the passage of legislation that provides modest drug coverage under Medicare, the high cost of medications places an increasingly large financial burden on the elderly. In addition, in recent years, Medicare reimbursements for health care have been cut back. Larger premiums and co-payments have meant that affluent Medicare patients experience fewer problems when they need medical care than do the less prosperous elderly, who find the required out-of-pocket expenditures, especially for increasingly expensive drugs, very burdensome. The Medicare Part D prescription drug benefit, which went into effect in 2006, covers cumulative drug expenses up to $2,250, but not between $2,251 and $5,100. This resulted in a $2,850 "donut hole" in coverage. The Patient Protection and Affordable Care Act (PPACA) seeks to ameliorate this problem over the long term. According to the Medicare website, "The ACA helps seniors in the donut hole until it is closed. Copayments required for brand-name and generic drugs are being phased down to the standard 25 percent by 2020. Brand-name drugs discounts from manufacturers increase each year in the coverage gap. Copayments for generic drugs are reduced by seven percentage points each year until the coverage gap is eliminated" (www.ncpssm.org /PublicPolicy/Medicare/Documents/ArticleID/1161/Closing-the-Medicare-Part -D-Donut-Hole).

Despite widespread coverage, existing forms of health insurance do not reach many people. A study published in the journal *Health Affairs* (Schoen et. al 2011) estimated the number of U.S. adults who were underinsured or uninsured in 2010. Using indicators of medical cost exposure relative to income, the authors found that 44% (81 million) of adults ages 19–64 were either uninsured or underinsured in 2010—up from 75 million in 2007 and 61 million in 2003. Adults with incomes below 250% of the federal poverty level accounted for sizable majorities of those at risk of becoming uninsured or underinsured. President Obama's PPACA, passed in 2010, may succeed in increasing the affordability of care for people in this income range but, as of this writing, it remains to be seen how much increased coverage is actually provided by this act. This and other issues related to health care access are discussed further in "Health Care Reform" below. Ongoing opposition of many states to signing on to a federally subsidized expansion of Medicaid coverage could significantly limit the PPACA's impact.

Barriers to access are only partly financial and there are also important non-financial impediments. These include discrimination and exclusion that may result from conscious or unconscious bias, overt racist attitudes, and racial stereotyping;

geographic barriers; and barriers imposed by differences in culture and language. As discussed below, however, removing barriers to medical services may not have as large an impact on reducing health inequalities as many have supposed. There are other equally, if not more important, causes of health disparities.

Private hospitals and academic medical centers have long assumed some of the responsibility for providing uncompensated care to the poor and indigent, but their budgets are steadily shrinking. This trend is due largely to the extension of prospective payment, spurred by the adoption of diagnosis-related groups (DRGs) for hospitalized Medicare patients. Likewise, preferred provider arrangements have eliminated cross-subsidies through which hospitals have covered the costs of providing uncompensated "charity" care by increasing charges for insured patients and those who pay directly out of pocket. Most managed care plans negotiate payment to the lowest level, making such cross-subsidies difficult.

Public hospitals continue to provide access to health care for those who cannot otherwise afford it but, under the pressure of fiscal crises, local and state governments have found such institutions burdensome to maintain. Both because of the resources available to them and the insurance status of their clientele, these institutions may be inferior to hospitals in the voluntary, not-for-profit sector.

Two other pockets in our health care system guarantee access to care in specific circumstances. Under the federal "antidumping" law, the Emergency Medical Treatment and Active Labor Act (EMTALA), patients who arrive at an emergency room in any hospital accepting federal funding must be assessed and stabilized before they can be transferred. Prisoners also have guaranteed rights to health care under rulings of the U.S. Supreme Court, although the quality of that care is regularly challenged in federal courts.

Mrs. Gomez's case illustrates the issues raised in a system that denies some people access to health care that it makes available to others. Health care institutions, especially those in poor or minority communities, are often considered to have a special obligation to provide health care to residents. When patients are uninsured or under-insured, staff sometimes feel the need to get around the rules by "gaming the system" in order to provide necessary care. In this case, the solution blurs the distinction between two types of care. *Emergency care* is limited to traumatic, unanticipated, often life-threatening injuries and illnesses that require immediate treatment. In contrast, *outpatient care* is planned, routine primary care, including the monitoring and treatment of chronic conditions. Because emergency care is episodic, it does not provide the continuity, comprehensiveness, and multidisciplinary resources so important in the ongoing prevention and treatment of chronic illnesses, such as renal disease.

It is reasonable to question whether the predictable need for emergency care justifies a practice of using the resource preventively. The routine proactive use of emergency resources may well impair the hospital's ability to provide care for true emergencies. Because public hospitals have historically covered care for the uninsured, the doctors might be able to refer Mrs. Gomez to a city hospital, where her condition could be managed on an outpatient basis as long as she receives regular dialysis. Given the increasing financial drain, however, even the municipal system may not be able to continue providing uncompensated care indefinitely. Moreover, the PPACA will not enable Mrs. Gomez to receive the care she needs, for the population composed of unauthorized immigrants is one of the largest groups of people excluded from access to insurance coverage under the PPACA. Providing care for undocumented immigrants is likely to remain a controversial social and political issue for some time to come.

As this brief review makes clear, there is no universal legally protected right to health care in the United States. Everyone in this country is legally free to seek health care and, when the proper arrangements are made, to receive it. But, with the noted exceptions, there is no recognized societal *obligation* to provide it. Instead, our society permits access to health care to depend on one's ability to pay or the source of one's health insurance. As a result, health care has not been equally available to all those who need it. This is an especially serious problem for the many uninsured in our nation, because full and successful functioning is, to a large extent, dependent on health status, which is, to a large extent dependent on access to health care. The socially sanctioned inequality of opportunity that deprives some people in this country of the health required to realize their potential fully has been a moral abdication that rises to the level of serious injustice.

JUSTICE AND HEALTH DISPARITIES

A health inequality is not necessarily a health inequity. A health inequity should be addressed as a matter of social justice; it is in some important sense unjust or unfair, or at least unnecessary. A health inequality, by contrast, is normatively neutral for, while all instances of health inequity are instances of health inequalities, the converse is not true (Ward et al. 2013). Two examples illustrate this. First, mortality rates of people ages 80 and over are greater than the mortality rates for people ages 18 to 65. This health inequality is not a health inequity if it is not due to differences in access to preventive services or treatments but to natural biological dysfunctions associated with age. Second, even when health inequalities result from differences in social status or position in a social hierarchy, they are not always unjust. For example, arguably excluding Medicaid coverage for cosmetic surgeries like liposuction is not unjust, even though people with private health insurance may have such procedures covered. In order to determine whether health inequalities rise to the level of health inequities, some account or theory of justice in health care is required.

That said, a number of studies have shown that significant racial and ethnic disparities in access to health care that *are* health inequities do exist. While there have been improvements in access to care for racial and ethnic minorities, numerous studies, including the 2012 Disparities Report from the Agency for Healthcare Research and Quality (Agency for Healthcare Research and Quality 2012), show that racial and ethnic disparities in health care, including diagnostic, curative, life-sustaining, and palliative care interventions, remain (Richardson and Norris 2010; Braveman et al. 2009; Shavers et al. 2012; Meghani et al. 2012). Racial and ethnic minorities suffer disproportionate morbidity and mortality from chronic diseases, including cancer, heart disease, diabetes, and stroke (Davis et al. 2007). They also tend to receive poorer care once they enter the health care system. Racial and ethnic disparities in children's health and health care have also been documented (Flores 2010). These disparities have remained relatively unchanged for decades in the United States, as has the average life expectancy of blacks, which is six years shorter than that of whites (Epstein and Ayanian 2001; Freeman and Payne 2000). According to one estimate, compared to the vast sums dedicated to improving medical technology in an effort to save lives, five times as many deaths could be averted if the disparities in health care were corrected (Woolf 2004).

Racial disparities in medical services suggest possible discrimination or bias, either deliberate or unintentional, by health care providers, including physicians and institutions. It is argued that the causes of the inequities implicate health care systems rather than just individual providers and will need to be addressed systemically (Meghani et al. 2012; Epstein and Ayanian 2001; Freeman and Payne 2000). Although the disparities in health care tend to fall along racial and ethnic lines, commentators caution against viewing the problem as stemming only from patients' cultural values and provider discrimination. Indeed, it has been suggested that the ultimate problem is the enormous inequality of income and wealth in our society that negatively impacts the health and health care of marginalized populations and erodes a common commitment to health for all (Daniels 2008). The PPACA may significantly expand access to insurance coverage in the United States, but it does not address the larger problem of what has been called the "socioeconomic gradient of health" (Daniels 2008, p. 22).

HEALTH CARE AS A REQUIREMENT OF JUSTICE

Given the limited legal right to health care in this country, discussed above, is there at least a moral claim that can be supported? The President's Commission for the Study of Ethical Problems in Medicine and Biomedical and Behavioral Research confronted this issue in its influential 1983 report entitled *An Ethical Framework for Access to Health Care*. According to the commissioners, health care is different from other consumer goods, such as televisions and automobiles, because it is crucially related to the length and quality of life. Moreover, like education, health care is necessary to achieve equal opportunity in society. Without decent access to care, health status is likely to suffer and poor health status prevents people from enjoying the range of opportunities that would otherwise be available to them.

Because the nation's health care needs are vast, sometimes unpredictable, and extremely costly, the President's Commission concluded that the free market alone cannot meet them adequately and society has an obligation to assume part of the burden. The commissioners cautioned, however, that this societal obligation is not unlimited; it must be constrained by the balance of costs and benefits to the population. Moreover, they argued, the fact that society is morally obligated to provide *some* care does not mean that everyone is entitled to an equal amount or quality of health care. In other words, not all *inequalities* in access to health care amount to *inequities* in access, and it is only the latter that justice requires us to eliminate. As long as everyone is guaranteed access to an *acceptable* or *decent* level of health care, the report maintains, society will have fulfilled its moral obligation. How to decide what is included in a decent basic level of care remains contentious. Efforts to specify and agree on what is included in a basic level of guaranteed care have typically appealed either to a list of categories of services considered essential or to a notion of an average level of services (Daniels 2013).

The President's Commission self-consciously chose not to use the language of "rights" to frame its notion of a societal duty. Yet many bioethicists, using the same arguments presented in the commission's report, have concluded that each citizen has a moral right, as distinguished from a legal right, against the government to guarantee a decent level of health care.

HEALTH CARE AND HEALTH

In discussing justice, bioethicists have typically focused on problems of access to *health care* and have not considered the distribution of social goods that determine the *health* of societies and social groups. However, if our interest in health care derives from our concern to secure health for individuals and groups, then health care is too narrow a focus. The goods are referred to as the *social determinants of health* and there is a vast and growing literature on the relationship between health equity and its social determinants. Particularly noteworthy is the fact that universal access to health care in a society does not eliminate or even significantly reduce health inequalities in it (Sreenivasan 2008; Daniels 2008). There is substantial evidence from studies in the United Kingdom and other Western European countries that differences in access account for only a relatively small percentage of variation in health status within a given population (Adler and Ostrove 1999; Marmot et al. 1978). More closely correlated with health, and more significant in explaining health differences between advantaged and disadvantaged members of society, are socioeconomic factors that shape a person's relative social advantage. These factors include income, education, and profession and, while there is debate about exactly how these operate, numerous studies have documented that the greater the inequality in socioeconomic status within a society, the greater the inequality in health status (Daniels, Kennedy, and Kawachi 2000). Although this relationship is not simply a contrast between the health of the rich and the poor, the influence of poverty on health status is certainly significant, operating through such factors as inadequate housing, unhealthy diet and lifestyle, unclean environment, and unsafe living conditions.

Expanding our focus of concern about health to encompass its social determinants also means that access to health care is simply a special case of a right to have one's health needs met. The range of actions that impact the health needs of populations includes steps to combat the multiple effects of poverty, and not just measures to enhance access to health care for the poor. Because health care is not the only important determinant of health status, it is not necessarily unjust or unreasonable not to provide certain beneficial medical services if the resulting savings are invested in education or job training instead. There is, of course, no guarantee that savings in one area, such as health care, will find their way to another equally worthy area, such as education.

THEORIES OF JUSTICE

Answers to questions about access to health care and the distribution of social determinants of health presuppose some views on the nature of individual rights, social obligations, and notions of fairness, even if they are not articulated. If there is a *moral* right to health care or to the amelioration of health inequalities, it must be grounded in and justified by some more general theory about the nature of social justice. Generally speaking, a person is treated justly if he is treated according to what is fair, due, or owed. The specific term *distributive justice* refers to fair, equitable, and appropriate distribution of the benefits and burdens of social cooperation. Here we refer to the equitable distribution of the benefits and burdens of health care resources and the broader determinants of health. Three theories of distributive justice—libertarian, utilitarian, and egalitarian—dominate current thinking, and each has very different implications for the right to health care in particular.

In the libertarian theory of justice, espoused most prominently by Robert Nozick and Tristam Engelhardt (Engelhardt 1991; Nozick 1974) individuals have moral rights to life, liberty, and property, which a just society must recognize and respect. In this view, the sole function of government is to prevent these rights from being interfered with and to protect the individual's life, liberty, and property against force and fraud. Everything else in society is a matter of individual, not societal or governmental, responsibility. For the libertarian, there is no moral right to health care and no societal obligation to provide it.

The utilitarian theory of justice, articulated by John Stuart Mill and Jeremy Bentham, is committed to maximizing the common good. Acts, practices, and rules are to be judged better or worse, right or wrong, according to how effectively they promote this goal. Whereas libertarians stress freedom from government interference, utilitarians are more disposed to government welfare programs because these may be necessary to promote the good of society as a whole. For utilitarians, there is a moral right to health care insofar as its provision contributes to the overall good of society's members.

The egalitarian theories of justice reject libertarianism because it fails to include what egalitarians perceive as a fundamental moral concern: those who have more than enough should help those in need. Egalitarians reject utilitarianism because it fails to provide sufficiently strong support for individual moral rights. A leading twentieth-century egalitarian theorist, John Rawls, maintained that inequalities in the distribution of "primary social goods" (e.g., income, opportunities) are justified only if they benefit the least-well-off members of society. Norman Daniels (1981, 1985, 2008), drawing on Rawls's theory of justice, extends his principle of fair equality of opportunity to argue for some form of universal access to health care and, more broadly, health.

RATIONING

It is hard to deny that individuals in this country are not equal with respect to the availability of health care. Beyond concerns about the costliness and inefficiency of the nation's health care system, disparities in access to care raise fundamental questions about whether the system is fair and just. Given the number of competing goods that require the investment of societal resources, such as housing, jobs, education, and defense, it appears that guaranteeing all citizens access to even beneficial health care must compete with obligations to perform a broad range of social actions, many of which also impact health. This follows when we enlarge our focus from health care to include the social determinants of health, for then an obligation to promote health does not necessarily neatly translate into an obligation to invest in health care. Accordingly, it is necessary to confront the challenge of health care rationing and recognize that, while some forms of rationing are morally justifiable, others are not.

Rationing Defined

In the ongoing debate about health care, *rationing* has become a highly charged term with moral overtones. The basic ethical problem is how to structure our health care system so that it *fairly* distributes limited resources and provides *equitable* access to health care at *manageable cost*. To accomplish these various and sometimes conflicting tasks, many now call for the adoption of some explicit form of societal rationing or limit setting. As noted earlier, much of the U.S. health care system already involves a kind of implicit or covert rationing—that is, rationing by ability to pay and level of personal resources. Rationing on this basis is objectionable because of the special nature and importance of health care as a *good*, making its deprivation an injustice. The notion of rationing has several meanings, according to Daniel Wikler:

- trimming: "cutting back on services that few people want and no one needs" (e.g., targeting inefficient and ineffective care)
- cutting: "refusing genuinely needed and wanted care on the grounds that the cost is 'too high'" (e.g., a practitioner's decision not to provide a nonexperimental organ transplant to a medically suitable candidate based on a payer's refusal to reimburse for it)
- tailoring: "eliminates care which is (1) of questionable effectiveness, even though it may be popular or even standard, or which has marginal effectiveness relative to risk; or (2) care which prolongs conditions which are marginally endurable" (e.g., using expensive medical technology to sustain patients who are in a persistent vegetative state or have an extremely poor quality of life) (Wikler 1992, p. 399)

Cutting, that is, withholding care expected to be of net benefit to the patient, is the most ethically troubling form of rationing and the one that both proponents and opponents of rationing chiefly have in mind when they use the term. Commentators disagree about whether cutting is really necessary, except in special circumstances. Some commentators optimistically hope that trimming and tailoring, the adoption of an ethic of waste avoidance that counsels against spending on interventions that do not benefit patients, will for the most part eliminate the need for this more problematic form of rationing (e.g., Brody 2012). Others disagree, arguing that the aging of the population, the onward march of medical progress, and the limits of societal resources mean that the more extreme form of rationing is unavoidable (e.g., Singer 2009).

Societal versus Bedside Rationing

Rationing health care can be done on a societal or community level, through a process of public deliberation leading to general guidelines for limit setting as a means of cost containment. This approach is known as *macroallocating* resources. Alternatively, rationing can be done "at the bedside" by individual physicians making decisions to deny particular interventions to particular patients as a means of controlling health care costs. This process is known as *microallocating*.

An example of macroallocating, or societal rationing, is the Oregon Health Plan, officially enacted in February 1994. The Oregon plan originated in 1987 in a choice faced by the state legislature when it decided to invest its limited health care dollars in prenatal care for thousands of uninsured poor women rather than fund organ transplants of questionable efficacy for a relatively small handful of patients. The Oregon program involves the following elements: an attempt to guarantee universal access to health care through the expansion of the state Medicaid program to include every person officially defined as poor; recognition of the necessity of limits in the care that is provided to everyone on Medicaid, these limits to be determined by how much money the state can afford to spend on health care in any given year; and an open and democratic process for making these difficult decisions about limit setting. In a series of town hall meetings throughout the state, residents voted on the priority order of health care services, ranking what they considered essential basics, such as prenatal care, at one end and nonessentials, such as cosmetic surgery, at the other end. The cut-off for what was funded in any given year would be determined by the amount available in the Medicaid budget for that year.

The Oregon plan has been criticized on the grounds that it achieves the goal of cost control solely at the expense of those who are already disadvantaged, namely, poor women and children (Daniels 1991). On the other hand, the plan has been praised for making a social commitment to guaranteeing some level of health care for all poor people in the state and for relying on an open and publicly accountable system for making rationing decisions. It is generally agreed that health care rationing can only be morally acceptable if it results from a fair and transparent process for health care priority setting, the task then being that of specifying the key elements of such a process (Gruenewald 2012).

Microallocating is highly controversial. On the one hand, it is argued that bedside rationing is inevitable and that it is the responsibility of physicians to participate in cost containment in morally credible ways. Physicians, in this view, are the stewards of health care resources at the site of use and in the best position to assess both clinical and cost effectiveness. On the other hand, bedside rationing is criticized on several grounds: physicians may allow their personal biases to influence their decisions about which interventions are and are not worth the cost; variability from physician to physician means that there will be no uniform standards for limit setting or consistency in implementation; and physicians cannot be both agents of cost containment and advocates for the best interests of their patients. A middle ground would see some modest form of physician rationing as appropriate and, possibly, obligatory.

HEALTH CARE REFORM

Efforts to reform the health care system in the United States have proven controversial because of the difficulty of finding societal consensus on a general ethical rationale for comprehensive health care reform (Trotter 2012). Given the different conceptions of what justice requires, even when there is widespread agreement that our health care system is seriously flawed from the standpoint of justice, there is no consensus on why or what to do about it. Moreover, political agendas, notions of entitlement and governmental intrusion, and moral conceptions of character and social worth inevitably polarize the debate. Despite these challenges, important steps have been taken by the U.S. government to expand access to health care for large groups of people in our society, from the signing of Medicare and Medicaid into law in 1965 to the Patient Protection and Affordable Care Act of 2010, the single most important piece of social legislation affecting health care in more than 40 years.

The PPACA includes a number of provisions intended to make health care more accessible, affordable, accountable, cost and clinically effective, and just (Maruthappu, Ologunde, and Gunarajasingam 2013). The law's key provisions include

- requiring insurers in the individual and group markets to cover all persons who apply for insurance, regardless of health status;
- requiring insurers to cover preexisting conditions and set their premium levels independent of the insured's health status;
- permitting children to remain on their parents' insurance until age 26;
- requiring states to expand their Medicaid program to cover all citizens whose income is at or below 138% of the poverty level or risk losing federal funding;
- establishing an "individual mandate" that requires everyone who is not covered by an employer-sponsored health plan, Medicaid, Medicare, or other public insurance program, to purchase an approved private insurance policy, and including a financial penalty to encourage compliance;
- establishing insurance exchanges, where individuals can shop for approved private insurance policies that meet their health care needs at affordable cost; and
- providing federal subsidies to people with incomes close to the poverty line to help them purchase approved private insurance policies.

When the constitutionality of the PPACA was challenged in 2012, the U.S. Supreme Court held that the law's individual mandate is a constitutional exercise of Congress's taxing power but that states cannot be forced to participate in the act's Medicaid expansion under penalty of losing their current Medicaid funding. (See part IV for fuller discussion of this decision.) For multiple reasons, a number of states initially chose not to accept federal funding to expand their Medicaid programs, although a number have since reconsidered that decision. Making state Medicaid expansion optional in this way is likely to severely limit the law's impact on the number of persons nationwide who will be covered by health insurance.

To no one's surprise, the political response to the PPACA has been mixed. Many liberals have hailed the law as a significant and long-overdue step toward universal health care coverage, but not all were satisfied. Some still consider a single-payer system to be the only workable, rational, and equitable system for health care coverage, using Canada and European countries as models. Political conservatives, on the other hand, regarded the law as an instance of governmental overreaching and many have vowed to repeal "Obamacare" or, at least, obstruct its implementation.

Whether guaranteed universal access to quality, affordable health care is a requirement of justice depends on the particular theory of justice one adopts. This is not a requirement under a libertarian theory, and while a utilitarian theory is concerned about the health of the public, this does not guarantee that each and every individual has access to quality, affordable health care. Such a requirement is best explained by an egalitarian theory. From this standpoint, the PPACA must be judged to have made some progress toward a more just health care system.

REFERENCES

Adler N, Ostrove J. 1999. Socioeconomic status and health: What we know and what we don't. In Adler N, ed. *Socioeconomic Status and Health in Industrial Nations: Social, Psychological, and Biological Pathways.* New York: New York Academy of Sciences.

Agency for Healthcare Research and Quality. 2012. National Healthcare Disparities Report.

Braveman PA, Cubbin C, Egerter S, Williams DR, Pamuk E. 2009. Socioeconomic disparities in health in the United States: What the patients tell us. *American Journal of Public Health* 100 (S1):186–96.

Brody H. 2012. From an ethics of rationing to an ethics of waste avoidance. *New England Journal of Medicine* 3566(21):1949–51.

Daniels, N. 1981. Health-care needs and distributive justice. *Philosophy and Public Affairs* 10(2):146–79.

Daniels N. 1985. *Just Health Care.* New York: Cambridge University Press.

Daniels N. 1991. Is the Oregon rationing plan fair? *Journal of the American Medical Association* 265(17):2232–35.

Daniels N. 2008. *Just Health.* New York: Cambridge University Press.

Daniels N. 2013. Justice and access to health care. In *Stanford Encyclopedia of Philosophy,* http://plato.stanford.edu/entries/justice-healthcareaccess/.

Daniels N, Kennedy B, Kawachi I. 2000. Why justice is good for our health. In Cohen J, Rogers J, eds. *Is Inequality Bad for Our Health?* Boston: Beacon Press.

Davis AM, Vinci LM, Okwuosa TM, Chase AR, Huang ES. 2007. Cardiovascular health disparities: A systematic review of health care interventions. *Medical Research and Review* 64(S5):29S–100S.

Emanuel EL. 1991. *The Ends of Medicine: Medical Ethics in a Liberal Polity.* Cambridge, MA: Harvard University Press.

Emergency Medical Treatment and Active Labor Act (EMTALA), 42 U.S.C. §1395dd et seq.

Engelhardt T. 1991. *Bioethics and Secular Humanism: The Search for a Common Morality.* Philadelphia: Trinity Press International.

Epstein AM, Ayanian JZ. 2001. Racial disparities in medical care. *New England Journal of Medicine* 334(19):1471–73.

Flores G. 2010. Racial and ethnic disparities in the health and health care of children. *Journal of the American Academy of Pediatrics* 125(4):979–1020.

Freeman HP, Payne R. 2000. Racial injustice in health care. *New England Journal of Medicine* 342(14):1045–48.

Gruenwald DA. 2012 Can health care rationing ever be rational? *Journal of Law, Medicine & Ethics* 40(1):17–25, www.ncpssm.org/PublicPolicy/Medicare/Documents/Article ID/1161/Closing-the-Medicare-Part-D-Donut-Hole.

Marmot M, et al. 1978. Employment grade and coronary artery disease in British civil servants. *Journal of Epidemiology and Community Health* 32:244–49.

Maruthappu M, Ologunde R, Gunarajasingam A. 2013. Is health care a right? Health reforms in the USA and their impact upon the concept of care. *Annals of Medicine and Surgery* 2(1):15–17.

Meghani SH, Polomano RC, Tait RC, Vallerand AD, Anderson KO, Gallagher RM. 2012. Advancing a national agenda to eliminate disparities in pain care: Directions for health policy, education, practice, and research. *Pain Medicine* 13(1):5–28.

Mill JS. 1957. *Utilitarianism.* New York: Liberal Arts Press.

Morreim EH. 1989. Fiscal scarcity and the inevitability of bedside budget balancing. *Archives of Internal Medicine* 149(5):1012–15.

Nozick R. 1974. *Anarchy, State, and Utopia.* New York: Basic Books.

President's Commission for the Study of Ethical Problems in Medicine and Biomedical and Behavioral Research. 1983. *Securing Access to Health Care.* Washington, DC: U.S. Government Printing Office.

Rawls J. 1971. *A Theory of Justice.* Cambridge, MA: Harvard University Press.

Richardson LD, Norris M. 2010. Access to health and health care: How race and ethnicity matter. *Mount Sinai Journal of Medicine* 77(2):166–77.

Schoen C, Doty M, Robertson R, Collins S. 2011. Affordable Care Act reforms could reduce the number of underinsured U.S. adults by 70%. *Health Affairs* 30(9):1762–71.

Shavers, VL, Fagan P, Jones D, Klein WMP, Boyington J, Moten C, Rorie E. 2012. The state of research on racial/ethnic discrimination in the receipt of health care. *American Journal of Public Health* 102(5):953–66.

Singer P. 2009. Why we must ration health care. *The New York Times Magazine*, July 15.

Sreenivasan G. 2008. Justice, inequality, and health. In *Stanford Encyclopedia of Philosophy*, http://plato.stanford.edu/entries/justice-inequality-health/.

Trotter G. 2012. No theory of justice can ground health care reform. *Journal of Law, Medicine & Ethics* 40(3):598–605.

Ward A, Johnson PJ, O'Brien M. 2013. The normative dimensions of health disparities. *Journal of Health Disparities Research and Practice* 6(1):46–61.

Wikler D. 1992. Ethics and rationing: "Whether," "how," or "how much"? *Journal of the American Geriatrics Society* 40:398–403.

Woolf SH. 2004. Society's choice: The tradeoff between efficacy and equity and the lives at stake. *American Journal of Preventive Medicine* 27(1):49–56.

CHAPTER 12

Organizational Ethics

From bioethics to health care organizational ethics
Moral responsibilities of health care organizations
Organizational ethics and compliance
Ethics and the allocation of resources
Ethics committees and organizational issues
Developing an organizational ethics service

The asthma control program at Gotham Medical Center was started by the group physician practice (GPP) in 2000. The GPP is an example of a mixed economic model. Rather than a fully capitated practice, it participates in a health maintenance organization (HMO), but also provides care on a fee-for-service basis.

The asthma program was directed by a nurse administrator who was hired by the GPP and to whom referrals were made by physicians in the group. Her role was to work with patients to enhance their understanding and management of their medical conditions. Information was provided by phone and in person to both children and adults about symptoms, appropriate medications and when to take them, and how to manage asthma attacks without having to go to the emergency room for care. The asthma program seemed to have been clinically effective, based on the decreased number of Emergency Department (ED) visits for asthma treatment and the reports of improved patient and family satisfaction. The program had also been an important health care resource for the community.

Despite its benefits, however, controversy had arisen about the asthma program's financial implications. On one hand, the program's administrative costs had been borne by the GPP. In addition, the program's clinical success had resulted in fewer patient visits to physicians' offices and less frequent hospital admissions, decreases that had cut into the GPP's revenues. From the standpoint of the HMO, however, reducing physician and ED visits and hospital admissions had kept medical costs down, which was one of the HMO's primary missions. In 2002, the GPP decided to terminate the asthma program, based on the increased administrative costs and the decreased revenues.

What interests are in tension when organizations consider which health care services to provide? Do health care organizations have ethical, as well as financial and business, obligations that inform their decisions? What role can and should ethics committees play in organizational matters?

FROM BIOETHICS TO HEALTH CARE
ORGANIZATIONAL ETHICS

In the ever-widening scope of concerns addressed by health care ethics committees, organizational ethics is a relatively new consideration. Until the 1990s, the study of ethical issues in health care focused on moral problems and conflicts in the clinical setting that have been addressed in the preceding chapters of this handbook. Increasingly, however, clinicians and administrators have come to recognize that how a health care organization makes decisions directly affects the quality of the care it delivers. For your ethics committee to address both organizational and clinical issues, it is important to appreciate the relationship between the two areas of concern.

Largely as a result of efforts to limit the rapid and seemingly uncontrolled rise in health care costs, the care delivery system has changed radically during the past 35 years. New and often competing scientific, economic, and political imperatives demand attention. The clinical dynamic is no longer controlled by physicians acting more or less autonomously. Managers and administrators make and enforce policies that restrict the available options and the ability of physicians and patients to make choices about them. New analytic frameworks are necessary to meet current and future challenges in allocating health care resources and decision-making authority.

One response to skyrocketing health care costs has been a new environment in which medical practice is managed by organizations that impose economic discipline on clinical decision making. While fiscal concerns remain significant in the changing health care system, other factors, including heightened focus on quality of care and length of stay, have also promoted greater organizational control of clinical decision making. As a result of economic considerations, legislative agendas, and concern with improving clinical practice, there has been increasing emphasis on mechanisms of quality assurance and clinical effectiveness assessment in medical care.

The most significant change since the introduction of Medicare and Medicaid in 1965 is the Patient Protection and Affordable Care Act (PPACA) of 2010, discussed in chapter 11. While the overarching aim of the PPACA is to reduce the number of U.S. citizens without health insurance by requiring affordable health care insurance coverage for all, it, along with other health care reform efforts, has given impetus to fundamental changes in how health care is conceived, delivered, evaluated, and reimbursed. These new paradigms are reflected in the training of health care professionals and the responsibilities they assume, the reciprocal expectations of patients and their caregivers, and the missions and visions articulated by care-providing organizations. These seismic changes in the health care landscape require organizational responses that have profound ethical implications. What began as tentative steps by ethics committees to contribute to institutional policies and procedures must now become an essential part of their mission, as ethics is fully integrated into the examination of organizational decision making.

Organizational ethics introduces an *intermediate* level of analysis between the narrower set of clinical concerns and the broader societal policy issues. Health care organizations—hospitals, nursing homes, visiting nurse agencies, hospices, and facilities that provide specialized care for specific patient populations—make daily decisions about resource allocation, clinical priorities, conflicting interests, and community responsibilities, all of which have ethical implications. In this analytic perspective, the organization as health care provider assumes ethical rights and responsibilities similar to but distinct from those of individual health care professionals. Of central importance in distinguishing clinical from organizational ethics is the notion of moral agency. Traditionally, bioethics has examined the actions of *individual* agents—clinicians, patients, and family members—and held them accountable in light of ethical principles, norms, and obligations. In the intermediate anal ysis, the locus of moral agency differs from that of clinical ethics and the *organization* itself is seen as having obligations to adhere to certain norms of ethical behavior.

The successful operation of any multifaceted enterprise depends on the efficient recognition and resolution of problems in the most effective manner using the most appropriate resources. Thus, issues related to marketing, finance, risk management, legality, security, compliance, and human resources are referred to the respective departments with the relevant expertise. Likewise, in the clinical and research settings, disputes about diagnostic, therapeutic, and investigational protocols are addressed in a commonly accepted process. The analysis of ethical issues that arise on the organizational level involves a different orientation and requires its own process.

While clinical ethics consultation is the recognized and routinely accessed resource for resolving ethical conflicts in the clinical setting, ethical dilemmas in the organizational setting present challenges that do not entirely lend themselves to the clinical ethics consultation model. Application of ethics to patient-centered care typically focuses on the needs, rights, goals, values, and preferences of individual patients; the obligations of clinicians to those patients; the interests and wishes of family or other surrogates; and communication between and among these key parties. The common goal—perhaps the only thing shared by all parties—is promoting the best interest of the patient.

In contrast, ethical conflicts in the organizational setting implicate diverse goals and interests, hierarchies of power and authority, conflicting roles and obligations, public and private agendas, long-range plans, and decisions that affect populations, as well as individuals. Rather than informed consent, confidentiality, patient autonomy, decisional capacity, and care at the end of life, organizational issues are likely to include conflicts of interest and obligation, marketing practices, competition with other organizations, responsibilities to the community, staff loyalty, physician retention, reimbursement, and regulatory compliance. Thus, organizational ethics requires a different analytic framework, increasingly including stakeholder theory, which aims to balance the multiple and often competing interests of the interested parties. The Joint Commission standard requiring organizations to have a standing mechanism to promote ethical behavior in all aspects of organizational functioning adds strength to the persuasive argument that ethical analysis is an important resource in organizational deliberation and decision making (dos Santos et al. 2012; Bean 2011; Wlody 2007; Chen, Werhane, and Mills 2007; Wall 2007; Rorty, Werhane, and Mills 2004; Heitman and Bulger, 1998).

This perspective has particular relevance to ethics committees, which have traditionally functioned as their health care institutions' analytic and consultative resource on moral issues and conflicts. While some have suggested that ethics committees resist involvement in organizational policies to preserve their traditional focus on protecting patient rights (Cushman and Fiore 2012), this handbook argues that the committee's role can no longer be limited to considering the ethical aspects of individual clinical interactions, but should encompass scrutiny of how the organization creates an environment in which quality care is provided because ethically sound decisions are made.

MORAL RESPONSIBILITIES OF HEALTH CARE ORGANIZATIONS

Central Hospital is considering some innovations in an effort to make its operation more efficient. In the process, it is confronting a conflict between its role as a health care delivery system and its role as a risk-bearing entity. For example, one of the suggestions under consideration is the establishment of an observation suite in or near the ED. Sometimes when patients come to the ED, their presenting symptoms (chest pain, shortness of breath, abdominal pain, asthma) do not make it clinically apparent whether they need to be hospitalized. An observation suite would provide a place where they could be observed closely for up to 24 hours while their condition either stabilizes or changes and their medical needs become clearer.

From the risk perspective, the advantage is the opportunity for 24 hours of monitoring, which is much less expensive than a hospitalization. From the hospital's viewpoint, however, such a resource may not be economically advantageous because it would drive up the cost of an ED visit without generating additional revenue to offset the cost. Because most patients are not in the risk category, the hospital would only be entitled to reimbursement for an ED visit.

Organizational ethics draws its core notions from the disciplines of both business and health care ethics. Traditional bioethics views organizations merely as settings for encounters between individual patients and individual clinicians. Its focus on the ethics of professions, including medicine, nursing, psychology, and social work, does not address the organizational climate that promotes or impedes the ethical delivery of health care. Business ethics recognizes medicine as a business enterprise but fails to appreciate the distinctive nature of health care as a good and the special quality of the provider-patient relationship. What distinguishes organizational ethics is the notion that organizations are more than aggregates of individuals with their own roles and responsibilities. As we have argued at greater length elsewhere (Blustein, Post, and Dubler 2002, 2004), organizations can usefully be thought of as moral agents with interests, values, and obligations that inform their goals and the means they use to achieve them.

How these matters are considered has not only philosophical significance, but enormous practical significance as well, especially for health care ethics committees. Viewed simply as economic entities, the moral responsibilities of health care organizations may be quite limited. Businesses have obligations not to defraud their customers and to engage in fair competitive practices, of course. But whether and why they have moral responsibilities that extend beyond this rather minimal set has been the subject of considerable debate in the business ethics literature. Health care organizations, however, are not just businesses. They are agents with more robust moral responsibilities because of the special good they deliver, and they should be expected to develop a sense of what is morally acceptable and unacceptable practice and to manifest that sense in their policies and procedures.

It would be naïve to suggest that health care organizations can be guided only by their moral codes. Like other business entities, they have a parallel and often competing responsibility to remain fiscally sound to meet their obligations to patients, employees, and the communities they serve. Central Hospital's decision about establishing an observation suite, for example, pits the benefits of risk reduction and improved clinical care against the economic burden of creating an expensive and under-reimbursed service. Because hospitals have fixed budgets, the analysis will require a balancing of goods, considering the worth of this unit in relation to other programs that may have to be delayed, downsized, or eliminated altogether.

In an analogy to the clinical setting, it might be asked whether organizations have the *capacity* for morally responsible conduct or whether, like individuals who lack this capacity, they can only be kept in line by external regulation, such as compliance requirements. We argue that organizations can be motivated not only by economic self-interest, but also by a capacity to regulate their actions according to a set of moral imperatives. This position has important implications for ethics committees in determining the scope of their involvement in the goals, policies, and procedures of the institutions they advise. Of course, that determination must be followed by the equally important but far more challenging task of helping executive leadership and boards of trustees to see ethics as an indispensible resource in organizational planning and decision making.

Health care organizations can act in morally responsible ways only if they have a clear sense of their core values in relation to other organizational goals. These values, typically articulated in the organizational mission statement and code of ethics, become an essential part of an organization's identity. As examples of how institutions might express their governing moral philosophies, part III offers several sample codes of organizational and clinical ethics. These codes were developed by the institutions' respective ethics committees, endorsed by their administrations, and formally adopted by their boards of trustees. They appear on the institutions' websites as a revealing portrait of their organizational culture, defining values, and guiding principles. As discussed further in part III, the process of organizational introspection required to develop a code of ethics can be a powerful tool in promoting ethics as a valuable organizational resource.

Neither a mission statement nor a code of ethics is worth much if leadership, especially at the executive level, does not appreciate the need for monitoring and evaluating performance to determine the organization's effectiveness in light of its values and goals. The organization can only act as a moral agent through visible and authoritative individuals who use the organizational mission as a benchmark for assessing organizational behaviors. Although the mission should be taken seriously at all levels of the organization, executive leadership plays a special role in ensuring that organizational activities truly reflect its stated goals and values.

ORGANIZATIONAL ETHICS AND COMPLIANCE

Samantha Evans, an experienced neonatal ICU (NICU) nurse, began her shift by assessing the most recent admission, a neonate born at 26 weeks. She checked all the tubes and wires attached to his tiny body and was about to check his vital signs when the nurse manager came to the isolette and told her that she had been reassigned to another patient. When Samantha asked why, the nurse manager replied, "Because you're black. There's a note on the front of chart, 'No African American nurses to care for baby, per father's request.' You know how these things are, it's nothing personal, We don't want any problems caring for this sick baby."

The imperative to provide nondiscriminatory care is grounded in the tradition of healing professions, explicit instruction in professional codes of ethics, state and federal legislation, standards of accreditation bodies, and Patient Bill of Rights (American Medical Association Code of Ethics; American Nurses Association Code of Ethics; American Hospital Association; Joint Commission). Yet, until recently, little attention has been paid to what has been called an "open secret"—patient refusal to receive care from doctors or nurses of particular ethnicities, genders, or other defining characteristics—because these requests are often accommodated surreptitiously to avoid unpleasant situations (Chen 2013; Phippen 2013).

Recognizing that the transformation from fee-for-service to managed care presents ethical problems in addition to those that arise in clinical care, in 1995 the Joint Commission changed the name of its standards chapter from "Patient Rights" to "Patient Rights and Organization Ethics." The new standards require health care organizations to develop and operate according to a code of ethical behavior that addresses "marketing, admission, transfer and discharge, and billing practices" and "the relationship of the hospital and its staff to other health care providers, educational institutions, and payers" (Joint Commission on Accreditation of Healthcare Organizations 1998:55–56, Standards RI.4.1 and RI.4.2). Though not specifically addressed here, patient rights certainly do not include the right to exclude caregivers because of race, religion, sexual orientation, or other characteristics that are irrelevant to the sound practice of medicine.

Although the Joint Commission refers to its new standards as "organizational ethics," we use the term to distinguish a normative reach beyond the minimum required for adherence to laws and regulations. Compliance, a separate but related area of organizational scrutiny, focuses on those obligations whose nonfulfillment amounts to fraud and abuse, or lack of professional integrity, while organizational ethics is concerned with obligations whose nonfulfillment involves a much wider range of types of unethical conduct. Organizational ethics recognizes that organizations confront many ethical problems for which no applicable laws and regulations exist; in other words, unethical conduct may not be illegal. Moreover, because ethical problems often resist neat and easy solutions, they may demand a more nuanced analysis than the determination of whether compliance has or has not occurred.

Hospitals and other health care organizations have responded to legal and regulatory requirements by appointing people whose responsibility is monitoring institutional compliance. Working with the offices of risk management and legal counsel, compliance officers are charged with ensuring that institutional policies and procedures meet or exceed specified governmental standards. Your institution likely has an office of compliance dedicated to this essential effort. In contrast, your ethics committee's function is to provide the principled analyses and recommendations that will promote ethically sound organizational decisions and actions where violations may not be as easily discernible. Ideally, compliance and ethics collaboration provides a robust resource that educates the institutional community and promotes the highest standards of organizational and clinical functioning (Report on Medicare Compliance 2014; Nelson 2012).

Returning to Samantha Evans, her manager's effort to smooth over the situation, while, perhaps, well intended, is off the mark and entirely misses the ethical breach. From Samantha's perspective, this is a very personal as well as professional matter. She is being held to the same standards as her colleagues in the knowledge, skill, and commitment that characterize the care she delivers *without regard to her patients' race, religion, creed, gender, or socioeconomic status.* This level of professionalism is required by the nursing codes to which she is pledged, as well as by her hospital as a condition of employment.

Samantha has the right to expect a reciprocal organizational commitment. She has the right to expect that the organization will ensure a working environment that promotes the delivery of care in a manner that does not discriminate on the basis of characteristics unrelated to her abilities and performance. While her nurse manager might respond, "I want to protect my nurse from an unpleasant, demeaning, and, possibly violent situation," Samantha has the right to feel secure that the organization's commitment to her dignity is every bit as strong as its commitment to the dignity of the patients in its care. Creating and fostering an ethical environment that promotes a therapeutic dynamic is among the core ethical obligations of health care organizations.

ETHICS AND THE ALLOCATION OF RESOURCES

City Hospital has a 15-bed intensive care unit and, as usual, tonight the unit is fully occupied. When the ICU is full and the ED has also reached its limit, this hospital, like others in the region, typically closes its ED to ambulances because it cannot accommodate additional patients. Ambulances that would normally bring patients to this hospital are diverted to the nearest hospital with an open ED. On this night, all area hospitals have closed their EDs because they are filled to capacity. Patients picked up by the emergency medical service (EMS) must be taken somewhere, however, so City Hospital must admit a patient despite its saturation.

The last patient admitted to the ICU is a 45-year-old man with chronic schizophrenia with a high fever and overwhelming infections who has been brought in from one of the city's state-operated psychiatric facilities. Another bed is already occupied by a 96-year-old woman brought to the ED from a nursing home, where she had been found unresponsive. Efforts to restore her to consciousness have so far been unsuccessful.

A third patient in the unit is a 23-year-old woman, an IV drug user with 2 children, who presented in the ED with symptoms of *Pneumocystis carinii* pneumonia (PCP). Because of her pulmonary disease, she is in respiratory distress and needs to be stabilized before starting antiretroviral therapy. The remaining ICU beds are occupied by patients whose average age is 75 and for whom continued ICU treatment has been deemed essential.

The patient who has just been brought to the ED is a 63-year-old professor of internal medicine who has just had a heart attack. The university where the professor teaches recently endowed a new wing of the hospital.

Which patient, if any, should be removed from the ICU to make room for the professor? What criteria should be used in determining eligibility for ICU care? In what way do decisions about allocating ICU beds involve issues of justice?

Questions about resource allocation are among the most common and important in organizational ethics. (See also the discussion of rationing in chapter 11.) Allocation decisions are trade-offs, necessitated by the fact that health care resources and the economic assets needed for their provision are limited. Sometimes the trade-offs involve hard choices between doing things that would improve the health of a population in serious need and doing what is necessary to preserve the fiscal integrity of the organization and, thereby, its long-term ability to continue serving the needs of the community. More commonly, the trade-off is not between some needed program and institutional survival, but between a new program and those that are already in place meeting other needs.

Resource allocation decisions often have to balance and rank a number of competing considerations. For example, when budgets are limited, resources devoted to very costly cutting-edge treatments and technologies that might benefit a few patients diminish what is available for less expensive care that can benefit a larger number. Investing in large-scale marketing campaigns to attract more patients may result in less being spent on providing care to those who are already patients. A growing problem for organizations is determining how to budget for the care of undocumented persons, as well as citizens who are uninsured or underinsured. The mandates in the PPACA can be expected to have an impact on the number of people with no or inadequate health insurance and, to some extent, this might help health care organizations avoid otherwise difficult and controversial decisions.

In these and similar cases, the central questions are: Who wins? Who loses? What alternatives do the losers have for getting their needs met? Because resource allocation decisions confer benefits on some (the winners) at the cost of not conferring benefits on others (the losers), they raise issues of distributive justice. The distribution of the benefits and burdens inherent in resource allocation decisions should be done in a way that is fair to all concerned and does not discriminate against any group or individuals.

One distinction is between expensive and scarce resources. For example, in City Hospital, ICU beds are an *expensive* resource that is made into a *scarce* resource by an organizational decision limiting the number of beds. If the institutional budget permitted ICU expansion, more beds could be made available. In contrast, solid organs, such as hearts, are from the outset a scarce resource because of their finite supply. Because ICU beds are expensive and limited, not all persons who could potentially benefit from critical care can receive it in the ICU.

Another useful distinction is between rationing and triage. *Rationing,* discussed in chapter 11, is setting limits on spending to allocate limited resources among competing care and treatment needs, thereby denying beneficial care to some. *Triage,* the approach used in most EDs and ICUs, is determining the order in which care is provided, using as criteria the urgency of the care needs and the likelihood of benefit. Generally accepted medical criteria exclude from the ICU patients considered unlikely to benefit from critical care because it would be physiologically futile, patients who are in a permanent vegetative state (PVS), or those who have met the criteria for brain death. Priorities are established and patients with a greater likelihood of benefiting from ICU care are given preference over those who are less likely to benefit from care in that setting. The alternative to this approach is to increase the ICU census by admitting more patients and potentially decrease the quality of care.

Decisions regarding the allocation of limited resources in City Hospital should be based on sound medical and ethical criteria. It is reasonable to question whether giving the ICU bed to the professor, simply because his university has endowed a new wing of the hospital, is fair to the other patients who are already benefiting from ICU care. This might well be seen as an unjustified form of favoritism that has little to do with medical criteria, clinical benefit, or distributive justice. The ethics committee role in reviewing institutional policies would contribute a principled analysis to the guidelines for ICU admission, focusing on the just and clinically indicated allocation of a limited resource. Explicating the ethical foundation of this and other policies provides not only the justification, but also the transparency, necessary to build support. Likewise, the ethics committee can be an essential resource in preparing for and managing medical emergencies, such as the 2014 Ebola virus disease (EVD) outbreak, and in setting guidelines for response to actual or anticipated epidemics and pandemics, such as the 2009 swine flu pandemic. Ethics participation at the leadership level can ensure that all relevant policies, guidelines, and departures from routine standards of care are thoughtful, transparent, evidence-based, and both clinically and ethically justified.

ETHICS COMMITTEES AND ORGANIZATIONAL ISSUES

The Atlas Hospital medical director has brought the following issue to the Atlas bioethics committee for consideration. Especially during protracted hospitalizations, patients' conditions and, therefore, their medical needs change. Often patients who were admitted to one medical or surgical service subsequently need to be transferred one or more times to a different service for continued care. In each instance, the process requires the medical team on the first service to communicate with the medical team on the second service, explaining why the patient would benefit from the transfer. Depending on its evaluation of the patient's condition and its own clinical burdens, the second service has the option of accepting or rejecting the transfer. It has come to the medical director's attention that clinical services are avoiding accepting transfers for reasons other than clinical indication.

Atlas Hospital is also working to promote clinical efficiency and discourage unnecessarily long hospitalizations. Accordingly, when a patient either leaves the hospital or dies, the length of stay (the number of hospital days) is credited to the discharge service, not the admitting or transferring service. That means that, if a patient spends 60 days on a surgical service and is transferred to a medicine service for

2 days prior to discharge, the entire 62-day length of stay will be credited to the medicine service. Because the costs incurred during a hospitalization are applied to the clinical service caring for the patient, it is in each service's best interest to minimize lengths of stay. Under this system, it is also unsurprising that services are not eager to accept patients who have or are likely to have long lengths of stay.

The organization's ethics committee can serve a vital function by monitoring the consistency of the institutional mission and goals with the policies and procedures that guide them, and the administrative decisions that realize them. Its effectiveness requires the recognition that ethical issues arising in health care cannot be neatly compartmentalized and addressed separately from other institutional matters. Because clinical and business concerns are interrelated, decisions about them must be grounded in or consistent with the ethical principles and values that inform the organizational mission. As discussed below, an effective ethics committee's mission, composition, agenda, and the issues it considers should reflect this broader scope (Cesta 2011).

The interservice transfer issue is a good example of how ethics committees can influence organizational decision making and, thereby, promote better clinical decision making. The Atlas committee analyzed the situation in terms of the conflict between the obligation to promote patient best interest and the obligation to be responsible stewards of institutional resources. Patients are benefited by transfer if their treatment needs can be met more effectively in another clinical setting. Transfer burdens them if they are deprived of the clinical judgment, skill, and continuity of care on which they rely. The committee also recognized that even physicians who intend to act in their patients' best interests will be reluctant to make medically appropriate decisions that appear to disadvantage their clinical services. Organizational involvement and support are essential to developing solutions that are medically and ethically sound. The committee's ethical principles and suggested guidelines for interservice transfer appear in chapter 15.

DEVELOPING AN ORGANIZATIONAL ETHICS SERVICE

Your ethics committee's utility as an analytic and advisory resource is only as good as its access to and active involvement in organizational planning and decision making. Genuine integration of the ethics perspective in the formulation and execution of institutional policies and activities requires a fundamental and often difficult culture change. The significant differences between the clinical and organizational cultures challenge both ethics committees and organizational leadership seeking meaningful collaboration. Transparent and inclusive decision making, which is central to ethical process, may be seen by financial and business management as intrusive and inhibiting. Administrators may need the reassurance of sustained demonstration that ethical analysis and recommendation can enhance the efficacy and validity of organizational decision making without compromising its efficiency or security.

Leadership acceptance of and comfort with organizational ethics begins with introduction of the concept and education about its potential benefit. As in any important endeavor, a successful campaign requires meticulous planning and execution to create a favorable first impression. Quite simply, your ethics committee has one chance to do this well; otherwise, you'll be doing damage control.

The essential first step is gathering information about how and by whom decisions are made in your organization so that you have a clear picture of the lines of authority, communication, and responsibility. You also need to identify pockets of potential resistance and the reasons for uneasiness. Understanding your organizational structure and the composition of your ethics committee will help determine the most effective way to provide your ethics resource. Three basic approaches, as well as variations, have been suggested:

- Keep your ethics committee structure but expand the scope of its function to address both clinical and organizational issues. This would require revising the committee mission and supplementing the membership with management professionals who bring business, health policy, and financial expertise. The advantages of this approach include the respect and confidence your committee already enjoys and its existing skill in ethical analysis. Challenges include potential committee resistance based on members' lack of comfort with organizational issues and, depending on the frequency of meetings and the clinical responsibilities already on its agenda, the added workload.
- Create a separate ethics committee to focus on organizational issues. This would require recruiting members with the necessary business, financial, and policy knowledge and skills, as well as those with the complementary ethics expertise. Advantages include an agenda dedicated to organizational issues and a membership with the relevant expertise. Challenges include the need for members with the requisite knowledge and skills in ethics analysis, the risk of "silo thinking" when matters are labeled *either* clinical *or* organizational, and, because of the overlap in organizational and clinical issues, the potential duplication of effort.
- Retain one ethics committee with an expanded mission and a restructured function, creating two subgroups that focus on clinical and organizational matters. Advantages include the lack of confusion resulting from artificially designating issues as either clinical or organizational; the existing knowledge and skills base in ethics analysis supplemented by business, financial, compliance, and other organizational expertise; the built-in collaboration when concerns overlap; and continual reinforcement of the symbiotic nature of the clinical-organizational relationship.

The approach your committee chooses will depend on its size, clinical activity, frequency of meetings, available knowledge and skills resources, commitment to including organizational ethics in its mission, and the receptivity of senior management (Cesta 2011; Nelson 2008).

Engaging leadership interest and support will be facilitated by clearly presenting the committee's expanded mission, function, and relationship to organizational leadership and management. Just as clinical ethics committees had to reassure clinicians that they were not the ethics police, they must be equally reassuring that they are not the organizational ethics scolds. One useful strategy is creating a taxonomy of decisions, conflicts, or problems that potentially raise ethical issues and would be appropriate for ethics deliberation. These conundrums should be described in terms of the presenting situation; the key parties; the conflicting interests; the options for resolution with their respective benefits, burdens and risks; the likely outcomes; and the ethical analysis. (If that process sounds familiar, it's because it mirrors the way you prepare for a clinical ethics consultation.) Presenting a few sample cases enables leadership to see what types of situations would benefit from ethics involvement and how that involvement would facilitate the decision-making process. In addition to sample cases, you might also outline the process for requesting ethics consultation and what the response would entail. These issues, as well as strategies for addressing them, are discussed at considerably greater length in *Ethics for Health Care Organizations: Theory, Case Studies, and Tools* (Blustein, Post, and Dubler 2002).

Another opportunity for educating and engaging the people you hope to interest in an organizational ethics service is a series of grand rounds. Presented to leadership, these sessions can be very informative in demonstrating appropriate issues, their ethical implications, and how ethics involvement would be useful. The format might be panel discussions moderated by different members of your ethics committee. Panel members might include a member of executive leadership, a leader in the department where the issues do or might arise, and an outside guest who is an acknowledged expert in the area being discussed. Examples of three possible organizational ethics grand rounds with questions for discussion appear below.

Ethical Obligations to the Community: Decisions about the Choice of Clinical Services
Introduction by president/CEO
Potential panelists include vice president for planning; executive director of medical group; director/professor of health and science policy
- Do health care organizations have a moral obligation to determine the health needs of the community in order to develop a strategic plan for an institution? If so, what is its basis?
- What special responsibility, if any, do health care organizations have to provide community benefit?
- How are community health needs identified and defined?
- How should a profile of community health needs be folded into an organization's strategic plan?
- When organizations must ration scarce and expensive resources to provide care for uncompensated, inadequately reimbursed, and under- or uninsured populations, how should choices be made among competing health needs?
- How should members of the affected community be involved in the assessment, decision making, implementation, and evaluation of the strategic plan?

The Interplay between Clinical Care and Responsible Stewardship of Resources: Shortening the Length of Stay
Potential panelists include senior vice president and chief medical officer; director, critical care medicine; senior research scholar
- The following vignettes might be presented to illustrate ethical issues:
  - the family of an elderly patient with dementia tries to block discharge until the patient can be admitted to the nursing home of choice

- a patient is not considered appropriate for admission to the ICU
- a patient is resistant to leaving the hospital and refuses all discharge plans
- What is the basis of the organization's moral obligation to responsibly steward scarce and expensive resources?
- How should the organization balance the individual patient's interests against the previously determined plan to protect the institution's fiscal integrity, central to which is limiting length of stay?
- In addition to shortening length of stay, what other measures (cutting workforce, reducing or eliminating services, limiting access to care) can the organization take to promote fiscal integrity?
- How should the organization choose among these cost-saving options?
- How should criteria for critical care admission and discharge be evaluated from an ethical perspective?
- What are the organization's ethical obligations to those patients denied access to critical care?

The Ethical Issues in Quality and Patient Satisfaction
Potential panelists include vice president of operations, director of quality improvement and outcome analysis, director of service excellence
- Why has quality become such an important ethical issue in health care?
- What ethical obligations do organizations have to ensure quality of care and how should they be balanced against competing obligations, such as community benefit, physician authority, and responsible stewardship?
- How is quality defined and measured in the health care setting?
- How does the organization translate abstract notions of quality into programs and systems?
- Should sanctions be available for practitioners whose quality of care falls demonstrably below the accepted standard and do not cooperate with system-wide improvement measures?
- How does the increased emphasis on patient satisfaction, especially the link between patient satisfaction scores and hospital/physician reimbursement, affect patient care?
- What effect does the increased emphasis on patient satisfaction play in evaluating quality of care?
- How do organizations help practitioners resolve the tension between what patients need and what they want?

REFERENCES

Bean S. 2011. Navigating the murky intersection between clinical and organizational ethics: A hybrid case taxonomy. *Bioethics* 25(6):320–25.

Blustein J, Post LF, Dubler NN. 2002. *Ethics for Health Care Organizations: Theory, Case Studies, and Tools.* New York: United Hospital Fund.

Blustein J, Post LF, Dubler NN. 2004. Holding healthcare organizations morally accountable. *Keynotes on Health Care* 35(3):1–8.

Cesta T. 2011. Every day, the case management department faces multiple dilemmas over ethics; An ethical dilemma found in a case study; Solution: Committees on organizational ethics. *Hospital Case Management*: 118–21.

Chen DT, Werhane PH, Mills AE. 2007. Role of organization ethics in critical care medicine. *Critical Care Medicine* 35(2)(Suppl.):S11–S17.

Chen P. 2013. When your patient's a racist, what's a doctor to do? *The New York Times*, August 1.

Cushman R, Fiore RN. 2012. Hospital ethics committees: The case for limiting policy work. *American Journal of Bioethics* 12 (11):23–24.

dos Santos RA, de Hoyos Guevara AJ, Amorim MCS, Ferraz-Netto B-H. 2012. Compliance and leadership: The susceptibility of leaders to the risk of corruption in organizations. *Einstein* 10(1):1–10.

Emergency Medical Treatment and Active Labor Act (EMTALA), 42 U.S.C. §1395dd et seq.

Hall RT. 2000. *An Introduction to Healthcare Organizational Ethics*. New York: Oxford University Press.

Heitman E, Bulger RE. 1998. The healthcare ethics committee in the structural transformation of health care: Administrative and organizational ethics in changing times. *HEC Forum* 10(2):152–76.

Joint Commission on Accreditation of Healthcare Organizations. 1998. *Comprehensive Accreditation Manual for Hospitals*. Oakbrook Terrace, IL: Joint Commission on Accreditation of Healthcare Organizations.

Lo B. 2000. Conflicts of interest. In *Resolving Ethical Dilemmas: A Guide for Clinicians*. 2nd ed. Philadelphia: Lippincott Williams & Wilkins, pp. 231–82.

Nelson WA. 2008. Addressing organizational ethics: How to expand the scope of a clinical ethics committee to include organizational issues. *Healthcare Executive* 43 and 46.

Nelson WA. 2012. Comparing ethics and compliance programs. *Healthcare Executive* 27(4):46–49.

Nozick R. 1977. *Anarchy, State, and Utopia*. New York: Basic Books.

Pearson SD, Sabin JE, Emanuel EJ. 2003. *No Margin, No Mission: Health-Care Organizations and the Quest for Ethical Excellence*. New York: Oxford University Press.

Phillips RS, Hamel MB, Teno JM, Bellamy P, Broste SK, Califf RM, Vidaillet H, Davis RB, Muhlbaier LH, Connors AF, Lynn J, Goldman L—for the SUPPORT investigators. 1996. Race, resource use, and survival in seriously ill hospitalized adults. *Journal of General Internal Medicine* 11:387–96.

Phippen W. 2013. Hospitals balance a patient's request with a fair workplace. November 10, www.tampabay.com/news/health/hospitals-balance-a-patients-request-with-a-fair-workplace/2151836.

Post LF. 2007. Ethics and the delivery of palliative care. In O'Mahony S, Blank AE, eds. *Choices in Palliative Care*. New York: Kluwer Academic/Plenum Publishers.

President's Commission for the Study of Ethical Problems in Medicine and Biomedical and Behavioral Research. 1983. *Securing Access to Health Care*. Washington, DC: U.S. Government Printing Office.

Report on Medicare Compliance. 2014. *Ethicist: Compliance programs are limited unless grounded in ethics* 23(18), http://aishealth.com/archive/rmc052614-04 (accessed August 2014).

Rorty MV, Werhane PH, Mills AE. 2004. The *Rashomon* effect: Organization ethics in health care. *HEC Forum* 16(2):75–94.

Spencer EM, Mills AE, Rorty MV, Werhane PH. 2000. *Organization Ethics in Health Care*. New York: Oxford University Press.

Wall S. 2007. Organizational ethics, change, and stakeholder involvement: A survey of physicians. *HEC Forum* 19(3):227–43.

Wlody GS. 2007. Nursing management and organizational ethics in the intensive care unit. *Critical Care Medicine* 35(2)(Suppl.):S29–S35.

PART II

THE CREATION, NATURE, AND FUNCTIONING OF ETHICS COMMITTEES

In this portion of the handbook, we turn from the formal ethics curriculum to the body that will use the curriculum, namely, your ethics committee. We begin with an overview of the composition and functions of health care ethics committees, including a range of materials and strategies that we hope will enlighten and guide your ethics committee in addressing actual and potential ethical issues that arise in your organization. These materials include samples of the following:

- clinical cases with brief ethical analyses, three with sample chart notes
- opportunities and formats for ethics education, as well as sample educational materials
- sample organizational policies that ethics committees typically draft or review

We want to stress that much of part II is included for illustrative purposes. You may not find all of these materials useful, appropriate, or feasible for your institution, but we hope that they will at least give you an idea of the variety of things that an ethics committee can do to carry out its mission.

CHAPTER 13

Profile of Ethics Committees

Origins
Committee functions
Membership
Expertise in ethics
Leadership
Securing a foothold

ORIGINS

The history of health care ethics committees, sometimes known as clinical ethics committees or bioethics committees, was briefly reviewed in chapter 1. As noted there, these committees have at least four ancestors: (1) dialysis patient selection committees that arose in the 1960s after long-term dialysis became available but was both costly and in relatively short supply; (2) prognosis committees, as in the well-known 1976 New Jersey case of *In re Quinlan*; (3) abortion selection committees that existed in hospitals in many states prior to the 1973 *Roe v. Wade* Supreme Court decision; and (4) institutional review boards (IRBs), which were charged with reviewing all federally funded medical research to ensure that they conformed to ethical standards.

Though very different from today's health care ethics committees in a number of respects, all these committees had this in common: their chief responsibility was to oversee decisions about issues that went beyond the narrowly technical or medical and involved professional, cultural, religious, or ethical values. (This was true even about prognosis committees, which were not merely concerned with factual questions.)

That said, there is enormous variation in how and with what resources and institutional authority ethics committees address evaluative issues. Ethics committees, as they have evolved since the 1970s, vary from institution to institution along every significant dimension, including the number and qualifications of members, types of committee activities and responsibilities, the visibility of those activities, and the committee's perceived quality and utility. Across the country, some committees flourish while others fail to thrive. New committees, as well as those of long duration, can assess and change a variety of factors that may improve their chances of survival and add to their success in supporting the ethical practice of health care at their institutions.

COMMITTEE FUNCTIONS

Traditionally, health care ethics committees have addressed some or all of three functions: education; policy development and review, and guideline recommendations; and case review and consultation. It is each committee's obligation to define for itself which of these activities it will take on, what portion of its time it will devote to each, and how it will address them. In each of the three domains, the responsible committee members should clarify their goals and assess how they might attain them feasibly and effectively. In setting out your committee's agenda, it is crucial to be selective, based on an assessment of your institution's ethics needs; your committee's collective interest, knowledge, and skills; and the available resources. Beginning with a modest plan and gradually adding to it is infinitely better than being unable to provide the services in an overly ambitious agenda.

For instance, if the ethics committee will provide ethics education, the committee should define its educational goals and how it will work to achieve them. A discussion aimed at improving educational efforts might focus on questions like the following: Toward whom should education be directed and in what format(s)? Should its efforts be confined to self-education and education of hospital staff only, or should it also sponsor educational outreach to the larger community and, if so, what form should that outreach take? Do committee members have sufficient expertise to teach ethics? Can they improve their knowledge base through continuing ethics education? If the hospital is affiliated with a medical school, are ethics committee members involved in teaching students? Can faculty who teach students medical ethics join the committee and lend their expertise to other groups within the institution? Are teaching activities geared to the needs of the institution? For instance, have members met with various disciplines and departments, such as nursing, social work, pastoral care, outpatient clinics, and the Emergency Department to see if they encounter challenging cases or have other specific requests for ethics teaching? Is there a set of basic topics in ethics in which the committee can offer instruction? Are there helpful articles and other prepared materials to distribute as part of the educational effort? What methods of evaluation should be adopted to learn which topics, formats, and instructors are well received and useful?

Similarly, in the case of writing and reviewing policies and issuing guidelines, the committee should assess its options, goals, and the needs of the institution. If other groups also handle policy development, the ethics committee might collaborate in some cases or take the lead in others, depending on the policy in question. For instance, the ethics committee might serve as consultant to colleagues in palliative care for policies on pain control at the end of life, but might have primary responsibility for revising a policy on do-not-resuscitate orders. The ethics committee should not attempt to duplicate work that is already handled well elsewhere, particularly in the domain of policy development. Rather, designated committee members can reach out to other divisions within the institution so that ethics expertise may be incorporated into policies throughout all hospital departments.

Health care ethics committees do not only function within acute care hospitals. Increasingly and as reflected in the expanded curriculum in part I, they are becoming commonplace in other types of care-providing institutions and organizations, such as nursing homes, home care agencies and visiting nurse services, psychiatric facilities, and hospice programs. (See chapter 17 for a selection of sample policies for different types of organizations.)

Though certain types of ethical issues, such as end-of-life decision making, may be common among a number of different institutions or organizations, each of them will also have its own programmatic, resource, and patient needs that require individualized attention. In addition, ethics committees are not always associated with a particular institution or facility. As noted in chapter 1, a single ethics committee might serve a number of different institutions or might make some of its members available for onsite ethics assistance at a particular facility. In each case, ethics committees should assess the particular needs of the institutions they serve and should develop policies tailored to them.

MEMBERSHIP

The committee should examine its composition and determine whether its membership reflects sufficient diversity to represent the entire institution. While some early ethics committees were constituted entirely of physicians, a committee with such a limited range of members is unlikely to be an effective resource to the institution's diverse disciplines and departments because it might only represent the physician perspective. Thus, a committee composed only of doctors may not be best qualified to understand, support, and provide ethics expertise for nurses, social workers, and other health care practitioners. These distinct health care professions adhere to specific codes of ethics and confront dilemmas that may differ from those faced by physicians. A well-designed ethics committee will reflect the multidisciplinary composition of your institution's team of health care professionals. An ethics committee consisting of diverse care professionals is also likely to do a better job of case review and policy development than a committee that has access to the views of only one or two disciplines.

Likewise, committee membership should reflect the fact that ethical issues arising in care-providing institutions are not limited to the clinical setting. As discussed in chapter 12, the health care organization itself is a moral agent with ethical obligations that inform its decisions and actions. Accordingly, the perspectives of departments such as Compliance, Human Relations, Consumer Affairs, Legal Counsel, Risk Management, and Employee Relations will enhance committee discussions.

Some committees, though by no means all, include one or two community representatives as a way of bringing the patient and family voice into the committee's deliberations. These members may be former patients or their relatives, members of the board of trustees, or individuals interested in bioethics. Community members who participate in discussions regarding patients' clinical care must understand that this is protected information and offer the same guarantee of confidentiality as health professionals.

Ethnic and cultural diversity is also an important element of committee membership. A significant number of consults stem from differences in religious practices and cultural expectations. For example, patients and family members from many cultures fear that full disclosure of a diagnosis of cancer or other serious condition will rob patients of all hope (Powell 2006). An ethics committee member from the same community serves as an educational resource to colleagues and a helpful liaison to patients, professionals, and the committee.

Another consideration that might influence decisions about committee membership is the importance of institutional perspective, support, and buy-in. Decisions that might be thought of as chiefly financial, administrative, organizational, or human resource questions often also have an ethical dimension, and administrators and institutional leaders may be able to provide a viewpoint that other committee members who have a more patient-oriented focus lack. Inclusion of senior officers might also lend the committee institutional legitimacy and traction that can facilitate the acceptance and cooperation of other health professionals with the work of the committee.

As much as an effective committee requires diversity, it also needs stability. A frequently changing membership decreases the ease with which colleagues can identify those with ethics expertise. Moreover, the committee cannot build on the experience and continued training of its membership if it is constantly changing. Committees with a high rate of turnover (or a significant proportion of no-show members) should view this as a sign of failure to thrive; busy professionals will not devote their time to a group that accomplishes little or whose work is of poor quality. In contrast, committees known for effective and skillful work enjoy a flow of volunteers seeking to join. Poor meeting attendance and a high drop-out rate signal the immediate need for intervention. The committee must address frankly every aspect of its functioning, from who chairs meetings and how effectively they are run, to whether the committee's goals are clear, realistic, useful, and adequately met.

Membership diversity also provides the committee with important access to a broad range of knowledge and skills. The American Society for Bioethics and Humanities has produced an invaluable report entitled *Core Competencies for Health Care Ethics Consultation*, now in its second edition, and a companion volume, *Improving Competencies in Clinical Ethics Consultation: An Education Guide*, which ought to be required reading for all ethics committee members. Though specifically geared to the task of ethics consultation, these core competencies are also a useful benchmark for ethics committees that provide education and policy development. The skills and knowledge described need not all be present in each individual. Indeed, a great benefit of the multidisciplinary character of the committee structure is that collective expertise can surpass that of any one person. Likewise, committee deliberations will benefit from a range of analytic viewpoints. If the overwhelming majority of members view issues through liberal lenses, the lonely member with a conservative orientation may hesitate to speak out, thereby depriving the committee of a valuable perspective.

Some of the skills noted in *Core Competencies for Health Care Ethics Consultation* include the abilities to identify and analyze values conflict, facilitate meetings, listen and communicate well, and elicit the moral views of others. Necessary knowledge and skill areas are quite broad and include moral reasoning and knowledge of bioethics issues, institutional policies, relevant health law, and familiarity with the beliefs and perspectives of staff and patients. Members who wish to further enhance their knowledge and skills might consider enrolling in one of the several one-year certificate programs, which provide in-depth study of bioethical theory and consultation techniques, and their application in the health care setting.

Committees that function at a high level continually monitor their strengths and weaknesses in expertise and skill, and address identified gaps by adding skilled members and encouraging continuing education for individual members and the group as a whole. In addition to providing ongoing education for members, a committee can also devise an orientation manual and a set of educational expectations for new members. Such a manual might include a list of useful reference works and journals in medical ethics, as well as copies of relevant institutional policies. Mentorship by a senior committee member to whom questions may be addressed and information about continuing education opportunities are also valuable. Providing a useful orientation for new members can be particularly helpful to those committees that have suffered from high turnover or low interest. Sitting through a series of meetings without having a clear role or understanding of the goals can lead new members to drift away instead of staying and contributing to the success of the committee.

EXPERTISE IN ETHICS

Ethics committees perform a unique function within a health care institution by virtue of the fact that they possess expertise in the area of ethics, an expertise that other bodies in the organization generally lack. Their role is well described as "the representation of those values and practices that define the health care institution as a moral community . . . first and foremost a community of caring" (Blake 1992, p. 297). Doubts may be raised, however, about whether there is such a thing as ethics "expertise" and, hence, whether any individual or group can possess it. The notion of expertise in ethics strikes many as objectionable on at least two grounds: (1) it presumes that there are objectively right or wrong ways of resolving ethical problems, whereas ethics is inherently subjective and relative; and (2) it may be perceived as an elitist notion since it presumes that there are certain select individuals— philosopher-kings—who, because they alone possess this expertise, are wiser and more knowledgeable about ethical matters than the rest of us. It is critical, therefore, to characterize accurately the sort of expertise that ethics committees can offer.

Ethics committees, at their best, do embody a kind of ethical expertise that involves several components, and they should not shy away from thinking of or defining themselves in this light. Knowledge of general ethical concepts and principles and some understanding of ethical theory are important requirements, but not all committee members need have extensive philosophical training in ethics. Every committee, however, should have among its members an ethicist or at least someone with some formal background in this area who is conversant with the relevant ethics literature and can educate other committee members in the fundamentals of ethics. In addition to familiarity with principles and concepts, committee members should be able to identify issues that might benefit from ethics consultation or committee attention, and distinguish them from issues more appropriately addressed by social work, consumer affairs or patient advocacy, pastoral care, risk management, or legal counsel. Finally, committee members should be able to differentiate issues about which there is consensus in the literature from those that are controversial, think about ethical problems in a critical and analytic fashion, and be sensitive to and knowledgeable about cultural differences and power asymmetries in clinical practice. Clearly, there is much that committee members have to learn and, for this reason, committee self-education must be an ongoing process rather than a one-time effort.

Skills are also important ingredients of the expertise that ethics committees possess, and they too require practice and continual honing. Requisite skills include the abilities to discern the existence and nature of particular ethical problems and dilemmas, communicate effectively and educate others, and facilitate discussion and mediation of ethical conflicts. There are widely accepted ethical (to say nothing of legal) principles that limit the options available for resolution of ethical problems and, whatever one's views about ethical relativism as an abstract philosophical theory,* there is consensus in the medical and ethics literature on specific issues. Even when ethics committees confront cases involving patients and families from different backgrounds, relativists and non-relativists alike can agree that cultural sensitivity should inform the analysis.

Further, there is no basis for the charge of elitism if it is understood that everyone on the committee can make a valuable contribution to the identification, analysis, and resolution of ethical issues. The democratic makeup of ethics committees, deliberately including individuals from different backgrounds with discrete personal and professional perspectives, as well as varying knowledge and skill sets, does not represent an objectionable form of elitism. On the contrary, the distinctive contribution of an ethics committee grows out of the conviction that an open exchange of ideas among persons with different backgrounds, values, and experiences is likely to result in a better *ethical* decision than one imposed by any single individual or profession.

LEADERSHIP

Committee leadership is of crucial importance in shaping the nature and success of the committee. The committee chair's tenure should be long enough for both organizational leadership and clinical and administrative staff to identify the leader with the ethics committee and its work. Though some committees have adopted a rotating chair, this strategy has the disadvantage of diffusing authority and decreasing visibility. On the other hand, some chairs do not provide effective leadership and an effort to support term limits may be a way to bring new energy to such a committee.

While the ethics committee chair should be a person respected within the institution, as well as someone with ethics expertise, not every facility has a person who fits this ideal description. Committees whose chair has great institutional credibility but limited formal training should be especially conscientious in continual self-education and efforts to enlist ethics professionals with formal training. A committee whose chair offers formal ethics expertise but limited clinical experience or

* Ethical relativism is the theory that all ethical judgments and principles are relative to the cultures, societies, and communities that accept them. In other words, there are no overarching universal moral norms and values from which one can criticize the judgments and principles they accept.

institutional recognition is hampered unless she builds collegial relationships with clinicians and administrators. Recognizing that most committee chairs will not have all the desired qualifications, the appointment of a co-chair who brings different knowledge, skills, and perspectives can supplement the strengths and make up for the weaknesses of a solo chair. The co-chair, or vice chair, also ensures that, in the chair's absence, the committee is not without leadership.

A strong, committed, knowledgeable, and well-respected committee chair is critical to ethics committee survival. The ethics committee chair functions as liaison between the committee and the rest of the institution. When the committee finds that a difficult recommendation is nonetheless the right one, a chair with strong collegial ties to leadership can help present the committee's views effectively. A committee chair who antagonizes colleagues with judgmental or arrogant pronouncements about what is and is not ethical undermines or at least marginalizes the work of the committee and may even cause its demise. In contrast, a chair who mediates conflict and addresses ethical tensions effectively and respectfully is an invaluable asset to the committee and the institution. Toward that end, the chair might arrange to serve on one or two strategic committees, such as the IRB, conflict of interest, or academic affairs, which provides visibility and the opportunity to form productive collaborations.

SECURING A FOOTHOLD

The ethics committee should be situated within the overall structure of hospital governance. Whether the committee reports to the medical board, the board of governors, or directly to the hospital leadership, a clear reporting structure creates accountability for the ethics committee, as is appropriate for any standing work group in the institution. The reporting structure can also affect how the committee is perceived within the institution. Reporting to the chief medical officer or the medical executive board may give the committee traction with physicians, while reporting to the Compliance or Legal Departments may create the impression that ethics is governed solely by laws and regulations. The reporting structure also shows the committee where it may turn for additional support, which may be financial, for example, funding for a lecture series, or may be political, as when the committee wants to address a sensitive topic like questionable billing practices in one hospital division or invite a controversial speaker to keynote a symposium.

An ethics committee will not flourish and may not even survive in a useful way unless it has visible, enthusiastic, and sustained institutional support from both leadership and staff. Senior leaders committed to ethics reflect that commitment in large and small ways, from including ethics representation on influential committees to placing the bioethics committee or service in a prominent place on the institutional website and in the brochure that describes the institution. In contrast, if a key leader, such as the chair of a powerful department, doubts the value of ethics endeavors, the institution will follow that lead and ethics activities will be peripheral to the organization's mission and low on its list of priorities.

New committees and those hoping to improve their efficacy need to assess and monitor their level of institutional support. Keeping in mind that directors of hospitals and other health care organizations face extraordinary demands on their time, attention, and financial resources, the ethics committee may wish to consider ways in which support might be strategically increased. Before approaching leadership to ask for support in the form of space, money, or other resources, the committee should define what it offers the institution in exchange. The notion of *value added* should frame how the committee presents itself to leadership. An ethics committee that can show how its current or planned services are or will be effective and add value to the institution is far more likely to win initial or sustained support than a committee that assumes executive backing. Clearly defining the committee's purpose, demonstrating its accomplishments and how they benefit the institution, and articulating its goals and action plans for achieving them are essential to earning organizational support.

Support does not come only from above. A committee that enjoys strong backing from leadership but fails to win the respect of colleagues will not thrive. Every bit as important as winning the confidence of senior leadership is gaining a broad base of support from staff in the various departments, disciplines, and roles. The delicate balance here is to avoid intruding while providing easy and useful access to ethics expertise.

The most effective way to earn support, of course, is to provide a valuable and visible service. A committee that actively seeks out or creates opportunities to usefully assist in resolving ethical problems will earn recognition, credibility, and repeat business; an ethics committee that sits alone in the boardroom waiting for consult requests will fail. Do not expect staff to come knocking on your door, especially if your committee is still trying to establish a presence in your institution. You must be proactive.

Identity is crucial. Assume that clinical and administrative staff do not know what an ethics committee is or how it might be useful to their work. Make your first task clearly defining your committee's purpose, responsibilities, and scope of services. If your budget permits, consider creating a pamphlet that briefly defines bioethics and explains what your committee and consult service offer. A brief introduction to the work of your committee might look something like this:

Bioethics at the Medical Center

When decisions about health care raise ethical issues in the clinical or organizational setting, the ethics consultation service and the ethics committee serve as useful resources to the medical center.

Ethics Consultation Service

The ethics consultation service is available to meet with patients, families, or designated representatives, and caregiving staff to help clarify and resolve ethical dilemmas. Anyone involved in patient care—patient, family member, health care agent, or professional care team—with an ethical concern or problem can directly access the consultation service. Some of the issues typically considered in bioethics consultations include

- How and by whom is a patient's ability to make health care decisions evaluated when consensus on capacity is lacking?

- Who should make health care decisions for patients who cannot decide for themselves or communicate their wishes?
- Why are advance directives important in health care and how are they used?
- What should happen if there is uncertainty or disagreement among the patient, family, and care team about what is best for the patient?
- What should happen if the patient or family rejects recommended interventions or care plans?
- What should happen if the family insists that the patient not be given clinical information, including diagnosis and prognosis, or be included in care decisions?
- What should happen if the health care agent makes decisions that appear to conflict with the patient's living will?
- When should life-prolonging measures, such as feeding tubes or ventilators, be started, continued, or stopped?
- What should happen if palliative measures seem to risk hastening a patient's death?
- What should happen if the care team's treatment recommendations conflict with the patient's ethical, cultural, or religious beliefs or traditions?

Clinical ethics consultations can be requested by contacting [name of committee chair or chair of consultation subcommittee] at 123-456-7890. This service is available Monday through Friday, from 8:00 a.m. to 4:30 p.m. Requests for ethics consultation during evening and weekend hours can be referred to the administrative head nurse on call through the operator. Requests will be responded to within one working day or immediately in case of emergency.

Ethics Committee
The ethics committee is a multidisciplinary body that meets monthly and on an as-needed basis to address ethical issues that arise in the clinical and organizational setting. Rather than a decision-making body, the committee is a forum for study, policy and case review, and recommendation. The committee functions to

- identify and consider ethical issues that arise in the clinical and organizational health care settings;
- explore different approaches to health care decision making in the medical center and provide recommendations for resolving ethical dilemmas in patient care;
- participate in developing and reviewing medical center policy when matters of ethics are involved;
- assist in consultations when requested by the ethics consultation service and provide consultation assessment; and
- provide educational programs about bioethical issues, within both the medical center and the wider community.

All deliberations of the consultation service and committee are confidential and all information and records are protected. There is no charge for these services.

The next task is to make your committee and its services visible, familiar, and credible. Some ethics committees and consultants make rounds with medical teams as a means of increasing visibility and offering real-time assistance. The benefit of this approach is that it brings ethics into the daily fabric of clinical care, which is where it belongs. Consider having interested committee members each adopt one ICU or other unit and join its rounds once a week. As cases are discussed, ethical issues that might have gone unrecognized can be identified and potential problems can be addressed proactively. Sometimes, the ethics representative may have little or nothing to contribute; on other occasions, a member of the care team may say, "I wasn't planning to contact the ethics committee but, as long as you're here, let's talk about this situation."

At the same time, consultants and committee members must avoid the urge to please colleagues by providing quick answers that lack depth. For example, consultants who make rounds with medical and surgical teams must have the confidence and experience to note when a situation requires a more lengthy and in-depth resolution process than can be provided during rounds. Ensure follow-up by saying to the nurse, resident or other clinician responsible for the patient, "Let's talk further after rounds so I have all the relevant information and we can give this matter the attention it deserves."

In summary, ethics committees that flourish have several elements in common. Their goals are clearly defined, and continual efforts are made to improve the ways in which these goals are met. Membership is professionally and culturally diverse, and includes significant expertise in ethics. The committee fosters a genuine exchange of ideas and beliefs, and does not try to impose an artificial uniformity on the group's deliberations. It seeks to build strong collegial relationships with both leadership and colleagues. A committee that provides effective ethics education, policy development, case review, and consultation supports the delivery of excellent health care at its institution and helps ensure that it remains "first and foremost a community of caring" (Blake 1992, p. 297).

REFERENCES

American Society for Bioethics and Humanities. 2007. *Improving Core Competencies for Ethics Consultation: An Education Guide.* Glenview, IL: American Society for Bioethics and Humanities.

American Society for Bioethics and Humanities. Task Force on Standards for Bioethics and Humanities. 2009. *Core Competencies for Health Care Ethics Consultation: The Report of the American Society of Bioethics and Humanities.* 2nd ed. Glenview, IL: American Society for Bioethics and Humanities.

Blake DC. 1992. The hospital ethics committee and moral authority. *HEC Forum* 4(5):295–98.

Fox E. 2002. Ethics consultations in U.S. hospitals: A national study and its implications. Paper presented at the Annual Meeting of the American Society of Bioethics and Humanities, October 24, Baltimore, MD.

Powell T. 2006. Culture and communication: Medical disclosure in Japan and the U.S. *American Journal of Bioethics* 6(1):18–20.

Ross JW, Glasser JW, Rasinksi-Gregory D, Gibson JM, Bayley C. 1993. *Health Care Ethics Committees: The Next Generation.* American Hospital Association.

CHAPTER 14

Clinical Ethics Consultation

This is the part that you've been waiting for—where ethical theory meets clinical reality. A key function of ethics committees is providing clinicians with an analytic framework for identifying and resolving ethical dilemmas that arise in the clinical setting. As discussed in part I, these challenges often reflect the inherent tensions between and among the ethical obligations incumbent upon health care professionals. Sometimes the situations are matters of life and death, with elements of high drama. More often, they concern the rights and responsibilities of patients, families, and caregivers as they struggle to make decisions that are clinically, ethically, and legally valid. In that process, the perspective of the ethics committee is an invaluable resource.

This chapter begins with a conceptual overview, discussing the fundamentals of clinical ethics consultation, including three models that balance skills, resources, efficiency, and effectiveness. "Building an Ethics Consultation Service: Critical Success Factors" is not, despite what you may have hoped, a kit that guides you through construction of a consultation service. Rather, it sets out the constituent parts of an effective and credible service, including consultants, their competencies, the prospect of certification, and the evaluation of consult services, and examines the essential elements of integration, leadership support, expertise, staff time, access, accountability, credibility, organizational education, and evaluation. "Analytic Approaches to Clinical Ethics Consultation" reviews two paradigms for the analysis and resolution of ethical issues and conflicts. "Selecting the Best Clinical Ethics Consultation Service Model for Your Institution," as the title suggests, invites your committee to consider all these elements in light of your institution's needs and resources, and your committee's strengths and limitations, and to determine how to most effectively provide clinical ethics consultation. The sample "Access to Bioethics

Consultation" in chapter 17 illustrates how your committee can structure the way its services can be made available.

OVERVIEW OF ETHICS CONSULTATION

Our goal in this chapter is to provide an introduction to health care ethics consultation, beginning with a conceptual overview. Ethics consultation is a structured method of helping patients, care professionals, families, and other parties resolve ethical concerns in clinical settings and is now widely recognized as an essential part of health care delivery. The vast majority of U.S. hospitals have active ethics consultation services, usually a function of the institutional ethics committee, but these services vary widely in their approach, intensity, and effectiveness (Fox 2002). Ethics consultation has been endorsed by numerous governmental and professional bodies, and is legally mandated under specific circumstances in several states (Tulsky and Fox 1996).

By providing a forum for discussion and a method of careful analysis, effective ethics consultation promotes health care practices consistent with high ethical standards, helps to foster consensus and resolve conflict in an atmosphere of respect, honors participants' authority while respecting their values and preferences in the decision-making process, educates providers to approach current and future cases according to agreed-on principles, and fosters the notion of justice by ensuring that like cases will be treated in similar ways. Ethics consultation has also been shown to save health care institutions money by reducing the provision of nonbeneficial treatments, as well as decreasing certain hospital lengths of stay (Schneiderman et al. 2003; Schneiderman, Gilmer, and Teetzel 2000; Dowdy, Robertson, and Bander 1998; Heilicser, Meltzer, and Siegler 2000). Research also suggests that an effective ethics consultation service may even reduce staff turnover when nurses and social workers perceive accessible and effective support in addressing ethical issues in the clinical setting (Ulrich et al. 2007). While these positive instrumental byproducts of bioethics consultation should be welcome, especially to organizational leadership, it must be remembered that they are not the primary goal, which is to promote sound health care decision making, with respect for clinicians, patients, and families, and support for caregiver concerns.

Early in ethics committee development, most case consultation was retrospective, and that often remains the approach today for committees just starting to do consultation. Increasingly, as committee members gain experience with each other and with the ethical norms in their institution, and as the committee becomes comfortable with reflective analysis, real-time consultation becomes more customary. Thus, ethics committees and consultation services, to one degree or another, are involved in retrospective review either of a case on which the consultation service has consulted or a case handled without ethics participation; and prospective case consultation that involves members of the ethics consultation service intervening to affect the outcome of an active case or even address a potential issue proactively. This chapter focuses on prospective consultation on active patient cases or potential ethical problems.

THREE MODELS OF CLINICAL ETHICS
CONSULTATION SERVICES

Clinical ethics consultation is a particularly challenging function and is managed differently in different institutions. In some cases, consultation is handled by a standing team or revolving subgroup of the ethics committee, while in other facilities an entirely separate group or a single individual provides consultation and reports back to the committee for its review (Fox 2002). If the ethics committee will take primary responsibility for ethics consultation, it needs to provide requisite training and support for consultants. If the committee's function will chiefly be case review, it needs to provide training to committee members in how to assess the consultant's work. This handbook begins with an educational curriculum in part I that provides ethics committee members, as well as ethics consultants, with an introduction to basic bioethical theory, and ends with a hypothetical illustration in part V of how an ethics committee might actually conduct a review of a clinical case and an institutional policy. Members who are interested in enhancing their skills in clinical ethics consultation may also wish to consider some of the training programs available across the country.

Clinical Ethics Consultation

225

Whether ethics committees assume responsibility for conducting clinical consultations on an ad hoc or rotating basis or periodically review the work done by a dedicated consultation service, members need a foundation in ethical analysis and a sense of why similar cases invoke certain reasoning. While consultation considers each case individually, the ethical concepts and principles that inform the process, presented in part I, provide analytic clarity and consistency. Committees may also find it useful to compile a library of cases that can serve as analytic models so, in addition to the case examples in part I, chapter 16 provides sample cases and the type of analyses they might receive in clinical ethics consultations.

Clinical ethics consultations are typically performed by an individual ethics consultant, an ethics committee, or an ethics consultation team. Responding to the need for clarity on the core knowledge and skills competencies required to conduct clinical ethics consultation, in 2000 the American Society for Bioethics and Humanities (ASBH) published *Core Competencies for Health Care Ethics Consultation*. This comprehensive report examined the advantages and disadvantages, strengths and weaknesses, knowledge and skills requirements, and strategies for evaluating these three models. In the absence of licensing or certification standards, *Core Competencies for Health Care Ethics Consultation* became the gold standard for ethics committees and institutions to reference in shaping their consultation services. The second edition, published in 2011, updates, expands, revises, and clarifies the content, greatly enhancing its utility. This second edition and the companion volume, *Improving Competencies in Clinical Ethics Consultation: An Education Guide* (American Society for Bioethics and Humanities, 2007), should be required reading for ethics committees and consultants.

As discussed below, each of the three models has advantages and disadvantages. Although some ethics consultation services might rely exclusively on one of these three models, it is also important to recognize that each has its effective application under different circumstances, so some combination of them might best serve the needs of your institution. Consultation services should determine which model is most appropriate for each consultation, depending on the ethical and clinical issues raised, the parties involved, the consultation skills required, and the staff available. That said, a given institution may prefer one or another consultation model and methodology and be structured to facilitate that mode most easily.

Individual or Solo Consultant Model

In this model, one person—either an independent "solo" consultant or a member of an ethics consultation team or committee—is assigned to perform a consultation alone. The advantages of the individual ethics consultant model are that it provides fewer logistical hurdles (e.g., scheduling meetings) and facilitates quick response to urgent consultation requests. The disadvantages are that the consultant must possess all required knowledge and skills to perform the consultation, he may not be able to maintain sufficient control over all aspects of the consultation process, and there are fewer checks and balances to protect against the intrusion of the consultant's own values and biases. One way to deal with some of the disadvantages is to have the consultant's initial meeting with the entire health care team, making the collective knowledge and skills of the team available as the baseline for the consultation. Depending on the particulars of a case and consultant availability, working as a pair may be advantageous. For example, the bioethics mediation approach, described below, typically utilizes an individual consultant on each case. Whenever possible, however, the consultants may prefer to work together so that they can co-mediate, a process that maximizes skills.

It is incumbent on the individual ethics consultant to recognize her strengths and limitations, and to get help when needed. The successful ethics consultant builds a web of strong, collegial relationships within the health care facility and network, and calls on others for assistance with particular clinical, ethical, legal, cultural, or religious concerns. Even the most highly trained and experienced ethics consultant benefits from confidentially discussing complex cases with other experts.

In addition, individual consultants should engage in systematic review of their consultations with colleagues. One approach is to share difficult cases with the other ethics consultants on the service and retrospectively with the ethics committee. Another check on the process comes from entering a note in the patient's medical record, where it can be read by clinicians, administrators, lawyers, and risk managers, alerting them to a developing problem. The note may be placed in the record before perspectives are solicited from other persons who have different roles in the institution and may provide useful information and feedback to the consultant.

Committee Consultation Model

In the second model, a standing interdisciplinary committee—that is, a relatively stable group of typically between 6 and 20 people—jointly performs the consultation. The advantages of this collaborative model are that it facilitates collective proficiency and includes ready access to diverse perspectives and multidisciplinary expertise. Its disadvantages are that it requires a great deal of staff time; is not well suited to situations that require a rapid response; and diffuses responsibility among committee members, which can contribute to "groupthink." Most important, the potential for patients and family members to feel intimidated by a large group of white-coated professionals works against the aims of a mediation approach, which seeks to "level the playing field." Eliminating white coats for consultants and using a small subset of the committee as the link between the committee and the patient or family can help to minimize this power imbalance.

The committee model may be especially useful for ensuring broad organizational input into difficult consultations, including those that might establish institutional precedent or end up in the media or the courts. In addition to solving the immediate problem, this sort of consultation helps to structure the situation if the problem gets magnified or blows up. This model may also be useful to facilities that are relatively new to ethics consultation, handle a low volume of consultations, or lack specialized ethics expertise. Most committees are good at talking; some are proficient in analysis; and some, with experience, can bring perspective and wisdom to the enterprise.

Team Consultation Model

In the team model, responsibility for the ethics consultation is shared by a small group of people selected from a pool of qualified consultants, typically members of the ethics committee, based on the knowledge and skills required by the circumstances of the case. The advantages of the consultation team model are that it lends itself to rapid responses and ensures diverse perspectives and expertise because the members of the team can vary to meet the situation. Small groups can be less intimidating for patients and families, and the team itself provides a natural forum for support and reflection. On the other hand, the team model is less efficient than the individual consultant model and provides fewer checks and balances than the committee model.

The team model allows tasks to be divided among members of the team, accommodates a wide range of situations and levels of consultant expertise, and is in some ways a compromise between the individual and committee models. It is the most common consultation model, used by more than two-thirds of hospitals in the United States (Fox 2002).

BUILDING AN ETHICS CONSULTATION SERVICE: CRITICAL SUCCESS FACTORS

Regardless of the consultation model(s) used, certain factors are critical for an ethics consultation service to achieve its goals and, for this reason, they should be formally incorporated into institutional policy. Ethics consultation services need to have integration, leadership support, expertise, staff time, and other resources. Access, accountability, organizational learning, and evaluation are also essential. These critical success factors are described below and, in greater detail, in the second edition of *Core Competencies for Health Care Ethics Consultation* and *Ethics Consultation: Responding to Ethics Concerns in Health Care* (Fox et al. 2005).

The successful ethics consultation service must develop and maintain positive relationships with the various individuals and programs that shape the health care organization's ethics environment and practices. Although your institution may have an ethics committee devoted to ethical issues that arise within particular services in the hospital, such as a neonatal intensive care ethics committee, an ethics consultation service should serve the entire institution, not just a particular clinical service. A fully integrated ethics consultation service responds to the entire range of ethics concerns faced by the organization, and more specialized ethics committees also contribute to the ethical culture of the institution as a whole.

The ethics consultation service should look for opportunities to forge strong connections with other departments and services within the organization, share activities and skills, and identify and work toward achieving mutual goals. The integrated service develops ongoing working relationships with programs and departments (e.g., pastoral care, patient advocacy, legal counsel, risk management, research, compliance, human resources) that commonly encounter ethics-related issues, clinical as well as non-clinical. Collaborating with different services and programs will enhance staff understanding of each other's skills and roles and contribute to the overall organizational efficiency.

One critical element in the notion of integration is access to the consultation service. If the service is to be available to all staff and patients, it is useful to have a policy that encourages any member of the staff—sub-interns to senior attendings, nurses and social workers—to request a consultation. Under such a policy, if the person calling for a consultation is not the attending of record, a call informing that physician about the consultation is an important early step in the process. It is also advisable as a matter of professional courtesy.

As with ethics committees, explicit organizational leadership support is essential if the goals of ethics consultation are to be realized. Ultimately, leaders are responsible for the success of all programs, and health care ethics consultation is no exception. Organizational leaders establish institutional priorities and allocate the resources to implement those priorities. Unless leaders support—and are perceived to support—the facility's ethics consultation service, its function cannot succeed.

Health care facility leaders should ensure that ethics consultation services have the requisite expertise, including the knowledge, skills, and character traits necessary to perform competent and effective ethics consultation. (See below for remarks on privileging ethics consultants.) Regardless of the consultation model used, the proficiencies outlined in the second edition of *Core Competencies for Health Care Ethics Consultation* must be represented on the ethics consultation service.

Ethics consultants need adequate dedicated time to perform consultation activities, the requirements of which will vary depending on the types of consultations handled. Even a straightforward ethics case consultation typically takes several hours, while more complex cases—especially those that are novel or precedent setting—may continue for more than a week, requiring 20 or more hours of effort by multiple individuals. In addition, consultation services, often supported by their ethics committees, handle a variety of other activities, including requests for general information or education, clarification of policy, review of documents, ethical analysis of hypothetical or historical ("non-active") cases or organizational ethics questions, and ethics teaching. Consultants should have a clear understanding with their supervisors that ethics consultation is not an optional or voluntary activity, but an assigned part of their jobs that requires dedicated time.

Ethics consultants need ready access to other resources, such as library materials, clerical support, training, and continuing education. Because many facility libraries lack a good selection of health care ethics references, a consultation service often needs its own core set of books and journals. A variety of useful ethics resources is also available online, making access to the Internet essential, as well. Finally, ethics consultants need training and regular continuing education to develop, maintain, and improve their knowledge and skills.

As indicated earlier, an effective ethics consultation service must be readily accessible to all patients, families, and staff. The service should be available not only in acute care hospitals, but in all care settings. Ethics consultation services should take steps to ensure that patients, families, and staff in the various sites of health care delivery are aware of the ethics consultation service, what it does, and how to access it.

Like any other important health care function, ethics consultation must have a clear system of accountability to organizational leadership and be plainly situated within the reporting hierarchy. To ensure accountability, responsibilities relating to ethics consultation should be explicitly described in the performance plans of everyone involved, from senior leaders to frontline staff.

Ethics consultants should contribute to organizational learning by sharing their knowledge and experience. Group discussion of actual cases (appropriately modified to protect the identities of participants) is an excellent way to engage and educate clinical staff. This can be done as an occasional or regular agenda item of ethics committee meetings or separately from them. With relatively little effort, a consultation service note can be reworked into a newsletter article that summarizes an important ethics topic. Policy questions handled by the service can be turned into "Frequently Asked Questions" and posted on a website. Efforts such as these not only increase staff knowledge, they also enhance the visibility, credibility, and relevance of the ethics consultation service.

The success of the ethics consultation service requires ongoing evaluation, defined as the systematic assessment of the operation and outcomes of a program compared to a set of explicit or implicit standards, as a means of contributing to the continuous improvement of the program (Weiss 1998). Evaluation efforts need not be elaborate or costly. Experts within the facility, such as quality managers, can assist in developing appropriate ways to assess these factors, ensuring that the measures used are valid and that data are collected and analyzed in a minimally burdensome fashion.

The question of how to evaluate ethics consult services has been a topic of considerable debate within the bioethics community since the inception of the practice. In the infancy of clinical ethics consultation, more than 20 years ago, there was considerable uncertainty about exactly what its goals were or should be and what academic and professional training should be required for its practitioners. The community is evolving toward consensus on the standards and methods for evaluating ethics consultation, although, given the nature of the activity, it is not surprising that some disagreement remains.

In part, this evolution is in response to larger forces in modern health care, including the patient safety movement, quality improvement practices, and pay-for-performance measures, which demand greater accountability from health care providers and organizations for the process and outcomes of their interventions. Ethics consultants are increasingly being required to demonstrate "deliverables," to show that the service they provide adds "value" to the institutions within which they work. In the quality- and cost-conscious environment of contemporary health care, they can no longer be taken seriously by health care professionals and administrators simply by appealing to vague notions of effectiveness. This evolution is also partly due to the fact that the bioethics community has gained a better understanding of consultation as a result of its growing acceptance and importance in health care institutions.

To properly evaluate ethics consult services, it is first necessary to specify their *goals* (Tarzian 2013; Dubler, Webber, and Swiderski 2009; Fletcher 1989). Primary among these is to help resolve uncertainties that arise in clinical care about the right thing to do, and conflicts between and among health care providers, patients, and families concerning the ethical care of patients. This is the particular expertise that clinical ethics consultants bring to the clinical encounter. Though conflicts are commonly what trigger requests for ethics consults, ethics consultants can also be useful in clarifying the values at stake in particular clinical situations and identifying and evaluating the various options that are available for addressing complex cases.

Further, consultants seek to promote ethical resolution of uncertainties and conflicts by providing *principled* analyses of the issues at stake, drawing on their analytic skills and relying on their knowledge of basic concepts and principles in the field of bioethics, as noted in the discussion of *Core Competencies for Health Care Ethics Consultation*, above. A principled ethical analysis is different from a mere expression of opinion, however serious and well intended the opinion may be, since the latter is not grounded in a body of principles that is consciously and consistently applied. The former analytic framework is what ethics consultants, or those who are qualified to act in this capacity, are specially trained to provide.

A second goal of ethics consultation is to provide all parties involved in the care of a patient—health care providers, family, and the patient, if able to participate—a safe space in which they can voice their views and concerns without fear of intimidation, marginalization or retribution. In an atmosphere of respect for each party, individuals who might not otherwise be heard are given the opportunity to contribute their perspectives and insights to decision making for the patient. In this way, ethics consultants seek to level the playing field and prevent any one party from dominating the discussion or the outcome. The rights and interests of the patient have priority, of course, but there are other stakeholders as well, and their views should be elicited and their relevance and import assessed. Consensus among all involved parties is not always possible or even desirable, so not all parties to the consult may be content with the outcome. But they can still be satisfied that the process has been respectful and that they have been able to effectively communicate their concerns, and this is chiefly what the consultant should aim to achieve.

A third goal of ethics consultation is to provide education for staff in how to analyze complex ethical issues so that they may become more adept at working through ethical disagreements on their own without the assistance of a trained ethics consultant. Ethics consultants should not be thought of as the "institutional conscience" because this sends a potentially invidious message that clinical care is the responsibility of the health professional and ethics the responsibility of the go-to ethics expert. There will, of course, always be situations in which the particular expertise of ethics consultants will be needed, but there are also many ethical issues that health professionals should be able to handle on their own. Among your committee's most important tasks is the constant reinforcement of the notion that ethics is a basic part of every health care professional's skill set.

Corresponding to these goals, evaluation of the ethics consultation should seek answers to the following questions: (1) Did the consultation appropriately formulate the ethical question? Did it promote a principled ethical resolution of the conflict or uncertainty in the case? (2) Did the consultant seek to and successfully establish a respectful and supportive process in which all involved parties were encouraged to express their views and concerns? These are the main questions, but another is of some importance as well: (3) Did the consultation process help to instill in other health care professionals greater understanding of and facility in discussing clinical ethics issues?

It is to be expected that a successful ethics consult will provide a principled rationale for limiting medical care when it is of marginal or no medical benefit to the patient. In addition to promoting high-quality, evidence-based clinical management, the intervention will inevitably have an impact on the costs borne by the hospital. This is especially true in the context of an ICU, where patients are the sickest and medical costs the highest. It is important to stress, however, that neither cost saving nor limiting care as such are properly goals of an ethics consultation. Rather, the goals are to ensure that only care that is beneficial to the patient is provided, thereby minimizing pain and suffering and not prolonging the dying process (e.g., Schneiderman et al. 2003).

The actual mechanics of consultation evaluation may vary from institution to institution. Measures such as reduction in the use of limited resources, decreased litigation, and fewer episodes of conflict are attractive metrics but susceptible to misuse since they might be achieved at the expense of ethical values of patient autonomy and well-being. Questionnaires and satisfaction surveys may be of some value, although their utility very much depends on the sorts of questions that are asked (Orr et al. 1996). Another approach is to establish an *external expert review process* in which consultants from other institutions are asked to evaluate the strengths and weaknesses of the consultation process in your institution, based on examination of a random selection of ethics consult notes in medical records. Examination of consult notes is obviously only an indirect measure of the effectiveness of the consultation itself, but it brings a degree of rigor and objectivity to the evaluation process.

Given the nature of the issues they address, it is not surprising that evaluating ethics consultation quality is a challenging task. Unlike medical interventions that often have specific measurable goals, success in achieving the goals of ethics consultations is not something that is readily quantifiable. It is difficult to assess whether a process has been respectful and supportive, whether care teams have acquired greater understanding of and facility in discussing ethical issues, and whether a successful resolution of an ethical conflict has been achieved. Indeed, one must first determine what counts as a "resolution" of an ethical issue, a question that is not amenable to precise measurement. Nevertheless, this does not mean that the value of ethics consultations is simply "in the eye of the beholder" and that there are no standards or criteria for assessing their quality. Fox and Arnold (1996) have proposed four such criteria:

- Did the practice, including both the process and the resolution, conform to established ethical standards? For example, a process that does not respect the rights of decisionally capable patients to informed consent and participation in decisions about their care is unacceptable.
- Did the participants find the intervention helpful? Would they request the service again (see also Schneiderman et al. 2003)?
- Did the participants perceive that the conflict was resolved in a principled manner?
- Did the participants, primarily but not exclusively health care staff, acquire new knowledge or capabilities as a result of the consultation?

No one criterion is sufficient for assessing the quality of ethics consultations (e.g., Schneiderman 2006) but, in combination, they can be a useful tool for your ethics committee, whether it conducts consults or reviews consults conducted by others.

Evaluation of the consultation process should be distinguished from evaluation of the credentials and qualifications of the ethics consultant. We turn to this next.

CREDENTIALING AND PRIVILEGING CLINICAL ETHICS CONSULTANTS

The proliferation of ethics consultation services and consultants in health care organizations has mainly been spurred by the requirements of the Joint Commission, the country's leading health care institution accrediting agency, that each institution establish an "ethics mechanism" to address ethical issues that arise in the course of patient care. The practice, however, has largely gone unregulated. It has proceeded without any clear or precise idea of who is qualified to do these consultations, what educational background and skills are required, and how they should be reviewed for quality. If the field of clinical ethics consultation is to legitimately be considered a "profession" and not merely an assortment of individuals with varying degrees of expertise, knowledge, and supervision, standards have to be developed. And, as with any profession, these standards must originate within the profession itself. They must then be supported by the institutions within which the consultants do their work through a process of privileging.

It is now generally accepted within the profession that ethics consultation and ethics consultants must be subjected to a level of scrutiny comparable to that of other members of the medical staff who see patients and write notes in the medical record. One proposal (Dubler and Blustein 2007; Dubler, Webber, and Swiderski 2009) is for a *credentialing* process that involves three basic components: participation in a formal training program, emphasizing the inculcation of a basic core of bioethical knowledge and proficiency in techniques of dispute resolution and mediation; completion of a one-year apprenticeship, similar to a clinical fellowship for medical specialties like oncology and critical care, under the direction of an experienced consultant-mentor; and verification of qualifications by appropriate documentation of the consultant's performance and fitness to do ethics consultations. For these measures to affect actual clinical practice, however, professional oversight is not sufficient. Hospitals must also take control of the process by establishiing methods for examining these individuals and making judgments about their preparation and training before they can be permitted to do consultations. This is the process of *privileging*, and ethics consultants no less than other medical practitioners should undergo it.

Recently, a task force of the American Society for Bioethics and Humanities, the professional organization that includes bioethics researchers, teachers, and clinical ethics consultants, proposed a two-step model for "quality attestation" for ethics consultants (Kodish et al. 2013). This is an elaborate process that involves assembling a portfolio consisting, among other things, of the following: a curriculum vitae, showing that the candidate has successfully completed at least a master's degree in a relevant discipline; a summary of the candidate's consultation education and experience; three letters of evaluation from individuals with responsibility for clinical oversight who are familiar with the candidate's work; and six discussions of case consultations that the candidate has led or co-led. If the candidate's portfolio passes muster, she is then eligible for an oral examination, which provides direct assessment of the candidate's interpersonal skills, bioethical knowledge, and ability to apply it appropriately. The authors of this report admit that their model is not a finished product and that quality attestation is a work in progress that will have to be refined over time.

One criticism of the model as so far developed is that it seems most suitable for major medical centers or teaching hospitals, not for smaller hospitals where few consultations are likely to be performed. Another is that the proposal seems premised on an individual ethics consultant model rather than a multidisciplinary team model of ethics consultation (Postema 2013). Adjustments will have to be made in the model to accommodate the diversity of both organizational contexts and consultation models.

ANALYTIC APPROACHES TO CLINICAL ETHICS CONSULTATION

The following two approaches to ethics consultation reflect the quite different natures of the institutions that use them, as well the perceptions of the professionals involved regarding their expertise, authority, and responsibility. Each structures the consultation process in different ways. In the CASES approach, developed for use throughout the Veterans Health Administration (VHA) system, ethics consultants are systematically guided through the process and practice of ethics consultations involving active patient cases. Bioethics mediation, the approach developed and used at Montefiore Medical Center, is based on the consult team's experience that calls for ethics consultations that are generally requests for help in resolving or managing conflict. Thus, it may be that the CASES approach will be very useful for certain medical centers or health systems, while the mediation approach may be more suited to others. Alternatively, some combination of these approaches or one of the several others not discussed here might prove useful, depending on the circumstances of a particular consultation and the resources of particular institutions and their consultation services.

We suggest that you use these two examples as just that—illustrations of possible analytic approaches to ethics consultation that may help guide you as you consider how to structure your ethics consultation service. You may wish to adopt elements of each and to explore whether and when each is appropriate for use in your institution.

The CASES Model—Kenneth A. Berkowitz, M.D.

The National Center for Ethics in Health Care is the primary office of the VHA for addressing the complex ethical issues that arise in patient care, health care management, and research. The mission of the National Center for Ethics in Health Care is to clarify and promote ethical health care practices within the VHA, the country's largest integrated health care delivery system. Toward this end, the National Center for Ethics in Health Care developed the CASES approach to health care ethics case consultation, a systematic step-by-step approach to providing consistent, effective, and standardized ethics case consultation at VHA facilities. Ethics consultants or committees wishing to learn more about the CASES approach and are considering its applicability are encouraged to consult the comprehensive discussion, including tools, templates, sample cases, and other resources, in *Ethics Consultation: Responding to Ethics Concerns in Health Care* (Fox et al. 2005).

The CASES approach involves five steps:

1. Clarify the consultation request
2. Assemble the relevant information
3. Synthesize the information
4. Explain the synthesis
5. Support the consultation process

These steps were designed to guide ethics consultants through the complex critical thinking needed to perform ethics case consultation effectively. They are intended to be used in much the same way clinicians use a standard format for taking a patient's history, performing a physical exam, or documenting a clinical case. Even when specific, observable action is not required, each step should be considered systematically as part of every ethics case consultation. Although the steps are presented in a linear fashion, *ethics consultation is a fluid process and the distinction between steps may blur in the context of a specific case.* At times, it may be necessary to repeat steps or perform them in a different order than presented here.

Clarify the Consultation Request

The first step requires the consultant to gather information from the requester to form a preliminary understanding of the circumstances and reasoning that prompted an ethics consultation request. Two initial questions should help the consultant confirm whether the request is appropriate for ethics consultation:

Question 1: Does the requester want help resolving an ethics concern, that is, uncertainty or conflict over which decisions or actions are ethically justifiable?

Question 2: Does the request pertain to an active patient case? *If the answers to both questions 1 and 2 are "yes, there is an ethical concern about an active patient case," the request should be handled through the CASES approach.*

Next, the consultant should formulate the ethics question, a sometimes difficult but essential part of ethics case consultation. Clarity about the ethics question allows all participants to focus on the same concerns and work efficiently toward resolution, while an imprecisely formulated question can sidetrack or derail the consultation process. Accordingly, the consultant should formulate the ethics question early in the consultation process and examine it again once all the relevant information is assembled.

Assemble the Relevant Information

Next, the consultant assembles the information necessary to develop a comprehensive picture of the circumstances and work through the case to facilitate an answer to the ethics question. The CASES approach builds on the work of Jonsen, Siegler, and Winslade (2002) in defining topics that should be reviewed in every ethics consultation, but reframes relevant information into four categories (medical facts, patient's preferences and interests, other people's preferences and interests, and ethics knowledge).

Considering the ethics question requires a review of the relevant ethics knowledge, which might include codes of ethics, ethical standards and guidelines, consensus statements, scholarly publications, precedent cases, applicable institutional policy, and law. The ethics consultant will be helped by familiarity with ethics-related journals and texts and an ability to perform computer-assisted information searches. Depending on the consultant's expertise, preparation may include selected readings or a literature review and sometimes discussion with a more experienced consultant.

Synthesize the Information

The consultant next analyzes and synthesizes the assembled relevant information into practical terms, applying the ethics knowledge to the other case-specific information and the ethics question. This difficult yet important proficiency requires a foundation of strong analytic skills, drawing on different approaches to moral reasoning and augmented by reading, study, and supervised practical experience. Based on the circumstances of the case, the consultant should determine whether synthesis would be promoted by a formal meeting of the parties, separate face-to-face discussions, or, in simple situations, telephone or deidentified electronic communication.

Explain the Synthesis

The completed synthesis should be made clear to others involved in the case through direct communication to key participants and documentation in both the medical record and consultation service records.

Support the Consultation Process

The consultant's final step is to support the overall process of ethics case consultation by following up with participants and learning what was done, completing a critical self-review after each case, soliciting feedback from peers, and assessing how the ethics consultation service is perceived by systematically surveying the participants in the case. Ethical issues that need to be addressed at the systems level should be brought to the attention of the appropriate individual or body.

Mediation: The Montefiore Medical Center Model—Nancy Neveloff Dubler, LL.B.

The following brief description is intended only to introduce bioethics mediation as one model for consultation services prepared to engage in the necessary training. Ethics committees wishing to learn more about bioethics mediation and are considering its applicability are encouraged to consult the comprehensive discussion, including case analyses and role plays, presented in *Bioethics Mediation: A Guide to Shaping Shared Solutions* (Dubler and Liebman 2004), where much of the material below appeared in an earlier form.

The Montefiore Medical Center bioethics consultation service was established in 1978 and, by the mid-1980s, the original bioethics consultants were responding to increasing requests for clinical ethics consultation. In time, it became clear that, rather than providing ethics directives or even analysis, the consultations offered some form of alternative dispute resolution or mediation.

In addition to a mastery of the rights, interests, and agreed-on principles of bioethics—an indispensable knowledge base—mediation adds techniques for managing and resolving conflict. Constructing a working hypothesis; framing and reframing issues; identifying underlying interests, concerns, and available options; supporting and stroking the parties; caucusing; and reaching incremental points of agreement are all skills that can be achieved through training. As mediation is increasingly valued for its effectiveness in resolving conflicts in many fields, its techniques are being taught in many forums around the country. Courses are given by mediation centers, as well as local and state bar associations, universities, and corporations trying to enhance employee productivity. The Internet provides an extensive array of options.

To further clarify this brief introduction to ethics mediation, consider the following questions:

1. What is mediation?

Mediation is a technique that is particularly well suited to conflict resolution in the health care setting. Bioethics mediation combines the clinical substance and perspective of bioethics consultation with the techniques of mediation and dispute resolution to

- identify the parties to the conflict (although disagreements between family and care providers are common, most conflicts have more than two sides);
- understand the stated (presented) and latent interests of the participants;
- level the playing field to minimize disparities of power, knowledge, skill, and experience (to the degree possible) that separate medical professional, patient, and family;
- help the parties define their interests;

- help maximize options for a resolution of the conflict;
- search for common ground or areas of consensus;
- ensure that the consensus can be justified as a "principled resolution," compatible with the principles of bioethics and the legal rights of patients and families;
- help to implement the agreement; and
- conduct follow-up. (Dubler and Liebman 2004, p. 10)

Bioethics mediation is different from bioethics consultation. *Bioethics consultation* refers to a directed substantive process. The consultant listens to the parties and helps move them toward a principled resolution of the dispute by explaining ethical principles and legal rules, applying them to the facts, and presenting the social consensus on the permissibility of different practices. *Bioethics mediation* refers to the use of classical mediation techniques to identify, understand, and resolve conflicts.

2. Why is bioethics mediation well suited to the resolution of conflicts in the health care setting?

In difficult cases, the real question is, which is the "least bad" process for drawing out and resolving the issues? Conflict must and will be resolved because the delivery of care demands that physicians, nurses, and other care providers be guided by a coherent plan. If necessary, that plan can be imposed by the medical or the administrative staff.

One of the greatest advantages of using the mediation process in bioethics disputes is its flexibility. The general structure of mediation can be altered and adapted to fit the needs of the participants and the clinical realities. One exception to the extended flexibility is the need to reach a "principled resolution." This requires that the rights of the parties, as distinct from their interests, be protected. Thus, it would not be possible to agree that a decisionally capable and adequately informed patient should be excluded from a decision about discontinuing life-sustaining treatment. It might, however, be possible to postpone that decision, until one or more of her family members has had time to adjust to the inevitable outcome. It is key to this intervention to remember that the process is a part of the product.

3. What are the limitations of bioethics mediation?

Bioethics mediation is not for every situation. Parties to a mediation must want to reach agreement. In some cases, the patient or family members may not have the emotional strength to face difficult facts or make hard choices.

4. Why should bioethics consultants try techniques of mediation?

In the experience of the Montefiore Medical Center bioethics consultation service, mediation often works for the reasons discussed above. Even when it does not work, it often helps to define and delineate the conflict. Finally, after the consultation service is experienced and has integrated mediation into practice, its collegial process may mean that medical staff will be more willing to call for help.

SELECTING THE BEST CLINICAL ETHICS CONSULTATION SERVICE MODEL FOR YOUR INSTITUTION

The foregoing discussion, as well as reference to the second edition of *Core Competencies for Health Care Ethics Consultation*, should assist your committee in shaping the clinical ethics consultation service that can most realistically and effectively meet the needs of your institution. Note the emphasis on *realistically*. In a perfect world, your ethics committee membership would include several individuals with broad and deep knowledge of bioethical theory, formal training in ethical analysis, collaborative relationships with organizational leadership and powerful clinical department chairs, and experience in conducting ethics consultation. If you live in that world, you may skip the rest of this chapter and move on to chapter 15.

More likely, however, your committee is made up of busy health care professionals with more interest in clinical ethics than knowledge or skills in addressing problematic ethical issues. The clinical and administrative staff in your institution may be unfamiliar with or have a negative association with ethics consultation; in either event, they may not be receptive to a new problem-solving initiative. Your organizational leadership may be skeptical, especially if the service is going to require resources. Your task, then, is to identify the ethics-related needs of your institution, assess the strengths your members bring, and determine what your consultation service can feasibly provide. Begin by considering a few questions:

- Which committee members have expressed interest in ethics consultation? Which disciplines do they represent? What are their current responsibilities?
- Do any consultants have formal or informal training in mediation, group dynamics, or other types of group interaction?
- Where do most ethical issues arise in your institution? Likely sites include ICUs, oncology units, emergency units, pediatrics, and neonatology. Do any consultants work in those areas?
- Will your consult team agree to read selected materials that provide a basic introduction to bioethics and ethics consultation, and meet on a regular basis to discuss assigned readings and engage in brief role plays or other exercises simulating consultation on ethical issues? The sample cases in chapter 16 can be useful as vignettes.

Deploying your consultants according to their knowledge, skills, availability, and preferences will require structure and the discipline to resist the temptation to promise more than you can deliver. Logistics also deserve attention, as indicated by the following questions:

- Recognizing that a group of consultants may be intimidating, would members of the consult team prefer to work in dedicated pairs or with any other available consultant?
- Does your committee, committee chair, or other member of the consult team have access to a full- or part-time secretary who can field consult requests, contact members of the consult service and key parties who should be included in the consult, and schedule meetings at mutually convenient times?

- What are the blocks of time during which your consult team can respond to consult requests? This requires a clear statement about how requests after hours, on weekends, or on holidays will be handled.
- Will consultants be on call on a rotating basis? Will there be a dedicated pager or an office number for requestors to call?
- If after-hours requests will be fielded by an administrative head nurse or other non-consultant, what information should that person obtain? Essentials include the patient's name, location and medical record number, name and contact number of the requestor, brief statement of the reason for the consult request, and the urgency of the issue.
- Do all members of your consult team have access to patient records for documentation of consults?
- How will follow-up be managed to ensure that the agreed-on resolutions are implemented?

Whichever model you decide best fits your institution's needs and your team's resources, be prepared to modify the process according to your consultants' experience and the feedback you receive from the consult participants.

ACCESS TO CLINICAL ETHICS CONSULTATION POLICIES

The effectiveness of any intervention depends largely on how well those requesting and participating in the intervention understand its purpose, procedure, accessibility, and appropriateness. This clarity is especially important in regard to clinical ethics consultation, which may not be a familiar resource to your clinical and administrative staff. For that reason, the structure, function, and processes of ethics consultation should be formalized in institutional policy that addresses

- the goals of ethics consultation;
- who may perform ethics consultation;
- who may request ethics consultations and the process for doing so;
- which issues are appropriate for referral to the ethics consultation service;
- which consultation model(s) may be used and when;
- who must be notified when an ethics consultation has been requested;
- how ethics consultations will be conducted;
- how ethics consultations will be documented;
- how participant confidentiality will be protected;
- who is accountable for the ethics consultation service; and
- how the quality of ethics consultation will be assessed and monitored.

Sample policies addressing access to clinical ethics consultation appear chapter 17.

REFERENCES

American Society for Bioethics and Humanities. 2011. *Core Competencies for Health Care Ethics Consultation: The Report of the American Society for Bioethics and Humanities.* 2nd ed. Glenview, IL: American Society for Bioethics and Humanities.

American Society for Bioethics and Humanities. Clinical Ethics Task Force. 2007. *Improving Competence in Ethics Consultation: A Learner's Guide*. Glenview, IL: American Society for Bioethics and Humanities.

American Society for Bioethics and Humanities. Task Force on Standards for Bioethics and Humanities. 1998. *Core Competencies for Health Care Ethics Consultation: The Report of the American Society for Bioethics and Humanities*. Glenview, IL: American Society for Bioethics and Humanities.

Dowdy MD, Robertson C, Bander JA. 1998. A study of proactive ethics consultation for critically and terminally ill patients with extended lengths of stay. *Critical Care Medicine* 26(2):252–59.

Dubler NN, Blustein J. 2007. Credentialing ethics consultants: An invitation to collaboration. *American Journal of Bioethics* 7(2):35.

Dubler NN, Liebman CB. 2004. *Bioethics Mediation: A Guide to Shaping Shared Solutions*. New York: United Hospital Fund.

Dubler NN, Webber M, Swiderski D. 2009. Charting the future: Credentialing, privileging, quality, and evaluation in clinical ethics consultation. *Hastings Center Report* 39(6):23–33.

Fletcher, John C. 1989. Standards for evaluation of ethics consultation. In Fletcher JC, Quist N, Jonsen AR, eds. *Ethics Consultation in Health Care*. Baltimore: Health Administration Press, pp. 171–84.

Fox E. 2002. Ethics consultation in U.S. hospitals: A national study and its implications. Annual Meeting of the American Society for Bioethics and Humanities. October 24, Baltimore, MD.

Fox E, Arnold RM. 1996 Evaluating outcomes in ethics consultation research. *Journal of Clinical Ethics* 7(2):127–38.

Fox E, Berkowitz KA, Chanko BL, Powell T. 2005. *Ethics Consultation: Responding to Ethics Concerns in Health Care*. Washington, DC: Veterans Health Administration. www1.va.gov/integratedethics/download/EthicsConsultationPrimer.pdf (accessed May 1, 2006).

Heilicser BJ, Meltzer D, Siegler M. 2000. The effect of clinical medical ethics consultation on health-care costs. *Journal of Clinical Ethics* 11(1):31–38.

Jonsen AR, Siegler M, Winslade WJ. 2002. *Clinical Ethics: A Practical Approach to Ethical Decisions in Clinical Medicine*. 5th ed. Columbus, OH: McGraw-Hill Medical.

Kodish E, Fins JJ, et al. 2013. Quality attestation for clinical ethics consultants: A two-step model from the American Society for Bioethics and Humanities. *Hastings Center Report* 43(5):26–36.

Orr, RD, et al. 1996. Evaluation of an ethics consultation service: Patient and family perspective. *American Journal of Medicine* 101(2):135–41.

Postema D. 2013. Does quality attestation come in only one size? *Hastings Center Report* 43(5):39–40.

Schneiderman LJ. 2006. Effect of ethics consultations in the intensive care unit. *Critical Care Medicine* 34(11):S359–S363.

Schneiderman LJ, Gilmer T, Teetzel HD. 2000. Impact of ethics consultations in the intensive care setting: A randomized, controlled trial. *Critical Care Medicine* 28(12):3920–24.

Schneiderman LJ, Gilmer T, Teetzel HD, Dugan DO, Blustein J, Cranford R, Briggs KB, Komatsu GI, Goodman-Crews P, Cohn F, Young EWD. 2003. Effect of ethics consultations on nonbeneficial life-sustaining treatments in the intensive care setting: A randomized controlled trial. *Journal of the American Medical Association* 290(9):1166–72.

Tarzian AJ. 2009. Credentials for clinical ethics consultation—are we there yet? *HEC Forum* 21(3):241–48.

Tarzian AJ. 2013. Health care ethics consultation: An update on core competencies and emerging standards from the American Society for Bioethics and Humanities' Core Competencies Update Task Force. *American Journal of Bioethics* 13(2):3–13.

Tulsky JA, Fox E. 1996. Evaluating ethics consultation: Framing the questions. *Journal of Clinical Ethics* 7(2):109–15.

Ulrich C, O'Donnell P, Taylor C, Farrar A, Danis M, Grady C. 2007. Ethical climate, ethics stress, and the job satisfaction of nurses and social workers in the United States. *Social Science & Medicine* 65:1708–19.

Weiss CH. 1998. *Evaluation Methods for Studying Programs and Policies.* 2nd ed. Upper Saddle River, NJ: Prentice Hall

CHAPTER 15

Ethics Education

Brown bag lunches
Journal clubs
Case conferences
Ethics grand rounds
Ethics modules in residency training and medical school programs
Ethics symposia
White papers, memoranda, guidelines, and protocols
Additional education opportunities

A key function of your ethics committee is providing education to your members and the clinical and administrative staff of your institution. The quality of committee deliberations reflects the depth and breadth of knowledge members bring to the consideration of ethical issues that arise in the clinical and organizational settings. The utility of committee recommendations about institutional practices depends on the ethical analysis that supports them. Explaining all this to administrators, trustees, and clinical staff members enhances broader understanding of the issues, their significance, and their resolution, as well as the value of the ethics committee as an institutional resource.

Ethics education can use many formats and we encourage you to experiment with interventions that are likely to get the best reception and have the greatest impact in your institution. Listed below are educational programs requiring varying degrees of time and effort commitment, only some of which may be suitable for you to consider. Depending on the interest, knowledge, and expertise of your committee members, as well as the size of your institution and the resources available, it is likely that your committee will undertake only a few strategies. Recognizing that membership on your ethics committee is an addition to rather than a replacement for your day job, the following is a list of formats from which you are invited to select one or two that seem appealing and feasible.

BROWN BAG LUNCHES

These informal sessions, sometimes known as "Lunch and Learn," may be held on a regular basis or whenever some ethical issue is particularly timely. They are typically open to the entire staff. An obvious appeal to busy professionals is the notion of multitasking—"Turn your lunch into an opportunity to eat *and* be educated."

Topics can range from the theoretical to the practical, focusing on national or local events, and addressing general issues or the particular needs of your institution. Major legal decisions, scientific advances, institutional protocols, and clarification of misperceptions are all appropriate topics for these meetings. For example, a discussion devoted to the implications of health care reform could be synchronized with the Supreme Court's decision about the constitutionality of the Patient Protection and Affordable Care Act, discussed in chapter 11 and summarized in part IV. A discussion about the ethics of cloning could be timed to coincide with revelations of scientific advances in stem cell research. These sessions can also provide opportunities to get input or feedback on new or revised policies and procedures. For example, if your ethics committee is reviewing a policy about conscientious objection, this would be an ideal forum in which to elicit clinicians' opinions and concerns.

One member of your ethics committee or a subcommittee that rotates the responsibility might organize and lead these lunches. The leader selects and becomes familiar enough with the topic to present a brief background and the salient points that make it relevant to the attendees. A lit search on PubMed or through your medical library should provide the necessary information. Because this is an informal discussion rather than a lecture, the leader may find it helpful to develop a brief outline, including key points and questions, to guide discussion. Depending on the topic and the resources available, optional handouts, including links to especially informative articles, might occasionally be useful. Because these sessions are informal and designed to promote education of staff and the ethics committee members responsible for facilitating discussion, the responsibilities of the leader(s) should not be unduly burdensome.

JOURNAL CLUBS

Regular journal club meetings to discuss recent and important issues in medical ethics are a good way to remain current with the literature. Selected ethics committee members could be assigned or volunteer to lead the discussions on a rotating basis. In addition to journal articles, chapters from significant books in the field, perhaps combined with relevant articles, might be assigned. Another valuable use of discussion groups is as a forum for presenting and getting feedback about works in progress by members of your ethics committee or other staff in your institution.

To avoid the perception of burdensome homework, readings should be selected based on relevance, intellectual accessibility, and length. The target group is likely not people with a deep background in bioethics, law, or philosophy. An article or chapter that is highly theoretical or arcane, textually dense or filled with jargon, or very long will discourage people from reading it and diminish their interest in future sessions. In contrast to other educational groups, journal clubs are most successful when participation is restricted to ethics committee members and special invited guests.

CASE CONFERENCES

An extremely effective way of making your ethics committee known and valued by your institution is working with particular departments and services to set up case conferences featuring ethically difficult cases, either on a regular or as-needed basis. These conferences should be distinguished from clinical ethics consultations, which, as discussed in part II, analyze the ethical issues raised by specific clinical cases with the goal of assisting in the resolution of ethical conflict or confusion. The participants typically include the patient, when able to engage in discussion and decision making; the patient's family or another surrogate decision maker when the patient lacks capacity; the members of the care team most directly engaged in the patient's care; and the ethics consultant. A summary of the clinical ethics consultation, including the recommended or agreed-on resolution, is entered into the patient's medical record.

In contrast, the cases presented at case conferences generally have already been resolved or at least significant progress has been made, so that there is no current need for ethics intervention. The purpose of the conferences is to debrief and educate staff about how to identify and analyze the ethical issues that arise in the course of their practice. These conferences are attended by chiefs of service, attending physicians, residents, interns, medical students, nurses, and members of other disciplines on the care team. Depending on the case, they may be conducted jointly with one or more departments or services, such as oncology, neonatology, pediatrics, internal medicine, geriatrics, palliative care, and family medicine. Normally, a member of the health care team involved in the case is chosen to present the relevant medical information, followed by the medical ethicist who analyzes the case from an ethical perspective, identifying the relevant ethical issues, the principles or obligations that may be in conflict, the implications for the therapeutic dynamic, and the options for resolution. Attendee participation is encouraged.

Case conferences do not have to be established de novo. Especially if the intent is to present them on a regular basis, it is often difficult for staff to make room in their busy schedules for yet another meeting. One solution is to piggy-back onto an already established regular meeting, such as morning report, patient safety committee, quality assurance (QA), or morbidity and mortality (M&M) conferences. The added benefit of this approach is that the ethics perspective is implicitly recognized as a valued contribution to the clinical deliberations. In other words, ethics is playing with the cool kids. That said, it might also be possible to create a new slot for ethics conferences on the calendars of one or more resident training programs (see "Ethics Modules in Residency Training and Medical School Programs" below) by linking up with a chief of service, department chair, or program director who is either on your ethics committee or believes that ethics is an integral part in clinical care. The importance of your ethics committee establishing mutually respectful collaborations with key members of the professional clinical community cannot be overstressed.

ETHICS GRAND ROUNDS

Among your ethics committee's most important contributions to your institution is introducing bioethics to the clinical and administrative staff, making ethical principles and concepts familiar, and keeping ethical issues on the institutional radar. One successful strategy is ethics grand rounds, a regularly scheduled forum open to the entire organization for discussion of ethics-related topics. Possible formats include presentations by members of your committee or outside speakers with expertise on a particular topic, debates, or panel discussions. Topics can include classic ethical issues like informed consent or truth telling; ethical dilemmas presented by challenging clinical cases or organizational situations; legal cases with ethical implications; articles in clinical journals; and ethics-related stories making local, national, or international news.

In developing a new bioethics service, one author (LFP) had three goals for the monthly ethics grand rounds:

- attract a broad representation of clinical, administrative, research, and academic attendees;
- instill the notion that ethics resides, not just in the bioethicist or the ethics committee, but in all disciplines and levels of responsibility; and
- engage attendees in actively deliberating the issues presented by the selected topics.

Accordingly, the format for this medical center's ethics grand rounds includes presenting an intriguing topic and inviting one or more professionals with relevant expertise to be guest speaker(s) on an informal panel. Guests have included physicians, nurses, and social workers; directors of the Compliance, Human Resources, Palliative Care, Risk Management, and Legal Department; hospital coordinators for hospice and the organ sharing network; and occasional outside guests with particular expertise. In addition to the opportunity to discuss provocative ethical issues, attendees and guest speakers are attracted by the continuing educational credits offered to physicians, nurses, and other professionals.

Preparation includes a flyer emailed to the entire medical center community several days before the rounds, listing the topic, guest speaker(s), and three objectives; the director of bioethics and guest speaker(s) reviewing a list of relevant articles suggested by a medical library lit search; and posting a selection of those articles on the Bioethics Library Link on the institution's intranet so attendees can access them either before or within six months after each session. The director begins each session with a three- to five-minute set-up, presenting a brief background of the topic and establishing the analytic context by answering the question, "Why is this an ethical issue?" Then, using a series of questions developed by the director and supplemented by the guest speaker(s), the panel considers and engages attendees in deliberating the ethical issues raised by the topic. A sample list of topics and guest speakers is presented below.

- The Ethics of a Marketplace for Organs (Director, Transplant Surgery)
- The Ethics of Palliation and Palliative Care (Medical Director, Pain and Palliative Care Service)

- The Ethics of Organ Donation after Cardiac Death (Director, Transplant Surgery)
- The Ethics of Saying, "I'm Sorry" (Head of Risk Management; Legal Counsel)
- The Ethics of Using Placebos in the Routine Care and Treatment of Children (Director of Pain and Palliative Care; Vice Chair, Department of Pediatrics)
- The Ethics of Health Care during Pandemics (Chairman, Emergency and Trauma Center)
- The Ethics of Futility: How Do We Define It? How Do We Identify It? How Do We Address It? (Four Critical Care Intensivists)
- The Ethics of Breaking Bad News (Head of Risk Management; Associate Legal Counsel)
- The Ethics of IVF-Induced High-Order Multiple Pregnancies (Chief, High-Risk Pregnancy; Chief, Neonatology)
- The Ethics of Post-Mortem Sperm Retrieval (Director of Reproductive Endocrinology; Chief, Department of Sexual Health and Infertility)
- The Ethics of Religion-Based Refusal of Medical Treatment (Coordinator, Bloodless Medicine and Surgery)
- The Ethics of Vegetative States and Other Disorders of Consciousness (Physician, Department of Neurology)
- Patient Satisfaction and Patient Care: Are These Goals Ever in Tension? (APN and Director, Nursing; Administrative Director, Service Excellence; Chief Compliance Officer)
- The Ethics of the Electronic Medical Record (Chief Medical Informatics Officer)
- The Ethics of Children as Organ Donors and Survivor Siblings (Vice Chair, Department of Pediatrics; Chief, Transplant Surgery)
- Whose Life Is It Anyway? The Ethics of Voluntarily Stopping Eating and Drinking (VSED) (Visiting Professor, Department of Preventive Medicine; Director, Center for Medical Humanities)
- There Is No Administrative or Two-Physician Consent: Who Makes Decisions for the Patient Alone? (Chief, Critical Care; Head, Risk Management; Associate Legal Counsel)
- Disney in the Nursery: Commercialization in the Clinical Setting (Chief, Neonatology)
- The Ethics of the National Drug Shortage (Clinical PharmD)

ETHICS MODULES IN RESIDENCY TRAINING AND MEDICAL SCHOOL PROGRAMS

Since 1999, the Accreditation Council for Graduate Medical Education (ACGME) has included ethics under professionalism in required competencies in residency programs. This means that, as a condition of accreditation, all residency training programs must include some ethics content. You can see why program directors might suddenly be interested in clinical ethics. Your committee can become a valuable educational resource by developing ethics modules to introduce into the residency training programs of clinical departments in your institution. The module can be taught in a more or less formal manner, ranging from lectures with regular readings and even short essay assignments to informal seminars devoted to ethical analysis of selected cases or issues. One author gives each program director a list of the topics that will be presented during the coming year so residents can identify and prepare summaries of two or three cases with relevance to each topic. Each session begins with 10 to 15 power point slides about the selected topic, followed by discussion of the illustrative cases presented by the residents.

Having read part I of this handbook, you already know that topics such as decisional capacity, informed consent, confidentiality, autonomy, and care at the end of life will be relevant to all training programs. Some material will have to be adapted to specialties, such as pediatrics, psychiatry, OB/GYN, and dentistry. The duration of the modules can vary, depending on how frequently the groups meet and the length of each session. You will need to determine how many committee members are interested in taking on this responsibility, as well as the knowledge and skills they each bring. Certainly, it makes sense to match a member who is a neonatologist with a program training residents in that field.

Begin by assessing the level and scope of interest. Some program directors may reach out to you, while others may need enticing. Consider sending an e-mail to program directors, letting them know that your committee can provide this service. Meet with the interested directors to determine the respective needs of their programs. Some are satisfied with an annual lecture on the basics of bioethics, while others are eager for their residents to meet quarterly or even monthly to focus on specific ethical issues. You will also need to work out logistics that are mutually convenient and comfortable (length of each session, meeting place, necessary equipment and other resources), recognizing that these are commitments for all parties. Family medicine and geriatrics residency programs may be good places to begin.

Hospitals affiliated with medical schools typically have third-year students rotating through selected clinical settings. This is an ideal opportunity to reach future doctors at the very beginning of their clinical experience and instill in them the notion of ethics as integral to the therapeutic dynamic. Depending on the level of interest, knowledge, and expertise on your committee, you may be able to arrange for one or more members to meet with small groups of students on each of their clinical rotations. One author has found that a successful format is to begin each session by asking, "What is it about [pediatrics / psychiatry / emergency medicine / obstetrics / internal medicine / surgery] that raises ethical issues that are different from those you might encounter in other clinical settings"? Because case-based teaching is typically more effective than didactics, students are encouraged to identify present relevant cases for discussion.

ETHICS SYMPOSIA

Another educational opportunity is a symposium, which enables both a broader and deeper examination of a topic than is possible in ethics grand rounds. The format may include at least one keynote address, ideally presented by a well-recognized authority with expertise in the topic; additional presentations that examine the issues from particular perspectives; one or more panel discussions(s); and break-out sessions in which small groups of attendees and speakers discuss selected aspects of the topic with an optional summary report to the full group of attendees. If you are able to engage two experts with divergent views on the selected topic, you may be able to present a stimulating debate.

Depending on the topic, the allocated budget, and the available resources, a symposium may be a full-day event, including a light breakfast, lunch, and afternoon snack, or a half-day event, perhaps with a luncheon for the keynote speaker(s), the ethics committee, and invited organizational leaders, and a break with refreshments for attendees. The program may be limited to invited professionals or be open to the lay public, as well. Admission may be complementary or require a modest registration fee. Publicity may consist of e-mailed flyers or brochures with information about the topic, speaker(s), agenda, and registration, as well as articles or announcements in targeted newspapers and professional journals. Your mailing list should target care-providing institutions and include ethics committee chairs and, depending on the topic, organizational leaders responsible for relevant areas, such as patient care, research, or marketing. Your list may also include schools of medicine, nursing, and other health-related programs; colleges and universities; and relevant service organizations and advocacy groups. Internal publicity may include posters, flyers, and screen savers throughout your institution. If possible, arrangements should be made to offer continuing education credits for physicians, nurses, social workers, and other attending professionals.

While the logistics of planning and presenting a symposium may seem daunting, with organization and repetition the process becomes easier and smoother. Keep your mailing list and modify it each year. Sending save-the-date messages and flyers with all the information by e-mail dramatically cuts printing and mailing costs. A few eye-catching posters strategically placed throughout the hospital, as well as screen savers and periodic reminders, can take care of internal publicity. Depending on your budget, you may want to ask your Marketing Department about an ad or press release in your local newspaper. The length and timing of the program and your budget will determine your food needs—light breakfast, lunch, or snacks. Recognizing that most well-known speakers have agents and schedules booked months in advance, and command significant honoraria, you should start planning very early and sharpen your powers of persuasion. The most important decision is the selection of a timely and provocative topic, and a sample list appears below.

- The Ethics of Healthcare Reform and the Patient Protection and Affordable Care Act: What Are Its Aims and Likely Accomplishments? What Are Its Strengths and Weaknesses?
- The Moral Response to Health Care Reform?
- The Ethics of Decision Making in the Care of Neonates, Children, and Adolescents
- The Ethics of the Electronic Medical Record
- Unexpected Revelations: When Children Are Not What Their Parents Anticipated
- Human Subjects Research: Prospects and Problems
- Getting Personal: The Ethics of Advances in Genomic Medicine

- Direct-to-Consumer Advertising (DTCA) in Health Care: Who Benefits? Who's at Risk?
- The Ethical Implications of Neuroimaging

WHITE PAPERS, MEMORANDA, GUIDELINES, AND PROTOCOLS

One way in which ethics committees can prepare for these functions is by research ing and writing about topics with particular relevance to their work and their institutions. Often, committees are asked to provide insights about an especially challenging issue. Sometimes, policy review or an untoward event triggers a closer look at how situations are or should be addressed. Occasionally, a topic in the news stimulates a desire to learn more about developments with ethical implications. Depending on the topic and the needs of the committee, these reports can take the form of detailed white papers or brief memoranda.

Because most committees are composed of busy health care professionals with interest but little formal training in ethics, your discussions will be more fruitful if members are armed with the background and key issues of selected topics, their significance in the clinical or organizational setting, the underlying ethical principles, and guidelines for implementing recommendations. While your committee is unlikely to need the breadth and depth of white papers on a regular basis, their time-consuming preparation can be most efficient and effective if a few members work together as a subcommittee whenever this level of attention is required. More often, an informational memorandum that states the issue, lays out a brief background and ethical analysis, and offers recommendations will provide useful structure for committee discussion.

In addition to preparing memoranda and the occasional white paper, ethics committees often develop guidelines and protocols that may eventually be formalized. These models are typically the result of clinical or organizational situations for which no plans of action or reasoning currently exist. Recognizing the likelihood that these scenarios may recur and wanting to avoid reinventing the wheel each time, committees find it useful to draft strategies for discussion and possible pilot testing.

The following are examples of materials developed by a medical center bioethics service, often with the help of one or two members of the ethics committee. To save time and enhance member familiarity with the issues, the documents were distributed to the full committee in advance of the meetings during which the topics would be addressed.

Two white papers ("Allocating Critical Care Resources: Keeping the Teeth in ICU Triage" and "Conflicts of Interest") and one memorandum ("Justice and Access to Unreimbursed Therapies") illustrate how selected topics can be researched and presented as useful committee resources. They can serve as discussion guides during deliberations and as the analytic framework for your committee's recommendations to the institution's clinical and organizational staff. "Guidelines for Transferring Patients between Services" and "Decision-Making Protocol for the Patient Alone" are examples of draft strategies to improve clinical and organizational processes. These working documents are offered as possible models for ethics committee response to selected situations that might benefit from structured appraisal and recommendation. They can also usefully inform clinical practice, ethics consultation, and in-service teaching.

Allocating Critical Care Resources: Keeping the Teeth in ICU Triage, by Jack Kilcullen, M.D., J.D.

More than almost any other clinical resource, the allocation of beds in the intensive care unit (ICU) generates controversy because it is both scarce and life-saving. Consequently, critical care physicians possess an ethical responsibility unique among their colleagues (outside the realm of organ transplantation) because they cannot advocate exclusively for any given patient, but must direct treatment in the ICU to the patients most likely to benefit. These decisions demand a thorough understanding of the complex interplay of a patient's underlying chronic illness and immediate threats to hemodynamic stability. Given the dangers of delay, these decisions must often be made quickly, knowing that there will now be one fewer bed available for the next patient seeking help.

Unlike the allocation of donated organs, the allocation of ICU beds is done without the authority of federal law, the safety of committee deliberation, or the methodical review among all competing preselected patients. It is often made only by a fellow and an attending, in the middle of the night and in the midst of other clinical pressures. More important than the lack of a waiting list is the fact that the patient for whom the ICU physician must save a bed could be the one still racing to the hospital. As unwilling as our society is to confront the concept that health care has limits, rationing is a long-accepted, yet always vexing part of critical care medicine.

To the family stunned by a loved one so close to death, the critical care staff has a special responsibility to provide understanding and compassion and to promote acceptance of painful clinical realities as they become inevitable. Palliative care professionals when available can help moderate the emotional pain for families with the offer of clear comfort-based measures for the patient, thus underscoring the reality that death is imminent.

Yet, complicating the already challenging process of triage is the rare patient's family members who, often with the involvement of their own physicians and senior hospital staff, bring pressure on the ICU attending to accept patients who lack any clinical claim to these beds. The effect is to undermine the ICU attending whose authority is established by specialized training and experience. The individual triage process becomes exponentially time consuming, distracting him from clinical responsibilities. The result of a forced admission, beyond depriving someone who might later need the bed, is a polluting of precedents established by more evidenced-based decisions, leading to further distrust within the institution and future demands for "special treatment." For the critical care attending, who has enough pressures to bear, this loss of institutional support can cut deeply into that shallow reservoir of morale.

The bioethics committee's purpose in considering ICU triage is to establish the proper institutional commitment to a just allocation of one of its most precious resources. For patients at the end stage of life, there are specific points that the committee should address:

- When brain death is strongly suspected, this determination shall be made while the patient remains at her current location, be it the emergency room (ER), the general floor, or the ICU. Patients in the ER determined to be brain dead may be admitted to the general floor to accommodate the family beginning to adjust to their loss. In no instance should the patient be admitted to the ICU once brain death has been determined.
- Patients with irreversible comorbid conditions who present with a potentially reversible acute deterioration may, after stabilization in the ER, continue to receive limited aggressive intervention on the general floor with consultation by critical care medicine in a manner consistent with the limits of floor nursing. Palliative care services will be incorporated with these limited interventions to support the patient and family during this difficult and ongoing acceptance process.
- Patients unknown to the medical staff who present with strong evidence of irreversible and rapidly progressive disease may be admitted to the ICU for stabilization and rapid confirmation of this dire diagnosis. They may, thereafter, be transferred to the general floor for palliative care.
- The ultimate authority for all ICU triage decisions by the ICU attendings rests with the director of critical care medicine.

Principles Related to Critical Care Placement

The following principles and guidelines use the term *triage* in reference to decisions about patient admission to, clinical management in, and transfer from critical or intensive care units. It is an ongoing active process integral to patient assessment that requires continual reexamination of the perceived need to be treated only in the ICU.

The Society of Critical Care Medicine published guidelines in 1999 for the allocation of ICU beds in an attempt to ensure they be reserved for those who have a reasonable prospect of substantial recovery. The Society encourages hospitals to articulate their own admission and discharge criteria in the light of their own available resources. The guidelines provide a classification system of descending priority. The highest priority is given to those requiring continuous and aggressive management in the face of ongoing instability (patients in shock or respiratory failure). The second priority goes to patients who need increased monitoring because they are at high risk for developing a life-threatening condition. The third priority is directed to unstable patients who have underlying terminal conditions that might be successfully stabilized but whose longevity is curtailed. Finally, there are those either too well to require ICU care or those who are so sick that, despite aggressive care, death is most likely imminent.

Brain Death

It would seem unnecessary to state that the threshold assessment of a patient newly arrived in the ER is whether she is alive. Yet, determining that neurological function has ceased down to below the brainstem is more involved than merely palpating for a pulse. This institution's policy requires an initial clinical assessment with subsequent confirmation by a physician credentialed by the Department of Neurology or Neurosurgery. A neurologist or neurosurgeon must then review the findings and, if necessary, specify whatever lab tests he considers necessary before attesting in the chart to the final outcome.

The state legislature, in recognizing that death can be defined as a permanent loss of brainstem function, gives considerable discretion to the hospital in how this determination will be made. As busy as the ER can become, it is still realistic to assume that its staff or others with appropriate credentialing could establish the necessary basis for a neurologist or neurosurgeon to make a determination in the vast majority of cases. Because a patient who has likely suffered brain death is considered clinically and legally dead, *admission to the critical care setting is never appropriate*. Such an admission would ignore established criteria for ICU admission, which require that the patient be likely to benefit from the critical care setting and, therefore, would be counterproductive to the family's acceptance of the death.

If a family has moral or religious objections to brain death as a determination of death, state law allows hospital admission to reasonably accommodate the family as it begins to accept the death or makes arrangements for transfer to a facility where cardiopulmonary support may be continued. These reasonable accommodations (e.g., not disconnecting the ventilator, continuing nutrition and hydration, continuing medications) should take place after transfer from the ER to another location in the hospital, but *not to the critical care setting*. The clinical staff should emphasize that the accommodations are for the benefit of the family, not the now-deceased patient.

Limited Aggressive Treatment outside the ICU
Acute Deterioration in a Patient with Irreversible Comorbid Conditions

The vast majority of terminally ill patients arriving in the ER are best described as "pre-hospice." They are stricken with profound disease, such as metastatic cancer or end-stage dementia, and often require substantial support to maintain life, including nursing home care, tube feeding, and mechanical ventilation. They come to the ER on multiple occasions with acute, often infectious, illness. Yet their families see the immediate deterioration as an isolated event and seek ICU admission, anticipating recovery sufficient to return them to their most recent setting.

On an informal basis, ICU admission rarely occurs. Critical care fellows and attendings need only invite a family member to describe the patient's previous six months in order to elicit how frequent these admissions have become. When the fellow observes that the patient appears to be at the end of life, most families see how easily this truth arises from their own words. Even though the patient in the ER has now been intubated and stabilized on vasopressors, families can appreciate that care on the general floor is more appropriate because it is more accommodating. They are explicitly told that the care plan is not to "do everything" and that floor nurses are not watching every patient at every moment. Still, they can agree that limited treatment (e.g., antibiotics) along with comfort measures can allow for the hope of recovery to be preserved while realistically letting "nature take its course." The inclusion of a professional palliative care service is invaluable in helping the family cope with whatever ensues. Nurses can turn over micromanagement of the ventilators to respiratory therapists. Any titration of infusions is handled by house staff. Thus, the general floor teams have become able to handle this limited aggressive care, knowing that the critical care physicians are always within reach.

Confirmation of a Dire Diagnosis

In unusual and compelling cases, a patient unknown to the hospital staff who is often only recently symptomatic may arrive in the ER with a subacute complaint, only to be found to have striking evidence of advanced terminal disease, usually a malignancy. Work-up may reveal multiple highly suspicious masses in both lungs or masses in the liver or scattered throughout the abdomen. For the family and patient, the news is completely unexpected and can be devastating.

When the patient is unstable and otherwise headed for the ICU, diversion to the floor because of a strongly suspected terminal diagnosis can further traumatize an already frightened family. Compassion would dictate that the patient be stabilized in the ICU and that a rapid tissue diagnosis be sought confirming the worst. Not only will the family be spared the immediate anxiety of the acute crisis, it will be possible to provide irrefutable evidence necessary to face the painful truth squarely. Transfer to the floor thereafter may be necessary for triage, especially if the patient has been stabilized hemodynamically. By that point some relationship of trust should have been established that would not otherwise have occurred had probability alone dictated the decision.

Final Authority for ICU Triage Should Rest with the Director of Critical Care Medicine

When the family of a patient at life's end stage becomes adamant in demanding ICU admission, the process risks disrupting the hospital. Often, the family's private physician may be asked to apply pressure on the ICU fellow or attending. Alternatively, the ER physician may feel targeted by the family's ire. Eventually, the case may reach the level of the medical director, who may be called on to intervene.

Ultimately, the decision ceases to be a medical one. If, over the objections of the director of critical care medicine, a patient is placed in the ICU, the decision invalidates the specialty nature of managing critically ill patients. It creates an adversarial climate and hinders the collaborative and trusting relationship essential for effective care. Most of all, it puts the patient's family in the role of physician, dictating the level and location of care.

No right exists to an ICU bed for every person whose life might be prolonged by unlimited medical care. Federal law, under the Emergency Medical Treatment and Active Labor Act (EMTALA), requires only that patients be evaluated and stabilized in the ER before the hospital transfers them elsewhere. Statutory and common law regarding malpractice requires adherence to a physician's general duty of care to a patient as physicians so define it.

Just as a heart transplant team cannot be expected to rescue every patient with a failing heart, the ICU staff cannot create beds where none exist. We risk denying a 30-year-old woman in eclampsia ICU admission because the last bed was just given to a 90-year-old demented man septic from his third bout of aspiration pneumonia. Justifying that decision to the husband of the pregnant woman is far more difficult than explaining to the man's daughter that critical care started in the ER will continue to a limited degree on the floor and not in the ICU. The role of the hospital medical director is to support the decision of the critical care medicine staff and explain to the family how the institution can properly care for their loved one through medical and palliative services consistent with the best standards of the profession.

Ethical Guidelines

The Medical Center Code of Ethics articulates the following overarching institutional commitment: "We recognize that our primary mission is to ensure the provision of high-quality, ethically based patient care."

The fundamental ethical principle of respect for patients underlies the health care institution's commitment to patient well-being and confers organizational obligations to promote clinical excellence, collaborative case management, and wise stewardship of resources. These institutional responsibilities require that patients be cared for in the most appropriate clinical setting, which, in the hospital, means the service with the most targeted skills and resources.

- Clinical decisions, including determinations of the most appropriate plan and locus of care, depend primarily on the patient's care needs, the therapeutic options, and the professional staff and technical resources available to provide the needed care. Particular attention should be given to the interventions that can and cannot be provided on each service.
- Triage criteria should be derived from evidence-based data about the clinical resources necessary to maximize therapeutic outcomes.
- Triage decisions should recognize that critical care is a resource and a set of clinical skills, not a location. Aspects of critical care can be delivered in non-ICU settings.
- The therapeutic objective is to provide only care that benefits the patient, without imposing unnecessary suffering or prolonging the dying process. When cure is no longer possible, the patient's comfort and dignity remain the focus, requiring close collaboration with the palliative care service.
- Patient requests for critical care and family or surrogate advocacy on behalf of patients should be considered but they are not dispositive in decisions about placement in ICUs. Decisions about admission to and transfer from ICUs are not to be dictated by patients or families. Care providers have an obligation to use clinical judgment, establish boundaries, and provide guidance and support in the triage process.
- Budgetary and bureaucratic concerns, while important to deliberations about resource allocation, must not impede or compromise the care of individual patients.
- Patients and families must be helped to understand the changing clinical picture and the goals, potential, and limits of critical care in order to prevent misunderstanding, unrealistic expectations, disappointment, and confrontation.

References and Additional Reading

Bone RC, McElwee NC, Eubanks DH, Gluck EH. 1993. Analysis of indications for intensive care unit admission: Clinical efficacy assessment project: American College of Physicians. *Chest* 104(6):1806–11.

Charlson ME, Sax FL. 1987. The therapeutic efficacy of critical care units from two perspectives: A traditional cohort approach vs. a new case-control methodology. *Journal of Chronic Disease* 40(1):31–39.

Emergency Medical Treatment and Active Labor Act (EMTALA), 42 U.S.C. §1395dd et seq. Examination and treatment for emergency medical conditions and women in labor.

Griner PF. 1972. Treatment of acute pulmonary edema: Conventional or intensive care? *Annals of Internal Medicine* 77:501–6.

Kalb PE, Miller DH. 1989. Utilization strategies for intensive care units. *Journal of the American Medical Association* 261(16):2389–95

Kollef MH, Canfield DA, Zuckerman GR. 1995. Triage considerations for patients with acute gastrointestinal hemorrhage admitted to a medical intensive care unit. *Critical Care Medicine* 23(6):1048–54.

Kraiss LW, Kilberg L, Critch S, Johansen KH. 1995. Short-stay carotid endarterectomy is safe and cost-effective. *American Journal of Surgery* 169(5):512–15.

Manthous CA, Amoateng-Adjepong Y, Al-Kharrat T. 1997. Effects of a medical intensivist on patient care in a community teaching hospital. *Mayo Clinic Proceedings* 72:391–99.

Mulley AG. 1983. The allocation of resources for medical intensive care. In President's Commission for the Study of Ethical Problems in Medicine and Biomedical and Behavioral Research. *Securing Access to Health Care.* Washington, DC: U.S. Government Printing Office, 3:285–311.

Multz AS, Chalfin DB, Samson IM, Dantzker DR, Fein AM, Steinberg HN, Niederman MS, Scharf SM. 1998. A "closed" medical intensive care unit (MICU) improves resource utilization when compared with an "open" MICU. *American Journal of Respiratory and Critical Care Medicine* 157(5):1468–73.

Oliver MF, Julian DG, Donald KW. 1967. Problems in evaluating coronary care units: Their responsibilities and their relation to the community. *American Journal of Cardiology* 20(4):465–74.

Ron A, Aronne LJ, Kalb PE, et al. 1989. The therapeutic efficacy of critical care units: Identifying subgroups of patients who benefit. *Archives of Internal Medicine* 149:338–41.

Society of Critical Care Medicine Guidelines for ICU Admission, Discharge, and Triage. 1999. *Critical Care Medicine* 27(3):633–38.

Conflicts of Interest

Introduction

During the past several decades, health care has undergone profound changes that have fundamentally altered the means by which care is provided. The once rather basic and singular relationship between doctor and patient has been expanded and complicated by teams of professionals, layers of bureaucracy, and limitations of contract. As new incentives and disincentives have emerged, the obligation to provide the best care for the patient has been modified by the obligation to operate within fixed and global budgets. Health care institutions, as well as individual clinicians, must respond to financial arrangements whose goal is to alter medical practice. Academic medical centers have singular problems in this environment as they try to fulfill their obligations to provide care, teach health care professionals, and conduct research.

The difficulties lie not only in the expanded cast of characters but also in the altered relationships and power balances. Physicians and other care providers have traditionally occupied positions of authority by virtue of their superior scientific knowledge and clinical expertise. The therapeutic relationship was not burdened, or at least not so obviously affected, by conflicting interests. Indeed, the legal and social presumption was that because of the fiduciary relationship, the care professional placed the best interest of the patient first and was, in fact, the patient's advocate.

The current health care dynamic has introduced new, contradictory, and potentially harmful imperatives. Prospective payment and full-risk contracts are designed to provide weighty incentives for limiting diagnostic and therapeutic interventions. The medical marketplace offers endless opportunities for professionals to benefit financially from the business of providing diagnostic and therapeutic services. Drug and medical device manufacturers aggressively solicit the attention and eventual loyalty of doctors in training, as well as their established seniors, through samples, gifts, and educational sponsorship. Private research dollars drive the clinical agenda and scientific discoveries are intellectual property.

Background

Conflicts of Interest Defined

The medical profession, once seen as noble and altruistic, is increasingly perceived— from without and within—as a commercial enterprise. The advent of the "health care industry" has brought new opportunities for personal and financial enhancement, opportunities that may become what are known as *conflicts of interest*. The legal definition of a conflict of interest varies from state to state, but generally refers to the relationship between those with public or fiduciary responsibilities and those in positions of reliance, specifically when the clash between their interests advantages the party in power and disadvantages or threatens to disadvantage the dependent party. A situation in which a fiduciary exploits her position for personal or financial gain is usually perceived to constitute a conflict of interest (*Black's Law Dictionary*, p. 299). Despite its generally negative connotation, a conflict of interest is a common circumstance in which an individual with responsibility to others, including professional responsibilities, might be consciously or unconsciously influenced by financial or personal factors that involve self-interest (Rothman 2008).

In the health care setting, the narrowest definition of a conflict of interest is a situation in which the patient's outcome is worse because the physician has either intentionally or unintentionally subordinated the patient's best interests to those of the physician (Lo 2000; Shalala 2000). A broader definition is that the physician's judgment or decision-making process is compromised, even though clinical outcomes are not impaired. A still wider definition includes even the *potential* for detrimental outcomes or compromised judgment, without evidence of actual harm (Lo 2000). Other definitions distinguish actual, apparent, and potential conflicts of interest. In defining conflicts of interest, this white paper argues that they raise ethical concerns because of the potential that they will *disadvantage vulnerable parties if they influence action inappropriately.*

Conflicts of Interest Identified

In the health care setting, three areas are especially prone to conflicts of interest: physician and institutional interactions with drug and device companies; medical research; and physician and institutional non-financial conflicts.

Physician-Industry Interactions

The relationship between physicians' contact with the health care technology industry and their clinical behavior has been the subject of considerable speculation, focused study, and, most recently, legislative action. Prior to the 1980s, pharmaceutical and device company outreach was fairly modest, providing practitioners with product information, samples, and token gifts to promote name recognition and loyalty. In time, company underwriting expanded in both scope and cost to include lavish gifts, travel expenses, and continuing medical education, "shifting the focus from providing information to providing incentives" (Tenery 2000, p. 391).

The interaction between physicians and drug and device representatives, known as "detail reps," begins in medical school and continues throughout residency training and subsequent practice. Among the favored techniques are providing drug samples, intended to promote recognition of, preference for, and prescription of the sample drugs, and gifts, ranging from pens and note pads with the company logo to meals and travel.

A considerable literature reveals that, despite physicians' beliefs to the contrary, these interactions with pharmaceutical and device company representatives demonstrably affect their professional behavior. Clinicians have repeatedly been shown to prescribe sample drugs, even when they differed from their drugs of choice or when other drugs have been shown to be more effective (Wazana 2000; McCormick et al. 2001; nofreelunch.org; Page 2000; Bero 1998; Orlowski 1992; Sutherland 1993; Tenery 2000; Campbell et al. 1998).

Institutional Interactions with Drug and Device Companies

Institutions, as well as the professionals who work in them, confront conflicting interests. A compelling organizational goal, especially for the academic medical center, is to enhance its reputation as a center of research and academic achievement. Institutional conflicts of interest exist when the academic medical center, its senior or midlevel officials, institutional review board (IRB) members, or members of its governing board hold financial interests in companies that provide drugs or devices for clinical use or sponsor research studies. Organizational decisions about allocation of resources, contracting with outside firms, and planning for growth and development are susceptible to actual or perceived influence created by these interests.

Another area of concern is industry-sponsored programs for resident education and continuing education for practicing physicians. With less available government and private funding, educational support from the drug and device industry has filled the void, leading to concerns about increasing industry influence and control (Wazana 2000; Tenery 2000; DeAngelis 2000).

Medical Research

Industry-sponsored research creates actual or potential conflicts of interest. The drug or device company's goal is to demonstrate that its products are safe and effective, especially when compared to existing or competing similar products. Researchers are motivated by the desire for intellectual fulfillment, professional recognition, obtaining or maintaining grant support, and the satisfaction of contributing to medical progress. These interests may conflict with their duties as researchers, and the potential for harm grows in proportion to the amount of control the company has in the design and conducting of research studies, and the interpreting and reporting of study results.

Researchers' conflicting interests are exacerbated when industry makes available additional incentives. Academic ambition and the desire for professional advancement already tempt researchers to publish too much and promote their positive results. Research investigators may also receive biomaterials, support for students, and research equipment that is essential to their research. Researchers report understanding that their gifts often come with restrictions, such as prepublication manuscript review or expectations that they would be acknowledged in publications reporting their research. With heightened commercialism of the medical-research community, stock options, equity interest, and other forms of direct payment to clinical investigators have also grown in popularity (Relman 1989).

Responses to Conflict of Interest

Two very different responses to conflicts of interest described by the Institute of Medicine have been used as models—one based on *prohibiting* any relationship with the potential to create a conflict of interest and one based on *managing* such relationships through disclosure and peer review. The prohibition model formed the basis of the National Institutes of Health guidelines, proposed in 1989 and later rejected by the scientific community, academic medical centers, and universities alike for being too sweeping, prescriptive, and unacceptably intrusive into matters of faculty behavior traditionally reserved to academia and the professions.

This opposition led to quick withdrawal of the proposal and the subsequent issuance of more relaxed guidelines, which were proposed by the Public Health Service and the National Science Foundation in 1994 and became effective the following year. These guidelines, based on the managing model, allowed research institutions considerable discretion in managing conflicts of interest, requiring that the existence but not the details of conflicts be disclosed to funding agencies. The most prescriptive element of this framework was the establishment of a federal threshold to define "significant financial interest" (McCrary et al. 2000).

In light of the deep and extensive financial entanglements that may exist between medical school researchers and industry, commentators questioned whether the federal guidelines were sufficient, arguing that disclosure alone might not suffice for purposes of institutional management and public reassurance (Korn 2000). It was suggested that, instead of focusing only on the work of those who may have conflicts of interest, more intense scrutiny should be directed toward all papers and work developed and produced in the research setting (Rothman 1993).

These two approaches to handling conflicts of interest appear prominently in the literature. Most ethicists argue that, at the very least, situations posing conflicts of interest should be disclosed (Cho et al. 2000). All financial ties between researchers and the products or procedures they are investigating should be fully revealed to the institutions sponsoring the research and to the journals publishing the results. When appropriate, the facts should be published in a footnote, but not revealed to the referees while the article is being reviewed (Relman 1989).

Many journals were unsatisfied with simple financial disclosure, however, and refused to publish review articles or editorials written by an employee of a company whose product figured prominently in the article or a company making a competitive product. The reasoning was that, when authors have financial as well as scientific interest in their subjects, questions inevitably arise that cast doubt on their objectivity (Rothman 2008).

The disclosure model has also been adopted as part of the Patient Protection and Affordable Care Act (PPACA), one goal of which is to increase transparency in health care. In December 2011, the Centers for Medicare & Medicaid Services (CMS) issued proposed regulations intended to increase public awareness of drug and device industry payments to physicians and teaching hospitals in the United States. These regulations respond to requirements, known as Sunshine provisions, in the PPACA. The purpose of the provisions is expressed in the preamble to the rule: "Close relationships between manufacturers and prescribing providers can lead to conflicts of interest that may affect clinical decision making. Increased transparency of these relationships tries to discourage inappropriate relationships, while maintaining the beneficial relationships" (P.L. 111–148, Sec. 6002). As required by the Sunshine provisions, CMS will publish on a public website "transparency reports," disclosing all industry payments to physicians and hospitals. The reasoning is that, informed with information interactions between care providers (individual physicians and organizations) and the drug and device industry, potential patients will be equipped to make more knowledgeable decisions about where and from whom they receive care.

Some commentators (e.g., Lo) suggest that, rather than trying to manage or reduce these conflicts of interest, the goal should be to prohibit them, banning all financial relationships between members of research teams and industry. Others (e.g., DJ Rothman) respond that such policies are a sweeping form of censorship, in addition to being unworkable and unenforceable.

Studies of how academic medical centers and other research institutions manage conflicts of interest reveal considerable variation in their policies and procedures, and a lack of specificity about the kinds of relationships with industry that are permitted or prohibited. Studies conducted in the 1990s and early 2000s concluded that current standards were likely inadequate to maintain the appropriate level of scientific integrity in research, protect the welfare of research subjects, prevent the erosion of public trust, and promote the high quality education of health care clinicians and researchers (Cho et al. 2000; Morin et al. 2002; McCrary et al. 2000; Bodenheimer 2000; Angell 2000; Emanuel and Steiner 1995; Boyd and Bero 2000; Lo, Wolf, and Berkeley 2000; Korn 2000). More recently, a comprehensive review of medical schools found that only 30% of the responding institutions had adopted policies that address institutions' financial interests, while 55 to 69% had adopted policies applicable to the financial interests of senior and midlevel officials, and members of the IRBs and governing boards (Ehringhaus et al. 2008).

Ethical Analysis
Conflicts of Interest, Harm, and Professional Integrity

Situations of conflict of interests can usefully be pictured as a dual continuum on which concern grows with the *likelihood* that self-interest will govern one's actions and the *degree* to which such behavior will compromise the interests of others. The critical point is that conflicts of interest raise ethical concern because of their *potential* to cause harm if they influence action in inappropriate ways. For this reason, perhaps the most useful definition of conflicts of interest would be "situations where one's profession, professional judgment, or professional code is in conflict with other demands or influences that, *if acted upon*, would compromise professional judgment" (Spenser et al. 2000, p. 73, italics added).

Conflicts of interest may also be distinguished from conflicts of commitment, which have been defined as "those sets of role expectations where competing obligations prevent honoring both commitments or honoring them both adequately" (Spenser et al. 2000, p. 74, quoting Werhane and Doering 1995, p. 61). The distinction here is that conflicts of commitment arise when the demands of responsibility exceed the time and resources available to meet them. Professionals may find it impossible to attend to all their clinical, research, and teaching duties at the same time or in the same way. As a result, their patients, students, and families may not receive the quantity or quality of attention they want or even deserve. The difference is that, although some people may be disadvantaged by conflicting commitments, their interests have not been sacrificed in order to advantage the professional.

Conflicts of interest raise ethical concerns in the health care setting because of the potential harms that may result from the improper conduct of professionals. Patients may suffer physical harm if physicians base clinical decisions on what is best for themselves or third parties, rather than on what is best for the patients who depend on them. The integrity of medical judgment may be violated even though a particular patient suffers no clinical harm. If physicians violate standards of good practice to foster their own self-interest or the interest of third parties, future patients may suffer adverse clinical outcomes. Trust may be undercut when patients fear that, if physicians are willing to compromise their well-being in some circumstances, they will not act on their behalf in other situations (Lo 2000, p. 232). When investigators have financial interests in or are funded by companies with activities related to their research, the research is likely to be of lower quality, more apt to favor the sponsors' products, and more likely to have delayed publication or not be published at all. Without policies and procedures to regulate these activities, academic research institutions and their faculty risk losing the public's support, respect, and trust in medical discoveries and standards of practice (DeAngelis 2000).

Are Conflicts of Interest Always Ethically Problematic?

A conflict of interest by itself does not indicate wrongdoing—it merely refers to a setting in which factors exist that might influence one's conduct in problematic ways. All professionals, including physicians, researchers, attorneys, and business professionals, confront conflicts of interest and, despite the popular tendency to regard such situations as inherently scandalous, it is likely that they are intrinsic to professional life. It has been suggested that because these conflicts can never be eradicated, their very existence should not be equated with professional misconduct, but rather accepted as part of professional life that must be managed in appropriate ways (Korn 2000).

While disclosure may identify someone as having a conflict of interest, it does not reveal whether the individual's behavior is actually problematic. Not everyone who faces the temptation of putting self-interest above responsibility to others succumbs to that temptation. Matters are further complicated by the inadequate distinctions between scientists whose work is biased because of deliberate inducement and those whose results may be unintentionally influenced (Rothman 1993). Although identifying someone as having a conflict of interest does not constitute an automatic accusation, the label is so commonly used with the intent to discredit a person or a work that it is disingenuous to claim that no accusation is intended when describing conflicts of interest (Rothman 1993).

This white paper argues that what is of ethical concern is both the individual response to the conflict of interest and the environment that either fosters or inhibits that response. While it may not be possible to prevent the interests of parties from conflicting, the ethical principles that govern professional practice impose obligations that constrain the behavior of practitioners and institutions. Failure to fulfill those obligations at the clinical, research, academic, or organizational level is ethically problematic because of the actual or potential harm to patients, research subjects, the therapeutic or scientific relationship, and the integrity of the profession.

Organizational Response to Conflicts of Interest

The existence of conflicts of interest triggers both an individual and an institutional response, informed by the ethical principles that give rise to professional obligations and ground professional practice. The conduct of clinicians and researchers is governed by the principles of beneficence and nonmaleficence, which require promoting the well-being of patients and subjects, and protecting them from harm by placing their interests before the career or financial interests of the professionals. Professionals are recommended to exercise integrity and good judgment, identify and manage conflicts, and disclose them when appropriate (AAMC).

Likewise, health care institutions are responsible for ensuring that patient care, research, and teaching activities meet high standards and conform to fundamental ethical principles. In this endeavor, organizations are required to implement decisions, policies, and procedures that do not sacrifice the interests of patients, subjects, staff, trainees, and the community to the financial and business interests of the institution. Yet, the institution also has its own viability concerns, including critical economic interests, which may conflict with its primary mission of patient care, teaching, and research.

Conflicts of interest require organizational response precisely because institutions are in the best position to identify them, manage them, and limit their adverse effects. Individual clinicians, researchers, and academics, as well as individual departments, even those with the highest standards and the best intentions to monitor their own conduct, are susceptible to self-interest and self-deception. As the entity with the overarching perspective and responsibility, however, the institution has both the obligation and the opportunity to address conflicts of interest comprehensively and effectively. Accordingly, organizational codes of ethics (see part III) typically recognize the institution's ethical obligations to explicitly disclose information about relationships that create conflicts of interest, as well as its obligations to place the well-being of those who depend on its services above the interests of those who provide those services.

Organizational Guidelines for Managing Conflicts of Interest
Definition

Conflicts of interest arise when a professional's personal or financial interests conflict with the interests of those who place their trust in the professional. In these cases, elevating the professional's interests over those of the parties in positions of reliance compromises or detrimentally influences professional judgment and undermines that trust.

In health care, conflicts of interest may arise in the clinical, teaching, and research settings. They may occur, for example, when physicians accept substantial gifts from drug or device companies; when researchers have financial interests in the corporate sponsors of their clinical research; when reimbursement systems provide incentives to physicians to forgo beneficial health care interventions; and when physicians recommend services at medical facilities in which they have substantial financial investment. Conflicts of interest need not be financial in nature. For example, academic promotion or enhancement of one's reputation within the profession may be the factor motivating disregard of professional responsibilities.

- *Having a conflict of interest is not itself unethical, although it may raise ethical concerns.*

The existence of conflicting interests is not, by itself, ethically problematic. Rather, it is the professional's behavioral response that can trigger ethical concerns if it creates actual or potential harm. Placing one's personal or financial interests ahead of one's professional responsibilities in a way that is prejudicial to these responsibilities is unethical because it violates the trust placed in the professional. Thus, one may be in a conflict-of-interest situation that creates the potential for adversely affecting one's professional judgment and fiduciary role, without its actually doing so.

- *Conflicts of interests are pervasive and cannot be completely eliminated or avoided. Rather, they should be identified and managed in ways that safeguard vulnerable parties from harm.*

Because conflicts of interest occur in every part of life, as well as in all professions and public service, a purist approach that advocates eliminating or avoiding all conflicting interests in health care is unrealistic. Indeed, the suggestion that all conflicts of interest can and should be entirely eliminated may have the unintended effect of inhibiting participation in clinical or scientific activities, or discouraging transparency about the existence of conflicting interests. Rather, the ethical obligation is to be alert to potential conflicts of interest, avoid problematic situations when possible and disclose them when necessary, recognize the factors that influence behavioral response to the conflict, and avoid conduct that jeopardizes the well-being of those in positions of reliance.

- *Professionals may face both conflicts of interest and conflicts of commitment, which should be distinguished and responded to appropriately.*

Conflicts of commitment often arise because an individual simultaneously occupies a number of different roles with competing demands, for example, those of professional and employee, health care provider and researcher. When competing responsibilities exceed the available time and resources, professionals should alert the affected parties to their inability to meet their needs at the same time or in the same manner. These situations should be distinguished from conflicts of interest, in which the interests of vulnerable parties may be sacrificed in order to benefit the professional. Despite the distinction between conflicts of interest and conflicts of commitment, the former can often masquerade as the latter. The difference is that conflicts of interest carry the potential for promoting the self-interest of one party (typically, the one in a position of power and responsibility) at the expense of others (typically, those in positions of vulnerability and reliance). In the health care setting, this is seen in the nexus between personal interest and clinical benefit.

- *Conflicts of interest raise ethical concerns even when no harm actually results.*

Some situations present conflicts of interest without actual harm. For example, many physicians claim that small gifts from drug companies are harmless because they do not compromise professional judgment or prescribing behavior. That is, the physicians believe that they have not acted on the conflicting interests in harmful ways. Even the perception of a conflict of interest may be damaging, however, because it undermines trust in the professional and the profession. In the research context, the perception that researchers are putting subjects of color at risk of abuse, even if erroneous, needs to be taken into account and addressed.

- *It is important to identify which interests of patients, clinicians, academics, researchers, organizations, and other affected parties might come into conflict.*

The existence of conflicts of interest must be recognized and acknowledged if they are to be addressed in ways that protect all parties. To do this it is necessary to identify which interests of which parties are in conflict. For example, in order to determine whether a physician's financial self-interest places him in a conflict-of-interest situation, it is necessary to spell out what interests are being placed in jeopardy. Once a conflict of interest has been identified, the necessary next step is to identify what actions by the professional would constitute misconduct because they would harm one or more parties. Self-deception often prevents people from recognizing the existence or potential harm of their conflicting interests. For this reason, external oversight, such as the IRB, is important.

- *Health care institutions have an obligation to create a climate that identifies and addresses conflicts of interest prospectively to prevent misconduct and respond forcefully to misconduct when it occurs.*

Conflicts of interest can arise on both the individual and the organizational levels, reflected in the decisions made on behalf of particular patients or the institution. Organizational conflicts of interest include those faced by professionals and others working in or for the organization, and those created by the organizational structure, mission or climate. For example, a health care organization that alleges its mission is to serve patients, yet elevates profitability above patient care, places itself in an objectionable conflict of interest. An institution that does not control the access of drug and device company representatives opens itself and its staff to objectionable conflicts of interest.

The organization has an obligation to establish an institutional environment that recognizes conflicts of interest, the reasons they arise, the consequences of improperly acting on them, and the ethical imperatives to manage them. Fulfilling this obligation requires an organizational commitment to implementing policies and procedures that educate staff about conflicts of interest, monitor problematic situations, identify and disclose conflicts that arise, clearly articulate organizational expectations of transparency and professionalism, and create mechanisms to manage the conflicts and minimize the likelihood of inappropriate behavior. For example, the institution might limit the locations, hours, and activities within which drug and device company representatives may interact with house staff. Grand rounds and in-service programs can usefully focus on identifying and managing conflicting interests.

• *All conflicts of interest must be recognized and acknowledged; in some cases, the potential for harm and erosion of trust may be so substantial that the conflicts should be prohibited.*

Because they have the potential to compromise the interests of vulnerable persons, conflicts of interest are always problematic. The question in each instance is whether the benefit of eliminating them outweighs the harm. Some conflicts of interest do not rise to the level of serious ethical concern and are managed in more or less routine fashion by widely accepted norms of professional and organizational practice. These situations are those in which both the likelihood of misconduct and the magnitude of the potential harm are low. In other cases, however, the risk to patients, research subjects, and other vulnerable parties and the potential for bias and erosion of trust may be so great, that it would be prudent to prohibit certain actions and situations. For example, certain types of gifts and support from drug and device companies, and certain physician referrals to medical facilities in which she has a financial interest, may be so likely to trigger misconduct or even raise questions about bias and impropriety that they should be banned.

• *Disclosure of conflicts of interest is an important, but perhaps insufficient, way of managing conflicts of interest.*

An institutional climate of transparency fosters recognition and disclosure of conflicting interests to safeguard against intentional or unintentional bias, inadequately informed consent or refusal, and decisions that inappropriately benefit fiduciaries at the expense of those in positions of reliance. Situations that carry a significant potential for harm or loss of trust should be disclosed to all parties. For example, the rationale for disclosure in the clinical setting is that an informed patient who understands the medical situation and available options will be able to place the physician's recommendations in context and compensate for any bias resulting from a conflict of interest. It may be unrealistic, however, to expect patients, research subjects, and other vulnerable parties to adequately assess whether and in what ways their situations may be tainted by biased professional judgment. Therefore, in some circumstances, disclosure alone may provide them with inadequate protection.

• *Health care organizations should create and support staff use of appropriate forums to which questions and concerns about conflicts of interest can be brought.*

Because conflicts of interest arise in such a wide variety of circumstances and in so many different forms, it is not feasible or even desirable for a health care organization to implement a comprehensive oversight mechanism for conflicts of interest. Rather, emphasis should be placed on the responsibility of the organization and individual departments to educate their members about conflicts of interest, provide mechanisms for managing them, and offer support for addressing concerns about them.

References

AAMC. Guidelines for Dealing with Faculty Conflicts of Commitment and Conflicts of Interest in Research, www.aamc.org/research/dbr/coi.htm.

Angell M. 2000. Is academic medicine for sale? *New England Journal of Medicine* 342:1516–18.

Bero LA. 1998. Disclosure policies for gifts from industry to academic faculty. *Journal of the American Medical Association* 279(13):1031–32.

Black's Law Dictionary, Sixth Edition. 1990. St. Paul, MN: West Publishing Co.

Bloche MG. 1999. Clinical loyalties and the social purposes of medicine. *Journal of the American Medical Association* 281(3):268–74.

Blumenthal D, Nangyanne C, Campbell E, Louis KS. 1996. Relationship between academic institutions and industry in the life sciences—an industry survey. *New England Journal of Medicine* 334:368–73.

Bodenheimer T. 2000. Uneasy alliance—clinical investigators and the pharmaceutical industry. *New England Journal of Medicine* 342:1539–44.

Bogdanich W, Meier B, Walsh MW. 2002. 2 hospital purchasing groups face questions over conflicts. *The New York Times*, March 4, A1, pp. 18–19.

Boyd EA, Bero LA. 2000. Assessing faculty financial relationships with industry: A case study. *Journal of the American Medical Association* 284(17):2209–14.

Campbell E, Louis KS, Blumenthal D. 1998. Looking a gift horse in the mouth. *Journal of the American Medical Association* 279(13):995–99.

Cho MK, Shohara R, Schissel A, Rennie D. 2000. Policies on faculty conflicts of interest at US universities. *Journal of the American Medical Association* 284:2203–8.

Collins G. 1997. Sunbeam sues the A.M.A. on Voided Marketing Deal. *The Wall Street Journal*, September 9.

DeAngelis CD. 2000. Conflict of interest and the public trust. *Journal of the American Medical Association* 284:2237–38.

Ehringhaus SH, Weissman JS, Sears JL, Gould SD, Feibelmann S, Campbell EG. 2008. Responses of medical schools to institutional conflicts of interest. *Journal of the American Medical Association* 299(6):665–71.

Emanuel E, Steiner D. 1995. Institutional conflict of interest. *New England Journal of Medicine* 332:262–68.

Griffith D. 1999. Reasons for not seeing drug representatives. *British Medical Journal* 319:69–70.

Kassirer JP. 1997. Our endangered integrity—it can only get worse. *New England Journal of Medicine* 336:1664–67.

Kim A, Mumm LA, Korenstein D. 2012. Routine conflict of interest disclosure by preclinical lecturers and medical students' attitudes toward the pharmaceutical and device industries. *Journal of the American Medical Association* 308(21):2187–89.

Korn D. 2000. Conflicts of interest in biomedical research. *Journal of the American Medical Association* 284(17):2234–38.

Lo B. 2000. *Resolving Ethical Dilemmas: A Guide for Clinicians.* 2nd ed. Philadelphia: Lippincott Williams and Wilkins.

Lo B, Wolf LE, Berkeley A. 2000. Conflict-of-interest policies for investigators in clinical trials. *New England Journal of Medicine* 343:1616–20.

McCormick BB, Tomlinson G, Brill-Edwards P, Detsky AS. 2001. Effect of restricting contact between pharmaceutical company representatives and internal medicine residents on posttraining attitudes and behavior. *Journal of the American Medical Association* 286:1994–99.

McCrary SV, Anderson CB, Jakovljevic J, Khan T, McCullough LB, Wray NP, Brody BA. 2000. A national survey of policies on disclosure of conflicts of interest in biomedical research. *New England Journal of Medicine* 343:1621–26.

Morin K, Rakatansky H, Riddick FA, Morse LJ, O'Bannon JM, Goldrich MS, Ray P, Weiss M, Sade RM, Spillman MA. 2002. Managing conflicts of interest in the conduct of clinical trials. *Journal of the American Medical Association* 287:78–84.

Orentlicher D, Hehir MK. 1999. Advertising policies of medical journals: Conflicts of interest for journal editors and professional societies. *Journal of Law, Medicine & Ethics* 27(2):113–21.

Orlowski JP, Wateska L. 1992. The effects of pharmaceutical firm enticements on physician prescribing patterns: There's no such thing as a free lunch. *Chest* 102:270–73.

Page L. 2000. More clinics ban drug samples, citing cost, safety concerns. *AMNews* staff. October 16.

P.L. 96-517, Patent and Trademark Amendments of 1980. Amended Title 35 USC, by adding Chapter 18, Section 200–212.

Prentice ED, Mann SL, Gordon BG. 2006. Administrative reporting structure for the institutional review board. In Bankert EA, Amdur RJ, eds. *Institutional Review Board: Management and Function.* 2nd ed. Sudbury, MA: Jones and Bartlett, pp. 31–32.

Relman AS. 1989. Economic incentives in clinical investigation. *New England Journal of Medicine* 320:933–34.

Rothman DJ. 2008. Academic medical centers and financial conflicts of interest. *Journal of the American Medical Association* 299(6):965–67.

Rothman KJ. 1993. Conflict of interest: The new McCarthyism in science. *Journal of the American Medical Association* 269:2782–84.

Schlafly P. Congressional hearing exposes conflicts of interest, www.eagleforum.org /column/2000/june00/00-06-28.html.

Shalala D. 2000. Protecting research subjects—what must be done. *New England Journal of Medicine* 343:808–10.

Shimm DS, Spece RG, Jr. 1991. Industry reimbursement for entering patients into clinical trials: Legal and ethical issues. *Annals of Internal Medicine* 115(2):148–51.

Spenser EM, Mills AE, Rorty, MV, Werhane PH. *Organization Ethics in Health Care.* New York: Oxford University Press, 2000.

Stryer D, Bero LA. 1996. Characteristics of materials distributed by drug companies. *Journal of General Internal Medicine* 11:575–83.

Sutherland M. *Advertising and the Mind of the Consumer: What Works, What Doesn't and Why.* Sydney: Allen & Unwin, 1993.

Tenery, RM, Jr. 2000. Interactions between physicians and health care technology industry. *Journal of the American Medical Association* 283(3):391–93.

University of Minnesota. www.research.umn.edu/ethics/modConflict.html.

Wahlbeck K, et al. 1999. Sponsored drug trials show more favorable outcomes. *British Medical Journal* 218:464.

Wazana A. 2000. Physicians and the pharmaceutical industry: Is a gift ever just a gift? *Journal of the American Medical Association* 283:373–80.

Werhane P, Doering J. 1995. Conflicts of interest and conflicts of commitment. *Professional Ethics* 4(3–4):47–81.

Westfall JM, McCabe J, Nicholas RA. 1997. Personal use of drug samples by physicians and officestaff. *Journal of the American Medical Association* 278(2):141–43.

Wynia MK, Cummins DS, VanGeest JB, Wilson IB. 2000. Physicians' manipulation of reimbursement rules for patients. *Journal of the American Medical Association* 283:1858–65.

Justice and Access to Unreimbursed Therapies

The following memorandum had its origins in discussions with the medical center heart transplant program about justice issues related to access to ventricular assist devices (VADs). In researching these issues, however, it became apparent that VADs were but one instance of the following generic problem confronting the medical center and other health care institutions: an expensive technology that can potentially benefit large numbers of people has recently received or is likely to receive FDA approval, but there is a time delay between approval and Medicare reimbursement for its use. How should the lack of reimbursement enter into organizational decision making about providing the therapy? The same question arises for many new pharmaceuticals that are awaiting or have recently received FDA approval. The issues and reasoning in this memorandum, therefore, have much wider application than to VADs alone.

Background

A recently completed study, Long-Term Use of a Left Ventricular Assist Device for End-Stage Heart Failure—dubbed the REMATCH (Randomized Evaluation of Mechanical Assistance for the Treatment of Congestive Heart Failure) study—compared the device with the latest drugs for patients with the most severe heart failure. The study found that the risk of death was 48% lower among patients who received the device, compared with those who received the most potent cardiac drugs. Although mortality was statistically reduced, few of the study patients who received the assist device survived longer than two years. The authors of the study conclude the following: "The use of a left ventricular assist device in patients with advanced heart failure resulted in a clinically meaningful survival benefit and an improved quality of life. A left ventricular assist device is an acceptable alternative therapy in selected patients who are not candidates for cardiac transplantation" (Rose et al. 2001, p. 1435).

Cardiac assist devices are extremely expensive, and this remains true even though the costs have dropped somewhat with the new generation of these devices. Costs of the first generation of VADs were in the range of $68,000 to $71,000 for the device itself and about $160,000 for the pre- and postsurgical and medical care during the 25- to 30-day hospital stay required for left ventricular assist devices (LVADs). Balanced against the costs of the technology are the possible savings from factors like reduced need for hospital admissions and years of life gained.

The FDA has approved the use of ventricular assist devices as a bridge to transplant and, as of November 2002, as a destination therapy as well. The important distinction is that a bridge therapy is used as a necessary support only until a more permanent or destination therapy, in this case, heart transplant, is available. Prior to its FDA approval as a destination therapy, the use of VADs for that purpose could not be reimbursed by Medicare or private insurance. But once they received FDA approval, Medicare decided to provide coverage for the use of VADs as a destination therapy in October 2003. Hence there was nearly a one-year time interval between FDA approval and Medicare coverage for this therapy.

VADs are but one example of a new generation of cardiac devices that hold out the prospect of benefiting large numbers of patients. Two other recent examples are implantable cardiac defibrillators (ICDs) and drug-eluting stents.

A recent study, entitled Multicenter Automatic Defibrillator Implantation Trial II (MADIT II), found that the death rate in patients with a prior myocardial infarction and advanced left ventricular dysfunction can be reduced by more than 30% with small devices called implantable defibrillators. The study also expanded considerably the number of patients for whom ICDs could be indicated. Estimates of the number of patients who meet the criteria of the MADIT II trial are between 400,000 and 600,000 (Moss et al. 2002). At the same time, the device itself costs about $20,000 and the surgical costs are around $10,000. With the number of new patients each year who could benefit from the device plus the three million patients who already have had serious heart attacks and could be helped, the total potential costs are enormous. The FDA approved the device for this large patient group in July 2002 and after extensive debate, the Centers for Medicaid and Medicare Services (CMS) decided to extend coverage to a select subgroup in July 2003. The decision to limit Medicare coverage was based on the belief that the government could not afford to pay for implantable defibrillators in all Medicare patients who meet the criteria set out in the MADIT II trial.[†]

The newest device in this area is the drug-eluting stent. Studies seem to indicate that this new type of stent is significantly better than bare-metal stents in preventing restenosis. Hospital administrators and device manufacturers are predicting that there will be a rapid conversion from bare-metal to drug-eluting stents and a slightly less rapid conversion from coronary artery by-pass graft (CABG) to the new devices. These next-generation stents cost three times as much as uncoated stents. Two drug-eluting stents received FDA approval for sale in the United States, one model in April 2003 and another in March 2004. Codes for Medicare funding became effective July 1, 2003. Although the time interval between granting FDA approval and assigning the Medicare codes was relatively short, only a few months, actual reimbursement did not begin immediately thereafter.

The Problem of Delayed Reimbursement

LVADs, ICDs, and drug-eluting stents share a number of common features and raise similar ethical problems. In each case, when the number of patients appropriate for the device is multiplied by the costs of the device and the care associated with it, the total expenditure is considerable. This inevitably raises the question of rationing: how much should government be expected to pay for these new therapies, given that its total budget for health-related services is not unlimited? This issue, while critical from a social justice standpoint, is not the topic of this memorandum, however.

The issue is of more immediate concern to health care organizations. In each case, there is a temporary issue of reimbursement because the decision by Medicare to cover the device does not occur until after FDA approval, anywhere from a few months to nearly a year later. Even after FDA approval, reimbursement may be delayed because each new device is typically assigned a unique ICD-9 billing code, which is used to compile one year of cost data in order to determine appropriate coverage. As a result, hospitals must often wait a long time, sometimes years, for reimbursement that adequately compensates for the costs associated with these technological breakthroughs. This delay places hospitals in a financially precarious and ethically uncomfortable position. They must consider whether and to what extent

---

[†] In July 2002, the FDA approved the MADIT II indications for the first ICD, and, in June 2003, the Centers for Medicare and Medicaid Services (CMS) approved coverage for a select subgroup of MADIT II patients. The FDA has since approved several other ICDs, and CMS has expanded its coverage.

they are prepared to take a financial hit by providing patients with FDA-approved devices before Medicare and other insurance reimburse them.

Ethical Principles

The issue raised by VADs, ICDs, and drug-eluting stents is essentially one of responsible and prudent stewardship of limited health care resources. In accordance with the principle of responsible stewardship articulated in its code of ethics, the medical center needs to consider how it should respond to these new technological breakthroughs, not just one at a time but from a broader perspective. This task is made more difficult because of the rapidity and frequency with which these new technologies become available. Discussions of this memorandum by the medical center bioethics committee generated the following guidelines:

- When there is a time lag between FDA approval of a new therapy and its coverage by public or private health insurance, the medical center should evaluate on a program-by-program basis how and to what extent it can absorb the cost of the new therapy.

  Explanation: Every new decision involving nonreimbursable care has to be considered on its merits and not merely as an adjunct to a decision that has already been made. For example, providing VADs as a bridge to transplant does not obligate the medical center to provide VADs as a destination therapy, if the latter is not reimbursable.

  This guideline is compatible with the following:
- The medical center should take a proactive stance with insurance companies to ensure speedy and adequate payment for new devices.
- The medical center should pursue creative strategies for making FDA-approved devices available to patients who can benefit from them without having to take a financial hit for doing so.

  Finally,
- The principle of informed consent requires that patients be fully informed about which cardiac devices are available to them and the conditions under which they will be provided.

Conclusion

New and challenging ethical issues arise when new therapies become available but are not yet reimbursable by public or private health insurance. The Medical Center will need to decide whether and to what extent it will offer FDA-approved but not-yet-reimbursed therapies. Such decisions necessarily involve trade-offs, specifically determining what other services and programs will need to be forgone or curtailed as a result of providing these new treatments. The problem of reimbursement will become even more pressing as new or modified devices improve upon the current generation of VADs and other cardiac devices, such as ICDs and drug-eluting stents, receive FDA approval and are clinically indicated for more patients.

References

Barold HS. 2003. Using the MADIT II criteria for implantable cardioverter defibrillators—what is the role of the Food and Drug Administration approval? *Cardiac Electrophysiology Review* 7(4):443–46.

Bigger JT. 2002. Expanding indications for implantable cardiac defibrillators. *New England Journal of Medicine* 346(12):931–33.

Centers for Medicare & Medicaid Services. 2003. Medicare announces its intention to cover ventricular assist devices as destination therapy. *Medicare News*, www.cms.hhs.gov /apps/media/press/release.asp?counter=881 (accessed May 11, 2006).

Groeneveld PW, Matta MA, Greenhut AP, Yang F. 2008. The cost of drug-eluting coronary stents among Medicare beneficiaries. *American Heart Journal* 155(6):1097–1105.

McClellan MB, Tunis SR. 2005. Medicare coverage of ICDs. *New England Journal of Medicine* 352(3):222–24.

Moss AJ, Zareba W, Hall WJ, Klein H, Wilbur DJ, Cannom DS, Daubert JP, Higgens SL, Brown MW, Andrews ML. 2002. Prophylactic implantation of a defibrillator in patients with myocardial infarction and reduced ejection fraction. *New England Journal of Medicine* 346(12):877–83.

Rose EA, Gelijns AC, Moskowitz AJ, Heitjan DF, Stevenson LW, Dembritsky W, Long JW, Ascheim DD, Tierney AK, Levitan RG, Watson JT, Meier P. 2001. Long-term use of a left ventricular assist device for end-stage heart failure. *New England Journal of Medicine* 345(20):1435–43.

U.S. Food and Drug Administration. 2003. FDA approves drug-eluting stent for clogged heart arteries. *FDA News* P03–31. www.fda.gov/bbs/topics/NEWS/2003/NEW00896 .html (accessed May 11, 2006).

Guidelines for Transferring Patients between Services

Patients are transferred between clinical services based on where their care needs will be most effectively met. The determination of when, how, and where transfers take place has been the subject of controversy in some instances when services have refused to accept transfers that the original treating services considered to be in the patient's best interest. This type of dispute may compromise patient care.

Because interservice transfer has both clinical and organizational ethical implications, the bioethics committee was asked to consider the issues, identify the relevant principles, and propose a set of guidelines as a way to preempt disputes over patient transfers and resolve conflicts if they occur.

Ethical Principles

The medical center code of ethics articulates the following overarching institutional commitment: "The medical center recognizes that its primary mission is to ensure the provision of high-quality, ethically based patient care." The code expressly articulates this commitment by recognizing that the institution's responsibilities include

- promoting continuity of care by coordinating services among providers
- promoting collaborative clinical management and supporting the authority of specific multidisciplinary teams
- supporting attending physicians' professional judgment and authority, while requiring institutional oversight and joint clinical management and imple-

menting a plan of care that reflects the patient's best interest, regardless of financial compensation

- promoting cost-effective care through cooperative clinical decision making that uses resources wisely
- supporting a principled dispute resolution system that addresses treatment and interpersonal conflicts, strives for consensus and is based on ethical, medical and legal principles.

The fundamental ethical principle of respect for patients underlies the health care institution's commitment to patient well-being and confers organizational obligations to promote clinical excellence, collaborative case management, and wise stewardship of resources. These institutional responsibilities require that patients be cared for in the most appropriate clinical setting, which, in the hospital, means the service with the most targeted skills and resources. Because the delivery of high-quality patient care requires institutional direction and support, the organization must take ownership of facilitating appropriate interservice transfers.

- Clinical decisions, including determinations of the most appropriate plan and locus of care, depend primarily on the care needs of the patient, the therapeutic options, and the professional staff and technical resources available to provide the needed care. Particular attention should be given to the interventions that can and cannot be provided on each service.
- Transfer decisions should recognize that relocation between services or even units within services may not be in the patient's best interest and should not be considered without compelling clinical reason(s).
- Transfer criteria should be derived from evidence-based data about the clinical resources necessary to maximize therapeutic outcomes.
- Budgetary and bureaucratic concerns, while important to deliberations about resource allocation, must not impede or compromise the care of individual patients.
- Physicians have a responsibility for the care of their hospitalized patients that transcends financial considerations or length-of-stay imperatives.
- Plans of care that respond to patients' treatment needs may require that individual physician case management be replaced by collaborative case management. This may require transfer to services that provide different types of care.

Interservice Transfer Guidelines—Draft Policy
Clinical Guidelines

- Transfers should be initiated with a request by the patient's attending or house staff for consultation by the service that is being asked to accept the patient. The request should specify the patient's clinical condition, diagnostic or treatment needs, and the reasons why transfer is considered necessary, including the resources and interventions that may be provided more effectively on the receiving service (e.g., wound debridement, psychiatric treatment).
- Within 24 hours, the consultation request should be answered by a physician who evaluates the patient for transfer, communicates with the requesting physician, and enters a note in the chart reflecting the transfer decision. If the

clinical situation is urgent, the request should be answered within one hour. Both the discussion and the note should address the patient's care needs, the transfer criteria, and the available resources. The note should clearly explain why the patient will or will not benefit from transfer to a different service.

- Upon transfer, further care of the patient becomes the responsibility of the accepting service, including the determination of type, level, and location of care.
- If, after discussion, there is disagreement about whether the patient should be transferred—if the patient's current service believes that transfer is appropriate and the consulting service refuses to accept the patient—the matter should be escalated to senior physicians on each service. The lines of communication should be resident-resident, service attending-service attending, and service chief-service chief. In this way, the matter is escalated to physicians of comparable experience, expertise, and authority on each service.
- Additional consultations from other services should be requested at any point if the deliberations would benefit from different perspectives and expertise.
- If disagreement remains, the matter should be referred to the medical director for resolution. If the clinical situation is urgent, the medical director's decision will be binding.
- The entire process of consultation, escalating discussion, and appeal should be expedited as much as possible. If the situation is urgent, the question of transfer should be resolved within two hours. If the situation is not urgent, the question of transfer should be resolved within 48 hours.

Organizational Guidelines

- Institutional policy should recognize that interservice transfer decisions should be based on (1) the patient's best interest, and (2) whether specific services have the clinical resources and skills to meet the patient's health care needs.
- The institution should take steps to promote efficient and effective transfer decisions, and to minimize administrative barriers, including length-of-stay consideration and attribution.
- Institutional policy should articulate and support conflict resolution mechanisms that address the care needs of patients and the resource needs of clinical services.

Decision-Making Protocol for the Patient Alone

Adult patients are presumed to have the capacity to make decisions about their health care. In the clinical setting, decisional capacity consists of the ability to

- understand the basic facts of one's medical situation, including current condition and prognosis;
- weigh the benefits, burdens, and risks of the presented treatment options, including the option of no treatment;
- apply a set of personal values;
- arrive at a decision that is consistent over time; and
- communicate the decision.

Patients determined to lack decisional capacity need treatment decisions made for them to promote their health and protect their rights of bodily integrity. Under most circumstances, guidance in making decisions for the incapacitated patient may come from an advance directive, expressing the wishes of the patient before losing capacity, or from family or even close friends with knowledge of what the patient would want or what would be in the patient's best interest. The notion of patient best interest is specific to the individual, but it is considered to include pain and symptom management, maintenance or enhancement of comfort and function, and amelioration of suffering.

Ethical Principles

Patients alone—those without capacity, advance directives, family, or friends—present special challenges because their wishes are inaccessible and the usual sources of information about them are unavailable. In the clinical setting, the responsibility for making treatment decisions for this vulnerable population necessarily falls to the clinical and administrative staff of the health care institution. This decision-making authority is grounded in the following principles:

- The health care institution has an obligation to provide high-quality care that responds to the patient's medical needs. The institution assumes additional fiduciary responsibilities to protect vulnerable patients who cannot act in their own interest, have provided no expression of their wishes, and have no one to advocate for them.
- The goals and plan of care are informed by the patient's condition and prognosis; the benefits, burdens, and risks of the therapeutic options; and an assessment of what is in the patient's best interest. These considerations receive heightened scrutiny when the patient is without capacity or personal supports.
- The best interest of a patient, especially one at the end of life, does not always require aggressive therapeutic or diagnostic intervention. The threshold determination should be whether the overall goal of care is cure, improvement, remission, maintenance, or comfort, and the plan of care should reflect the indicated focus.
- It is the responsibility of the attending physician, in consultation with the health care team, to make a medical assessment, including a determination of whether the patient is dying, develop a plan of care, and make medical recommendations.
- Respect for persons requires that their wishes about their own care be accorded as much deference as possible. Patients with decisional capacity who understand their treatment options and their implications should have their refusals of treatment honored so long as they understand the consequences of their decisions. Patients alone, although lacking the capacity to make care decisions for themselves, should not be subjected to treatment over their active objections. When the best interests of vulnerable patients are in tension with their "spoken choice," the institution has a heightened responsibility to exercise protective clinical and administrative judgment.
- In its dual role as health care provider and surrogate decision maker, the institution has a responsibility to use all appropriate clinical and administrative

resources in making and reviewing decisions that affect the treatment of patients alone.

- Because the following protocol is a multistep review of the medical need for one or more diagnostic or therapeutic interventions, it is not applicable in emergency situations when delaying immediate interventions will put the patient at unacceptable risk. In such situations, the well-settled doctrine of implied consent permits emergency treatment without consent.

Protocol

There is no such thing as administrative consent. Consent that is provided by a surrogate or a health care agent when a patient is not able to make his own medical decisions is a form of consent that is widely accepted as legitimate in a variety of situations. Administrative consent, however, is not a form of surrogate consent; indeed, it is not really any type of consent. What is misleadingly labeled *administrative consent* is actually a process of *review* by the medical director, or a physician designated by the medical director, to determine whether the medical case meets certain criteria. These criteria are discussed below.

The office of the medical director will perform the following functions:

- Consult with any attending physician who recommends that a patient without capacity, advance directive, or identifiable surrogate (a patient alone) undergo a specific procedure that requires signed informed consent. Review with the attending the proposed procedure, including its indications, the potential risks and benefits, and the alternatives, including no treatment.
- Request clinical consultations that may inform the decision by clarifying the goals and plan of care.
- Review efforts to identify a surrogate for the patient and, if indicated, make additional efforts, including contacting the patient's nursing home or prior treating physician(s).
- Ascertain whether
  - the patient alone is refusing recommended treatment or is merely unresponsive, especially the patient whose refusal appears focused and consistent;
  - ethical, clinical, or legal concerns, uncertainties, or disagreements have been raised by the patient's care team;
  - the decision generates conflict with administrative and clinical goals related to length of stay; or
  - disagreement exists within the health care team regarding the necessity of the intervention.

    In any of these circumstances, the office of the medical director will arrange for multidisciplinary case review by the medical director or designee, the patient's attending physician, another physician in the attending's department, risk management, the Legal Department, and the bioethics committee. This review may reveal the need for a dispute resolution process.
- Refer the decision to the medical director, or her designee, when no surrogate has been identified, no objections have been raised by the clinical team,

and the attending physician wishes to proceed. The medical director or designee will review the patient's medical record and examine the patient.

- If the medical director or designee *concurs* with the attending physician that the proposed procedure is medically indicated and in the patient's best interest, based on the options available to the patient at the time, the medical director or designee so indicates in the remarks section of the informed consent form. Administrative authorization to proceed with treatment is provided in lieu of the consent of the patient or surrogate.
- If the medical director or designee *does not agree* that the procedure is indicated or in the patient's best interests, she may discuss with the attending physician consideration of an alternative approach to treating/caring for the patient or request a multidisciplinary review, if needed, to clarify the issues further.

ADDITIONAL EDUCATION OPPORTUNITIES

Depending on your members' interest, knowledge, and skills, your ethics committee can provide education to your institution in additional ways. Consider creating a subcommittee that functions as a speakers bureau, making members available to provide information about the ethics service during orientations for new physicians and nurses. Offer an ethics perspective on standing committees or panels that are part of programs presented by other services or departments. Arrange for an interested member to serve on your institutional review board (IRB) and contribute to the protection of human subjects in research trials. Committee members who wish to further enhance their knowledge and skills may want to consider the one-year certificate programs, which offer more in-depth bioethics education.

Finally, the following blogs and websites (accessed September 2014) are just some of the online resources that provide a wealth of bioethics-related information and opportunities to interact with the bioethics community.

Institutes:
www.bioethicsinstitute.org (The Berman Institute)
http://rockethics.psu.edu/rockethics/bioethics (Pennsylvania State University)

Centers:
www.thehastingscenter.org (excellent bioethics materials from The Hastings Center)
www.ahc.umn.edu/bioethics (Center for Bioethics, University of Minnesota)
www.cbc-network.org (The Center for Bioethics and Culture Network)
https://cbhd.org (The Center for Bioethics & Human Dignity, Trinity International University)
www.practicalbioethics.org (Center for Practical Bioethics)

Other:
http://bioethics-international.org/index.php?width=1920&height=1080&show=index (The International Association of Bioethics)

www.nuffieldbioethics.org (Nuffield Council on Bioethics)

www.bioethics.gov (Presidential Commission for the Study of Bioethical Issues)

www.womensbioethics.org/index.php (Women's Bioethics Project)

www.ncbcenter.org (National Catholic Bioethics Center)

http://bioethics.net (blog, AMA's Journal of Ethics, Virtual Mentor)

http://globalbioethics.blogspot.com (international)

http://healthblawg.typepad.com (health care law blog)

www.ethicsweb.ca/resources (general ethics blog source—you can select health care, general ethics, and other relevant topics)

www.ethicsweb.ca/resources/bioethics/publications.html (list of bioethics publications available online)

www.bioethicsforum.org (has a nice list of additional blogs down the left side)

http://blogs.wsj.com/health (*Wall Street Journal* health care blog; not focused exclusively on ethics, but good for quick industry news)

www.eperc.mcw.edu/EPERC.htm (Medical College of Wisconsin website, including Fast Facts)

http://bioethics.od.nih.gov/academic.html (National Institutes of Health [NIH] website, very useful)

www.asbh.org (American Society of Bioethics and Humanities, very useful)

Sample Clinical Cases

The following sample cases are representative, but not exhaustive, of the kind likely to come before an ethics committee or consultation service. They appear as they would be presented for consideration, with a description of the clinical situation and an overview of the key ethical issues that would receive attention in an ethics consultation or case review. Three cases are supplemented by sample chart notes that illustrate how the ethics consultation might be documented in the medical record. To enhance their accessibility and utility, we have categorized the cases according to the issues they illustrate. Each category contains one detailed case with analysis, in some instances followed by a similar case that presents variations or raises additional issues. Further information about the concepts and principles discussed in the analyses, as well as other case examples, can be found in the relevant chapters in part I.

ADOLESCENT DECISION MAKING

Joey Barnes was a 15-year-old with Hodgkin's disease, a form of lymphatic cancer that is curable 90% of the time if it is discovered and treated promptly. But chemotherapy, the treatment that most often proves successful in fighting the disease, has a number of painful side effects.

After Joey began chemotherapy, his hair fell out, his jaw ached, and he was often left with a metallic taste in his mouth. He also complained of nausea and various aches and pains. These are common side effects of chemotherapy, in adults as well as adolescents, and Joey was told he could expect them when he began treatment. He agreed to continue the chemotherapy after consulting with the doctors and his parents, all of whom urged him to accept the treatment.

After a few months of treatment, however, Joey had a change of mind. The pain had become increasingly difficult for him to tolerate and he complained that it interfered with the things he liked to do most, like skateboarding, playing video games, and hanging out with his friends. He became withdrawn and depressed. He told his doctors and parents that he did not want to continue with chemotherapy. Against their advice, he ran off to a neighboring state so that he wouldn't have to undergo any more treatments. He spent roughly two weeks traveling, staying with fellow skateboarders he met and with families who took him in. While he was on the run, his parents received hundreds of letters and phone calls from strangers offering words of encouragement. Many former cancer patients who had been cured by chemotherapy offered testimonials. After two weeks, Joey returned home, but continued to refuse further chemotherapy. The doctors treating him sought court intervention to order Joey to continue with treatment. The court granted Joey's wish and allowed him to discontinue chemotherapy. After four months, Joey died at home, surrounded by his grieving parents.

As Joey's story and the case of James in chapter 5 illustrate, whether to accede to an adolescent's decision to forgo life-sustaining treatment is one of the most anguishing decisions that parents, as well as caregivers, can face. On the one hand, an adolescent like Joey still seems in many respects to be a child. While his interests, including skateboarding, video games, and spending time with friends, are age-appropriate, their significance seems much diminished when they are given as the reasons for a course of action that will end his life.

While Joey's interests are worthy of consideration and should not be ridiculed or dismissed, it would certainly be understandable if his parents told him that he is too young and inexperienced to be able to make a decision like this unilaterally and that, especially because the cure rate for his type of cancer is quite high with chemo, he will just have to tough it out. They might also, with some warrant, justify not acceding to his wish by predicting that, when the chemo is over and he has recovered, he will be grateful that they did not allow him to stop chemotherapy. Moreover, because Joey's desire to end treatment may be transitory, it has not withstood the test of time and become well settled, usually considered a requirement for these types of decisions. These points argue against acceding to Joey's wish to end treatment. It should also be remembered by all parties to the decision-making process that Joey has chosen to end *chemotherapy*, not *his life*, and efforts should continue to find a treatment regimen that, while less effective, may also be less toxic than chemotherapy and, perhaps, an option Joey would agree to try.

On the other hand, an adolescent's decisional capacity depends in part on his cognitive capacities, and these are more sophisticated than those observed in younger children. Adolescents Joey's age frequently demonstrate adult capacity, especially in cognition, although it may not be constant and their behavior may sometimes oscillate between childlike and adult behavior. They may often make rational decisions and choices just like adults and just as often display decisional immaturity.

Indeed, research has shown that middle adolescents like Joey do not generally underestimate risk any more than adults, despite the common view of them as impulsive and irrational. Add to this that Joey, unlike his parents or caregivers, knows firsthand what chemotherapy is like, and this might be grounds for crediting his decision with a degree of maturity that it might otherwise lack. These points speak in favor of acceding to Joey's wish.

The role of Joey's doctors is also complicated. There is strong reason to believe that treatment will be successful and that if Joey cooperates, they can help him get better. The doctors caring for Joey are trained to help prolong patients' lives, at least when those lives are of quality acceptable to the patients, and Joey's refusal presents an obstacle to this objective. His physicians should convey their reservations about his decision and attempt to dissuade him. The fact that they sought a court order to compel Joey to continue treatment should be explained as an expression of their concern, although it went beyond dissuasion.

Yet there are also grounds for respecting his decision if he is intellectually and emotionally capable of deciding. This is something that needs to be investigated in order to determine whether Joey's decision to end chemotherapy is reflective and not impetuous. It would also be advisable for Joey's physicians to consult with his parents, who are in the best position to assess the maturity of his decision.

Age alone cannot be decisive here and generalizations about adolescents are always precarious to some degree because there are enormous variations in cognitive and emotional capacities even among adolescents of the same age. By running away, Joey sought to terminate his relationship with his caregivers, but even if they acquiesce in Joey's decision, they should not abandon him or give him any reason to believe they have done so. They should continue to be involved at least to the extent of providing support to Joey and his family.

In the end, there is a sad truth that has to be faced: for chemotherapy to be effective, Joey must cooperate with treatment, and he is not doing so. Ethics aside, it is simply not feasible to force him to undergo chemotherapy against his will for an extended period of time.

ADVANCE DIRECTIVES

Mrs. Dunn is a 94-year-old woman who was admitted to the hospital from a nursing home for surgical repair of a hip fracture. Her baseline mental status was described by the nursing home as "moderate dementia with intermittent confusion and inattentiveness." The nursing staff says that she is usually vocal in refusing treatments and medications, and that coaxing is often required to obtain her cooperation for therapy.

According to the living will that Mrs. Dunn signed in 2004 when she was admitted to the nursing home, she has been a devout Jehovah's Witness for more than 30 years. The living will directs that "no transfusions of blood or blood products be given to me under any circumstances, even if physicians deem such necessary to preserve my life or health." At the same time she executed the living will, she also appointed her son, Tom, who is not a Jehovah's Witness, to be her health care proxy agent.

Although her health has been reasonably good, Mrs. Dunn has been hospital-ized several times during these years, for pneumonia, kidney stones, and appendi-citis. When she provided consent for the 2006 appendectomy, it was with the clear understanding that no blood transfusions would be given, and, fortunately, none was needed.

On admission to the hospital for hip surgery, Mrs. Dunn was evaluated and found to lack the capacity to make decisions about her treatment. She appears very un-comfortable, confused, and frightened. When attempts are made to examine her, she responds by pulling away and saying, "No, no!" Now that surgery is being con-sidered, her son, Tom, has been contacted to assume the decisional authority of her health care agent. When the clinical situation is explained, he says, "Do the surgery and give her blood if she needs it. At this point, she's too out of it to understand or object. The important thing is to give her the best chance to come through this safely and comfortably."

Dr. Lewis, the orthopedic surgeon, has requested a bioethics consult because of his expectation that she will need blood transfusions either during or after the sur-gical hip repair. If she needs blood and does not receive it, life-threatening com-plications (e.g., hemorrhage, heart attack) could result. If she does not have the surgery and the fracture is treated with bed rest, other complications (e.g., throm-bophlebitis, pulmonary emboli, pneumonia, pressure ulcers) could develop.

Dr. Lewis is troubled because he believes that surgery, with blood if necessary, is clearly the preferred option and that it is his professional responsibility to advocate for that approach. Yet, he also knows that Mrs. Dunn's living will is a legally enforce-able expression of her preferences. He questions whether a surgeon can be asked to undertake this type of surgery without giving blood if it becomes necessary dur-ing or after the operation. He also questions whether a surgeon may refuse to op-erate under those circumstances and, if so, what happens to the patient.

This is a case that cries out for a clinical ethics consultation. It invokes the prin-ciples of autonomy, beneficence, and nonmaleficence, and raises issues of decisional capacity, informed consent and refusal, advance care planning, and surrogate de-cision making. It involves the interests of a vulnerable patient, concerned family, conscientious physician, and responsible institution. It's practically a mini-course in bioethics all by itself.

Because the consult request comes from Dr. Lewis, his perspective is the ethics consultant's introduction to the case. His concern is that he may be asked to com-promise his professional judgment and obligations by withholding clinically indi-cated care, thereby putting the patient at risk. Knowing the likely complications of orthopedic surgery without blood transfusion, he is worried about Mrs. Dunn's well-being. He is also understandably nervous about his reputation and possible legal liability if foreseeable adverse events occur. How can he, as a responsible doctor, not protect his patient from likely harm? On the other hand, how can he abandon his patient by refusing to operate? Not surprisingly, the similar interests of the institution, represented by the offices of legal counsel and risk management, also reflect the organizational responsibilities to promote the patient's well-being and protect her from harm.

But the ethics consultant understands that this case presents multiple, sometimes competing, interests that need to be considered during the consultation meeting. While the concerns of the care professional and the institution are important, the central figures in this or any ethics conflict are the patient, the family, and, if available, the health care proxy agent.

Ideally, the capable patient is able to articulate her own goals and wishes in explaining her choice of a particular course of action. Clarity and consistency are especially important when the decision is to refuse potentially life-saving treatment. In this case, however, Mrs. Dunn is no longer able to advocate for herself and her wishes will have to be communicated through other means. Of course, this is where advance directives are critical in making sure that the voice of the now-incapacitated patient is still heard in the care planning. Perhaps anticipating that her religious beliefs would conflict with her medical needs, Mrs. Dunn's living will explicitly and unambiguously rejected blood and blood products under any and all circumstances, including the preservation of her life and health. The authenticity of this statement is bolstered by more than 30 years as a devout Jehovah's Witness, indicating a firm and settled adherence to the tenets of the religion. Her refusal of blood transfusions when she had the appendectomy suggests that she understood and accepted the risks of bloodless surgery, including possible death, making it likely that she would make the same decision now. Indeed, the theory underlying advance care planning is that respect for autonomy is demonstrated by continuing to honor the value-based wishes articulated and demonstrated by the patient when capable.

Her son, Tom, presents yet another perspective. His expressed goal is to protect his mother from what he perceives as foolish decisions that put her health and life in jeopardy. Because he does not share her religious beliefs, he sees them as a dispensable barrier to her well-being. He insists that his appointment as her health care agent empowers him to make decisions that respond to her current medical condition, even if they depart from her living will.

Tom is in a somewhat conflicted position because his two roles present competing interests and responsibilities. As a concerned son, his somewhat paternalistic approach is that advancing his mother's health and safety justifies overriding what he considers her self-destructive wishes. As a health care agent, however, his obligation is to represent what he knows of her wishes and values, unless they do not apply to her current situation. Unless he can demonstrate a reasonable likelihood that she would have changed her mind and accepted transfusions during the proposed surgery, her unambiguous living will and prior decision history argue forcefully for treatment that does not involve blood or blood products.

A clinical ethics consultation should surface these issues, explore the ethical reasoning, and help develop an appropriate care plan. Goals should include helping Tom to appreciate the importance of honoring his mother's long-held values. Skillful intervention should assist him in accepting that, while this would not be the decision he would want for himself or his mother, the refusal of blood is one of her core values, an essential part of who she is. His responsibility as her trusted agent includes being her voice and making the decisions that are authentic for *her*. He should be supported in making this very difficult decision and reassured that aggressive attention will be given to her medical needs, focusing on her comfort.

The consultation should also support Dr. Lewis's decision about whether he or another doctor should assume responsibility for Mrs. Dunn's care. He should be helped to understand that, if he cannot provide what he believes to be high-quality care within the limitations of the patient's wishes, he can meet his professional obligations by exploring alternatives. Considerations will include the potential for surgery without blood in this institution or transfer to a hospital that specializes in bloodless surgery. Because symptom management and end-of-life care will be important, a member of the palliative care service would be a helpful addition to the consultation. Additional guidance and support for Dr. Lewis might come from the institution's offices of legal counsel and risk management.

Mrs. Barnes is a 77-year-old woman who suffers from chronic obstructive pulmonary disease, peripheral vascular disease, and early dementia. During the six years that she has lived in the nursing home, her medical condition has remained fairly stable, although her cognitive status has gradually declined. Nevertheless, she is still able to interact with her family, care providers, and other residents, as well as make simple decisions about her daily activities. When she entered the nursing home, Mrs. Barnes completed a health care proxy document, appointing her daughter, Carol, as her primary agent and her son, Philip, as the alternate agent. A living will executed at the same time contains care instructions, including a statement that she would not want dialysis if she were terminally ill or permanently unconscious.

Recently, Mrs. Barnes complained of chest pain and shortness of breath, and exhibited a change in her mental status, becoming more confused and agitated. She was admitted to the hospital, where tests revealed that she had suffered a mild heart attack and was in acute renal failure. Her attending and a renal consultant have recommended a few dialysis treatments to improve her kidney function and possibly clear her mental status while the extent of her heart damage is assessed. When her care team determined that she was unable to make care decisions or provide informed consent to treatment, the clinicians turned to her appointed health care agent and alternate. Carol has consented to the recommended dialysis, but Philip argues that such a course would violate their mother's living will. Carol responds, "If Mom had known that temporary dialysis might improve her condition, especially while we are waiting to see about her heart, she certainly would have agreed to that. What she never wanted was to be dependent on long-term dialysis or to have it just prolong her dying."

An ethics consult has been requested to help resolve the conflict.

This case also presents an inconsistency between a patient's living will and the decision of the appointed proxy agent. Two critical differences, however, should be appreciated and highlighted by a skilled ethics consultation. First, the provisions of the living will may not apply to the patient's current clinical condition. Until further clinical assessments are completed, it is not possible to know whether Mrs. Barnes is in an irreversible or terminal condition that she would find unacceptably prolonged by dialysis. Until that determination is made, dialysis may enhance the possibility of a successful outcome.

Second, the statements in the living will may not accurately or fully express the patient's wishes. Carol's knowledge of her mother provides insights that are not available in the written instructions. As a result, she is able to interact with the care team, respond to a clinical situation the patient did not anticipate, and interpret what her mother would want in current or future circumstances. Ethics consultation can provide the explanation and support that will reassure all parties that the proxy agent's authority and knowledge and the patient's trust enable her to make the decision that the patient would make if she could.

AUTONOMY IN TENSION WITH BEST INTEREST

Mrs. Miller is an 88-year-old woman with obstructive and restrictive lung disease and severe chronically undertreated hypothyroidism. She was admitted to the hospital in respiratory distress, hypothermia, and hypotension and intubated in the ER. She has had several other admissions over the past six months for similar symptoms. She was extubated easily and is improving with treatment. She should be ready for discharge within the next week.

The staff is concerned about how Mrs. Miller's home situation has contributed to her medical condition. She lives at home with her 91-year-old husband, who has moderate dementia, and her 40-year-old son, Terry, who has psychiatric problems. Both Mr. Miller and Terry appear disheveled when they visit Mrs. Miller in the hospital.

Mrs. Miller appears to be neglected at home and is continually readmitted to the hospital in critical condition. Her colostomy has been poorly maintained, and it is uncertain whether the bruises on her arms are from senile purpura or physical abuse. She has some dementia even when she is receiving medication to keep her thyroid functioning normally and she seems unable to manage her care without help. After prior discharges, Terry has dismissed the visiting nurse service (VNS) or other help sent to the home.

Mrs. Miller's younger son, Larry, is her legally appointed health care proxy agent, but he does not visit and has been unwilling to be involved in her care. Attempted interventions by social service have been rebuffed. The family has been reported to adult protective services, but the results of that investigation are not known. In the past, when Mrs. Miller was treated and improved, she has stated consistently that she does not want to go to a nursing home. The care team is concerned about how to provide a safe discharge for her while respecting her wishes.

This case is a graphic illustration of the tension between honoring the patient's wishes and promoting her best interest. Arranging a safe discharge is the professional and legal duty of the health care team and the institution. Mrs. Miller's multiple and escalating care needs plus her limited ability to meet them mean that she should be in an environment, either her home or a skilled care facility, which provides assistance and support. Yet, she has clearly and consistently rejected the option of nursing home placement, choosing to return to a situation where her needs are not met and she is in jeopardy. In addition, the risk of elder neglect and abuse is substantial in this case, heightening the obligation to protect this vulnerable patient.

Capable patients have the right to make decisions about discharge, even decisions that appear to put them at risk. As the risk of harm increases, the level of capacity needed to understand the implications and accept the consequences is increased. Mrs. Miller's past decisions to remain at home, despite the apparent neglect that impairs her health and safety, require heightened scrutiny of her capacity to understand her risks and options. Because she was not receiving medication regularly, her thyroid malfunction resulted in periodic cognitive impairment. Her diminished or fluctuating capacity increases concern about her ability to assume responsibility for an unsafe living situation.

If Mrs. Miller is shown to lack sufficient capacity to make discharge decisions, that responsibility will fall to her health care proxy agent. The fact that Mrs. Miller appointed her son, Larry, indicates that she considered him the most reliable person to speak on her behalf. This trust should not be readily overridden unless the agent is shown to be incompetent, unwilling to make decisions, or acting clearly against the best interests of the patient. It would be important to encourage Larry's participation in the decision making. His lack of involvement may be the result of family dynamics, anger toward the patient, an estranged relationship, or incomplete understanding of his role as the proxy agent. He may need education and support so that he does not feel abandoned to make critical decisions alone.

Without an able and willing proxy agent, decision making for the incapacitated patient is challenging. One option is a court-appointed guardian. Drawbacks include the six to nine months the appointment process typically takes, during which she would be in an unsafe environment, and the guardian's lack of familiarity with her values and wishes.

The health care team's primary responsibility is to the patient, promoting her best interest and, if possible, respecting her wishes. While the team's function is not to do family therapy, minimizing the barriers to consensus can facilitate care planning. In cases like this one, bioethics consultation can perform a valuable mediation function by helping all involved parties to reach consensus on a discharge solution for the patient. Even if Mrs. Miller lacks the capacity to make discharge decisions, her assent to the plan would be critical to its success and to her feelings of self-determination. She considers nursing home placement unacceptable and, in attempting to balance her wishes with her safety, it would be important to explore with her the reasons she objects to residential care facilities and perhaps arrange for her to visit a few.

Social service involvement is necessary to discharge planning, which can touch on very intimate family matters, as well as resource issues. Psychiatric counseling may be useful as well. Without assurance that necessary care services will be available and accepted at home, however, nursing facility placement may be the only responsible option.

Ms. Powell is a 35-year-old woman who has been HIV-positive for 10 years, presumably due to her history of IV drug use. She lives alone in a single-room occupancy (SRO) building, but she has been incarcerated in the past. She has been in and out of detoxification programs 10 times and reports that her sister died of an overdose. She has not adhered to her antiretroviral regimen, but details of her HIV care were not available. At her last methadone clinic appointment, she was noted to have anemia and increasing renal failure, and she presented to the ER with cough, fever, and flank pain. She was admitted and, because there was also a question of tuberculosis, she was placed in isolation.

In the ER, Ms. Powell was initially noted to be agitated and showing signs of opiate withdrawal but, when the physician returned to complete the exam, she appeared lethargic. This pattern has continued in the hospital and appears to coincide with the appearance of certain visitors. The house staff suspects that she is actively using heroin in the hospital and, because she was also receiving methadone, they are concerned for her safety. When asked, she denies drug use in the hospital.

The case has been discussed twice at staff rounds and several issues were raised. The initial concern was how to deal with Ms. Powell's apparent active drug use while in the hospital. The staff believes that, if all visitors are barred, she will probably sign out against medical advice. Questions included whether staff could legally search her belongings and how to guard against a fatal overdose if she is using heroin at the same time she is receiving methadone. At the second meeting, the focus was on whether to place a shunt for hemodialysis when the patient is believed to be an active heroin user, knowing that the shunt could easily be used to administer drugs. Another question was whether staff could refuse to continue caring for a patient who would not adhere to a treatment plan and puts herself at risk.

This is another instance in which respecting the patient's wishes is in tension with clinicians' obligation to promote her best interest and protect her from harm. While no one is questioning Ms. Powell's capacity to understand the risks of her behavior, it might be suggested that her addiction makes her unable to control her behavior. In the continuum of capacity, the compulsion of an addict may become an impediment to understanding the risks and benefits of a proposed treatment or course of action. If a person can comprehend the risks intellectually but cannot behave in a way that demonstrates appreciation of the risks, the argument can be made that decisional capacity is lacking. Addicts are often well aware of the danger of their behavior and some genuinely do want to stop drug use. But the addictive nature of drugs prevents them from controlling their self-destructive impulses. Their capacity to understand is not translated into the behavior that would promote adherence to treatment or avoidance of risk. If this is the case, they are not deciding autonomously.

The conflicts here concern both the patient's behavior and the care team's responses to it, and an ethics consultation can be useful in unpacking and analyzing the issues. While the clinical interaction is always a critical element, some situations are especially difficult for professionals. Here, the team faces the problems of substance abuse, institutional policies, and the obligation to promote the best interests of a difficult patient who is resisting help.

Drug rehabilitation treatment is often associated with temporary success and frequent relapses. Detoxification efforts require patience and persistence. The expertise of specialists who deal with active drug users is needed in this situation. The house staff was expending time and energy attempting to deal with the problem in a logical fashion, while lacking the experience and resources to do so. Their frustration stems from their inability to implement a beneficial plan of care or protect the patient from self-inflicted harm.

Establishing a good and trusting clinical relationship may be especially difficult with some patients. They may not be candid about their medical history or adhere to appointments and treatments; they may engage in disruptive and self-destructive behavior. While it is important to be empathic, patient, and persistent, doing so can be frustrating. Often a contract approach can be effective in setting limits. If the contract is reasonable and fair, and all parties can agree to it, this approach may facilitate the treatment program.

Placing a shunt sets up a therapeutic dilemma. Used for its intended purpose, the shunt would allow regular dialysis to improve Ms. Powell's renal function. Providing her with venous access, however, greatly increases the possibility of drug abuse and possibly overdose, as well as bacterial infection. In dealing with a capable patient, staff should initiate a thorough discussion of the risks and benefits of the procedure and hope that the patient makes the prudent decision. If the staff believes that the shunt will place the patient at significant risk, alternatives should be explored.

Health care professionals have a well-established duty to treat patients in need of medical care and not abandon them. Withholding dialysis, which has a clear benefit to Ms. Powell, because of a highly foreseeable risk of nonadherence, misuse, and infection may be considered paternalistic. The obligation to protect the patient from likely harm justifies staff concern, however, and this is best addressed candidly with Ms. Powell to see if she wants to take the risk of the dialysis shunt.

Transferring the patient's care to another professional because the clinician's values conflict with those of the patient may be justified if the conflict poses a significant barrier to communication or care. This can be done when the reason is explained to the patient and accepting clinicians are available. Transferring the treatment responsibility because the patient is difficult and frustrating may be less easily justified and should be carefully considered.

CONFIDENTIALITY

Laura Chase is a 40-year-old woman who has been a source of anxiety to the ICU staff for 36 days, ever since she was admitted in severe sepsis and respiratory failure. According to the medical team, her condition is the result of a rare and virulent multi-drug-resistant infection that she developed in response to the multiple medications she takes for her HIV infection. Despite aggressive treatment, her condition has continued to deteriorate. In a relatively short time, she has gone from an active and healthy-looking woman to a patient who is intubated, sedated, and only intermittently aware of her surroundings. Her prognosis is very poor.

Mrs. Chase's unusual syndrome, young age, and rapid decline have made her the focus of considerable attention by the care team. Attending physicians, nurses, medical students, and house officers meet regularly outside her room to consider modifications in her treatment plan. Dr. Ewing, chief of the MICU, and Marianne Haber, clinical care coordinator, are particularly involved in managing her care and interacting with her family.

Laura's family consists of her husband, Frank, and her two sisters, Phyllis and Rita. Frank has been a constant and devoted presence at his wife's bedside. As her legally appointed health care proxy agent, he has taken an active role in learning about her condition and making decisions on her behalf. He and Dr. Ewing meet regularly to discuss Laura's prognosis and various treatment options. He has advocated using whatever drugs or other therapies might help her and give her a chance to beat this illness. Within the past week, however, especially as her condition has deteriorated, his daily visits have been getting shorter.

During one of their early meetings, Frank told Dr. Ewing that Laura's sisters are very worried about her and very angry with him. "They don't know that she's HIV-positive, so they cannot understand what is wrong with her. Laura never wanted them to know about her diagnosis and she has hidden it from them ever since she found out. She believes they would think she was worthless and she made me promise that they not be told. They know I'm not telling them everything and they think the worst."

Phyllis and Rita are very concerned about their sister and, as Frank indicated, very angry about what they perceive as people being less than candid with them. They suggest that Frank should be removed as the health care proxy because they believe he is a threat to Laura's safety.

Within the past few days, the care team has determined that the endotracheal tube should be replaced with a tracheostomy, which will be more comfortable and also lessen the risk of additional infection and bleeding. In this way, the intervention would both be palliative and potentially promote cure. When the recommendation was presented to Frank, he concurred with the reasoning but refused to consent to the procedure without the agreement of his sisters-in-law. Marianne has spoken at length with Phyllis and Rita, who appear to understand and even agree with the proposed trach but are adamantly opposed to anything that Frank approves.

Here, respecting the patient's autonomy by protecting her confidentiality has exacerbated a strained family dynamic and threatens to impede her treatment by interfering with decision making. The benefits of confidentiality include a respectful and trusting relationship between clinician and patient, and the patient's willingness to be candid about sensitive issues so that accurate diagnosis and effective care management can be achieved. Health care professionals have a duty to keep confidential any patient information learned in the course of the clinical relationship. Exceptions are usually related to situations that place others at imminent and significant risk of harm.

The capable patient can determine who should receive confidential information and under what circumstances. Laura has made it clear that she does not want her diagnosis shared with others, none of whom are placed at risk by her request. The proxy agent or surrogate is bound by the patient's wishes regarding health information. In this case, Laura has instructed her husband, who is her health care agent, that her HIV diagnosis not be disclosed to others and, unless others are placed at direct risk, her wishes should be honored.

Frank agrees to the recommended tracheostomy and feeding tube, but he wants the concurrence and support of Phyllis and Rita. His ability to act as Laura's decision maker is inhibited by the lack of consensus generated by their hostility. This intrafamilial conflict threatens to prevent or at least delay care that would clearly benefit the patient. While consensus among family members is a worthy goal, the primary responsibility of the health care team remains the patient. As Laura's appointed proxy agent, Frank is the person she chose and trusted to make decisions in case of her incapacity. Her wishes and values are to be expressed and implemented through him, although his job is made considerably more difficult by the constraints she has placed on what he may disclose. So long as he can competently and responsively function in this capacity, he should be supported by the team. The sisters' concern for the patient is also legitimate and should be acknowledged, but it cannot be allowed to interfere with care planning. In the event that consensus is not achievable, Frank may need support in consenting to the recommended treatment even without the concurrence of his sisters-in-law.

Bioethics mediation may be helpful in arriving at an appropriate plan of care and perhaps enhanced communication. The consult would seek to help Frank, Phyllis, and Rita focus on their shared concern for Laura and their mutual goal of identifying a care plan that promotes her best interest. Recognition that the care team supports Frank's decisions as responsible and beneficial may diminish some of the sisters' anxiety. Working to achieve these goals should not be confused with attempts to help the family resolve long-standing resentments and conflicts. Bioethics consultation is not family therapy and the focus should remain firmly on resolving the patient's care issues.

Mrs. Cole is a 32-year-old woman admitted to the ICU with bilateral pulmonary infiltrates and impending respiratory failure. Her hospital course has included treatment for AIDS-related opportunistic infections. While her clinical picture and past history are suggestive of AIDS, she has not been tested and has consistently refused to address AIDS as a possible diagnosis. She has required mechanical ventilatory support since admission. Prior to intubation, she told her mother, the nurse, and the social worker, "Don't let them label me with AIDS. I know they are thinking that and you can't let them do it." At this time, she also completed an advance directive that appointed her mother to be her health care agent. Mrs. Cole's mother, Mrs. Davis, and her 7 siblings have held a constant vigil during her 43-day hospitalization. Mrs. Cole's children, ages 10 and 12, appear to be in good health and visit often. Her husband of more than five years has been incarcerated for the past six months. Although Mrs. Cole is being treated for AIDS-related complications, her family has not been directly told her diagnosis because of her expressed wishes. Mrs. Davis, without asking the name of her daughter's illness, acknowledges that her immune system has been compromised. She has agreed to the use of AIDS-related medications if they are potentially beneficial to her daughter and, yesterday, consented to a DNR order. Mrs. Cole's death appears imminent.

Here, the confidentiality issue is complicated by the patient's fear and denial, and the threat posed to other parties at risk. Not only does Mrs. Cole not want her possible AIDS diagnosis revealed to others, she does not want to confront it herself. She is saying, "Don't tell my diagnosis to me *or* anyone else."

The duty of confidentiality precludes professionals from disclosing anything learned in the clinical interaction, whether from the patient or from diagnostic work-up. Based on patients' expectation of confidentiality, they are likely to feel safer seeking care and more comfortable discussing sensitive issues. Although she did not want to acknowledge her likely AIDS, on some level Mrs. Cole obviously recognized it as a possibility. Despite her anxiety, she sought treatment with the understanding that, if the dreaded diagnosis were confirmed, it would not be revealed to her or others. In other words, "Treat me for whatever I have, just don't say that it's AIDS."

Patients have the right not to know about their conditions if they request nondisclosure and treatment does not require an explicit label. Certainly, patients have the right to determine who has access to their personal information. Breaching confidentiality is justified only when withholding information places third parties at significant and imminent risk. The laws in many states include this exception to the confidentiality obligation to require notification of identified sexual or needle-sharing partners of patients with HIV/AIDS. The threshold at which confidentiality may be breached must be set fairly high to avoid casual disclosure of sensitive information.

Mrs. Davis, acting on behalf of her daughter, would likely have difficulty understanding the clinical situation or making sound decisions without complete medical information. Ordinarily, this would set up a conflict between the professional obligations of confidentiality and beneficence to the patient. Because she appears to recognize that her daughter has AIDS, however, she is providing consent without asking that confidentiality be breached. The implicit message is, "You don't have to tell me she has AIDS, just treat her for it."

Mrs. Cole's children, husband, and any other sexual or needle-sharing partners, however, are another matter because they are all at risk. Warning them (or, in the case of the children, those responsible for them) may afford timely diagnosis and treatment if they are infected and may also prevent further spread of HIV infection to unidentified third parties. The significant consequences justify breaching confidentiality and discussing with Mrs. Davis the need to test and potentially treat her grandchildren for HIV. How these sensitive issues are considered and handled will benefit from bioethics involvement.

In some instances, patients will discuss their medical conditions with their care professionals but insist that their diagnoses not be disclosed to their health care agents. These restrictions most commonly occur with stigmatizing conditions, such as HIV/AIDS. In such situations, every effort should be made to help the patient appreciate that the agent's ability to interact with the care team and make appropriate surrogate decisions will depend on her having the same clinical information that the patient would have in making decisions. Emphasis should be placed on the relationship of trust that underlies the proxy appointment and the agent's commitment to act in the patient's best interest.

Sometimes patients are more concerned about how the information will affect their relationship with the agent than they are with having it disclosed. Often the most distressing prospect is having to face the agent with information the patient may consider shameful. One approach is to ask, "Is there a time when you would feel comfortable having us tell your agent about your condition?" One patient with end-stage AIDS, whose mother was her health care agent, replied to this question, "When I'm too sick to see the disappointment in her eyes, then you can tell her."

DECISIONAL CAPACITY

Mrs. Andrews is a 77-year-old widow living in the community who was admitted via the emergency room encrusted with feces and covered with maggots. Her nutritional status was poor, and she was both malnourished and dehydrated. On medical examination she was found to have an umbilical hernia, bilateral knee contractures, urinary incontinence, multiple neurological impairments, and marked dementia. After surgery and physical and occupational therapy, her ambulation was improved but she remained incontinent.

In the hospital, Mrs. Andrews was noisy and disruptive and required a single room. When engaged one-on-one, however, she was charming and articulate. She was soon able to feed herself and after two weeks she is neither malnourished nor dehydrated.

Prior to her hospitalization, Mrs. Andrews had lived alone in an apartment in the same building as her son, his wife, and their three children. Her Social Security check is more than $1,200 per month. Her son has no apparent source of support, other than a $500 check every other month from Social Security disability. It is not clear whether he has been misappropriating her funds, but staff suspect that might be the case. What is clear is that Mrs. Andrews cannot care for herself and her family does not seem willing or able to provide the support that she needs to keep herself clean, well-fed, and ambulatory.

The care team believes that Mrs. Andrews needs to be placed in a nursing home, where she will receive consistent care. She has regularly refused this placement and said that she wants to return home. "What else does an old lady have in the world besides her children and grandchildren?" On other days she says, "I don't know what to do. Whatever my son says is fine with me." A liaison psychiatry consultation has concluded that "the patient has significantly impaired ability to form a judgment about her discharge plan."

Decisional capacity refers to the ability to process information, make decisions, appreciate their implications, and assume responsibility for their consequences. This ability is decision-specific because most people have the ability to make some but not all decisions. Capacity can be constant, diminished, or fluctuating. It can be exercised entirely by the patient, supported by others, or delegated by the patient to trusted surrogates.

Mrs. Andrews is a good example of a person with fluctuating capacity. Her ability to understand her situation and make decisions in her best interest appears to be affected by her medical condition, her dementia, and her anxieties about being in unfamiliar surroundings. She seems to benefit physically, emotionally, and cognitively from being in a setting where her care needs are met and she has regular interpersonal contact. Yet, she expresses the desire to return to her home and family, a situation that does not seem to promote her best interest and may put her at significant risk.

Discharge planning for Mrs. Andrews would require a benefit-risk assessment. If she goes home, she may not live as long as she could if she were to go to a nursing home, where she would receive the care she needs. Nevertheless, many elderly patients choose to return home, knowing that they may compromise the extent or the quality of their lives. The notion of "home" is powerful, encompassing one's possessions, memories, comfort, and sense of self. Even if the nursing home represents "better care," it can also be regimented, unfamiliar, and impersonal.

Yet, some patients who initially refuse placement eventually adjust to the nursing facility and do very well, especially in contrast to an unsafe home environment. Care providers need to advocate for the solution that they think is best for each particular patient and accept that, in some cases, patients will choose unwisely. Clearly, capable patients who make risky decisions are a source of concern to staff, even though their choices usually should be honored. The personal intellectual and emotional calculus of each patient is unique and not necessarily consistent with the rational, professional judgments of caregivers.

For many elderly patients, like Mrs. Andrews, however, there are moments of confusion or periods of diminished capacity. In these instances, consistency over time may be a substitute for total clarity. If every time the patient is clear, she answers the same way, this pattern of choice has weight in those times of some cognitive compromise. This is especially persuasive if her choices are consistent with her prior history of capacitated decision making.

The principles in tension are autonomy, beneficence, and nonmaleficence. Care providers have an ethical obligation to support the capable patient's exercise of autonomy. That obligation may, nevertheless, come into direct conflict with the obligation to promote the patient's best interest and protect the patient from harm, especially if she is vulnerable because of diminished or uncertain capacity.

Finally, there is a difference between autonomously consenting to or refusing a medical intervention and choosing a home care plan. In the latter instance, the rights and interests of others besides those of the patient are at issue. In the home care context, the principle at issue is *accommodation*, that is, how the patient's wishes and desires can be met or modified by the ability or willingness of those whose cooperation is needed to carry out the plan. In this instance, the degree to which Mrs. Andrews's family can or will provide needed assistance is very uncertain. With the help of social service, it may be possible for her to return home if a home care agency and adult protective services can monitor her progress. If she is unable to safely remain at home, the nursing facility option can be revisited.

Mr. Jeffers is a 58-year-old man with a history of diabetes, hypertension, coronary artery disease, peripheral vascular disease, and cocaine use. He is divorced and his family consists of his mother, with whom he lives, his sister, and three adult children with whom he has limited or no contact.

Mr. Jeffers has undergone several toe amputations and a femoral-popliteal bypass operation to stem the vascular damage related to his diabetes. He has consistently refused recommended coronary artery bypass surgery and left the hospital last time against medical advice. He was admitted this time with shortness of breath and right foot cellulitis. Because of the worsening peripheral vascular disease, a below-the-knee amputation (BKA) may not heal adequately and an above-the-knee amputation (AKA) might be required. He has refused amputation and all diagnostic measures. His sister can sometimes convince him to cooperate for an examination or test.

Mr. Jeffers's capacity has been difficult to assess because he refuses to complete an interview. During the most recent evaluation, he said that his "foot is very sick" and that he does not want to die; however, he terminated the interview after a brief time. Although he signed consent for the BKA, he refused testing necessary to plan the surgery and said that his foot "will get better by itself." His capacity to weigh the risks and benefits of the care plan is unclear. Moreover, these benefits and risks cannot be identified or assessed without the additional tests that he is refusing. A successful outcome will require his cooperation over a long multistep recuperative period; the care plan is complex and the prognosis, even under optimal circumstances, is guarded. The amputation is not considered to be an emergency at this time, but will likely become one in the near future.

In this case, the consequences of decision making by a patient without capacity are more immediate and serious. Unlike Mrs. Andrews, Mr. Jeffers does not have the opportunity for leisurely decisions or timed trials. Refusing amputation may lead to death, while having the amputation should greatly improve the length and quality of his life.

It is important to assess Mr. Jeffers's capacity to make decisions in light of his interests and values. The highly difficult decision about amputation has significant negatives, whichever course is chosen. To make an informed decision, he needs to understand fully the benefits and risks of both amputation and nonamputation. If he cannot make this potentially life-saving decision, he may still be capable of appointing someone, such as his sister, to be his health care proxy agent, with the authority to make the decision on his behalf.

Even if Mr. Jeffers lacks decisional capacity, he deserves care that demonstrates respect for him as a person. Forcing treatment, especially something as invasive as amputation, against his will poses serious threat to his dignity. Treatment over the objections of a patient, even one without capacity, can generally be justified only if there is a clear benefit to imposing the interventions. The less clear the benefit, the less acceptable the infringement of his right to noninterference. Here, the amputation may be the only thing that will preserve the patient's life.

Even if Mr. Jeffers is incapable of making informed decisions, he can and should be given the opportunity to provide assent, which also demonstrates respect for him as a person. If his sister can convince him to assent to recommended treatment, his cooperation with the care plan will facilitate surgery and recuperation. Without either his consent or assent, surgery may not be a safe or effective plan.

DISCLOSURE AND TRUTH TELLING

"I didn't know what to do," said Dr. Lewis, the intern. "I was about to go into Mrs. Gold's room to get consent for the colonoscopy when suddenly they were all there in my face saying, 'Don't tell Mama if she has cancer. Tell her anything else, but not that, not even that it's a possibility. It would kill her.'"

The "they" Dr. Lewis referred to were the grown children—a son and a daughter—of the patient, who had been admitted two days ago. Mrs. Gold is an 82-year-old woman who was brought to the hospital by her daughter after several weeks of fatigue, weakness, and gastrointestinal disturbance. Her history and physical strongly suggested colon cancer, and a colonoscopy would be necessary to establish the diagnosis and develop a treatment plan.

"I was so startled I just kind of nodded at them and mumbled something about not having anything definite to tell anyone yet," Dr. Lewis continued. "We all trooped into Mrs. Gold's room and they stood there while I explained that we needed her consent to do some tests to see why she is not feeling well. I don't know if I sounded as evasive as I felt. When I told my resident, Carol, what had happened, she was furious. She said that patients have the legal right to know their medical information and the family has no business telling us not to disclose it. When we made rounds the following morning, the family was waiting outside the patient's room and warned the team again. Carol explained about the patient's right to information and the son said, 'Listen, I'm a lawyer and I know all about rights. If you say anything that upsets or harms my mother, you'll find out firsthand what the law has to say.' Before things got even more tense, however, the attending, Dr. Martin, stepped in and assured the family that we would not do anything to put the patient at risk."

Mrs. Gold's tests have revealed that she does, indeed, have colon cancer. Dr. Martin put a big note on the front of the chart saying, "Patient is not to know her diagnosis as per instructions of family." There is considerable difference of opinion on the team about the appropriate way to handle the situation during the time she is hospitalized for surgery and subsequent treatment. The effort to avoid talking with Mrs. Gold about her condition has been very awkward for the house and nursing staff. Several people feel that they are being dishonest and are not spending as much time with her as she deserves. Others feel intimidated by the threat of a lawsuit if they disregard the family's instructions.

Because truth telling is a moral obligation, withholding the truth requires a morally compelling justification. Benefits of patients knowing their diagnoses and prognoses include adequately informed decision making, better adherence to treatment, and a more trusting clinical relationship. The burdens to the patient of disclosure (anxiety, sadness, or other types of stress) have been empirically shown to be normally outweighed by the benefits of knowing the facts. The therapeutic exception to the disclosure obligation is a rare instance in which the information is expected to pose a significant and imminent threat to a patient (such as suicide or serious destabilization of an already fragile condition).

More often, concerned and protective families, such as the Golds, wish to spare the patient distressing information. These requests usually reflect the family's sadness about the patient's condition and the belief that, while it may not be possible to protect her from illness, it may be possible to protect her from anxiety and fear. Because they see themselves as shielding her from harm, it is important to avoid the adversarial climate that would be created by focusing on the clash of "rights."

Rather, the family's devotion to and intimate knowledge of their mother should be acknowledged and supported. Efforts should be made to determine how the patient has handled bad news in the past and what approaches have been successful. In addition, the cultural norm of truth telling varies widely and the patient's background and family dynamics should be considered in determining how and to whom information is provided. Finally, they should know that, because multiple health professionals are caring for Mrs. Gold, there is no guarantee that the information can be successfully kept from her.

Mrs. Gold should be approached, independently of her family, and asked what she knows about her condition, what she wants to know, how much she wants to be involved in choices about her care, and how much she wants her family to participate in decisions. She should be reassured that she can choose to know or not to know, to make decisions or voluntarily delegate that task to her children.

A bioethics consultation can help put the focus on the goal, shared by the family and the care team, of doing what is in Mrs. Gold's best interest. A collaborative resolution may be achieved by explaining that the quality of care the family wants for the patient depends on a trusting therapeutic relationship that includes open communication. The family should be helped to understand that, while lying to the patient is ethically unacceptable for care professionals, if Mrs. Gold indicates that she does not want medical information, she will not be burdened with it. If she requests information, it will be provided in a way that minimizes her distress. She will not be subjected to massive amounts of painful or confusing information all at once. Rather, her questions will be answered over time as part of a process that includes adequate support.

Sample chart note
Re: Edna Gold
Reason for consultation: Family's request to withhold clinical information from patient.

Mrs. Gold is an 82-year-old patient who has colon cancer, as revealed by colonoscopy. She has not been told her diagnosis and her son and daughter adamantly refuse to permit the care team to discuss her diagnosis with her. As they put it, if she were to find out she has cancer, or even to suspect that she may have cancer, "it would kill her."

Cases like this are not uncommon. Family members have mixed motives for not wanting their loved ones to get bad news: it may be partly to protect the patient and partly to protect themselves. Family wishes regarding disclosure should certainly not be disregarded or discounted, but they need to be carefully and critically examined.

First, we must determine whether Mrs. Gold possesses or lacks decisional capacity. Decisional capacity is decision specific, so we have to inquire whether Mrs. Gold is able to make specific decisions about her illness—about whether and how it should be diagnosed and treated. There is no indication that Mrs. Gold is incapable of doing this. Ethically and legally, a capable patient normally has the right to receive information about her diagnosis and prognosis, and to provide informed consent to tests and treatment. Though Mrs. Gold was not told why the tests were being done, it is open to question whether the doctors were required at that point to inform her of their suspicions. But once the tests revealed colon cancer, the moral situation changed significantly. The patient should have the opportunity to decide what, if anything, she wants to do about her illness. There is also a practical concern: if the patient undergoes chemotherapy or radiation, how will the nature of her illness be kept from her?

When family members say the truth would kill their loved one, this is the start of series of questions. What evidence do they have for saying this? How has she responded to bad news in the past? Are they afraid that she will kill herself or give up the will to live, or just that she will be depressed? Depression is normal when bad news is disclosed, but depression itself is not life-ending. An important part of the discussion should also address whether the patient herself has any suspicions about the nature of her illness. If she suspects something serious is wrong, but is not told, studies have shown that this only increases patient anxiety and sense of isolation.

I would explain to the family that, while we respect their viewpoint, we need to assure ourselves that the patient herself does not want to know her diagnosis. This is a matter of professional ethics. Questions, such as "How much would you like to know about why you are here?" can be asked without the family being present and may reveal the patient's true preferences without inadvertently disclosing the nature of her disease. If the patient lets us know that she does not want to be involved or wants to be involved only marginally, this should be respected. To lessen the family's anxiety, they can be told that the word *cancer* does not have to be used with the patient since the word itself is frightening to many people.

Mr. Wernick is a 30-year-old recently married man with metastatic testicular cancer. In a patient this young, the cancer, although very aggressive, should respond well to treatment. The recommended plan would be an orchiectomy (removal of the testis), followed by a course of systemic chemotherapy, giving him an excellent prognosis. Dr. Bond also knows that this regimen carries a significant risk of impotence and infertility.

Mr. Wernick has told Dr. Bond that he and his wife should plan to begin a family as soon as possible. In fact, their shared love of children is one of the first things that attracted them to each other. Dr. Bond believes that knowledge of the likely side effects might well discourage the patient from undergoing the recommended therapy. His concerns are echoed by Mrs. Wernick, who stops him in the hall and says, "Just don't tell him about the possibility that he'll be infertile. We can always adopt. The important thing is to get him well."

In this case, the justification for disclosure is far more compelling. As a capable adult who has not waived his right to information, Mr. Wernick needs to assess what is in his best interest and make this important decision with full knowledge of the risks and benefits involved. Surviving cancer with a loss of function (impotence and infertility) may be an acceptable trade-off for some people but not for others. Armed with an understanding of the consequences, he may refuse potentially life-saving chemotherapy to avoid infertility, thereby increasing his risk of dying or he may choose life-saving therapy and alternative strategies for becoming a father. Manipulating information to influence his decision is unethical, preventing him from making an informed and autonomous decision.

Mrs. Wernick is deeply troubled by her husband's cancer diagnosis and what she fears will be his preference—to forgo life-saving treatment. Wanting him to accept chemotherapy and survive, she can encourage, persuade, and even pressure him.

Although Dr. Bond has a primary duty to his patient, which includes disclosing information material to his decision, the wife's concerns should be addressed, even if her request to withhold information cannot be honored. Dr. Bond can offer support and counseling, including advice on the issues she might raise with her husband.

END-OF-LIFE CARE

Lucy Ajuba is a 17-year-old from Kenya, who was diagnosed in January with a cancer that had invaded one kidney and metastasized to her bones, lungs, liver, and aorta. Given the extent of the metastases, her prognosis was determined to be poor. Lucy underwent surgery in June to remove the diseased kidney and began a non-experimental course of chemotherapy, but she showed no improvement. She was placed on an experimental chemotherapy protocol, but a scan done in July showed new metastases in her bones. By the fall, Lucy was experiencing significant abdominal pain, but the use of a fentanyl patch brought her some relief.

Shortly after her increased pain problems, Lucy was admitted to the pediatric critical care unit (PCCU) in renal failure. She continued to experience significant pain and, despite the fentanyl patch, she was often very restless and unable to lie still, although every movement was painful. She was also terrified because she was clearly getting worse instead of better. For example, her abdomen had become quite distended and she repeatedly asked, "Why my belly is so big?" After a few days in the PCCU, she was stabilized and transferred back to the floor, but her remaining kidney was found to be heavily infiltrated with cancer.

Lucy is emotionally immature for her age and unusually dependent on her parents, especially her mother. Before moving to this country, Mr. and Mrs. Ajuba had lost their only other child to malaria and they are very protective of Lucy. From the time of her diagnosis, they have insisted that she be told nothing about her medical status or prognosis. In spite of this, Lucy has indicated her awareness that her disease is serious and, more recently, that she is terminally ill. Both Mr. and Mrs. Ajuba are very religious and repeatedly express their faith that God will cure their child from what her father describes as a "white man's disease." They also insist that all aggressive measures be used to keep Lucy alive, although Mrs. Ajuba appears to be more realistic about her daughter's condition and prognosis.

Shortly after Lucy was transferred out of the PCCU, her oncologist recommended that, in light of her irreversible deterioration, a DNR order would be appropriate and that curative treatment should be replaced by aggressive palliation. After considerable resistance, her parents reluctantly agreed to the DNR, but the following day, her father rescinded the order. A few days later, Lucy's condition worsened and she was readmitted to the PCCU and intubated. Within the past 24 hours she has experienced four hypotensive episodes, each of which has been treated aggressively. She is receiving escalating support to maintain respiration, blood pressure, and other vital signs. In addition, she requires increasingly heavy sedation to manage her pain and agitation.

The treating team is concerned about continuing aggressive curative treatment that appears increasingly ineffective. Her oncologist has requested a bioethics consultation to engage the team and the family in considering appropriate end-of-life care.

Parents have discretion in making decisions about their children's health care because they customarily act in ways that promote the children's best interests. Their decisions usually are based on their own preferences and values because children are not mature enough to have developed long-range interests and goals. How best interest is defined depends on how the benefits, burdens, and risks are perceived and valued. In this case, the notion of best interest is disputed, with Lucy's parents arguing for continued life-sustaining treatment and the care team advocating a palliative approach.

Lucy's parents' wish to continue aggressive life-sustaining treatment may be multi-factorial, including misunderstanding of the clinical facts and unrealistic expectations that must be addressed. They may not be getting the information necessary to understand Lucy's clinical condition or they may be unable to understand the information because of their educational level, their cultural background, their fears and suspicions, or the emotional stress of caring for a critically ill child. An additional barrier may be their understandable inability to face the possible loss of another child. Care professionals are expected to be sensitive to the importance of cultural values and traditions in decisions about health, life, and death, and should provide information, especially bad news, in a supportive and accessible manner.

Here, the key parties include the patient, even though she is a minor. Lucy clearly has indicated awareness of the gravity of her illness and a sense of isolation and fear because she has been excluded from discussion about her condition. Involving the adolescent in information sharing and decision making in the face of likely death is both extremely important and challenging. Paternalism may be justified if an adolescent is not able to understand the information, or too immature to act in ways that would be beneficial. As the adolescent grows and matures, these justifications progressively weaken. Even if minors are not able to exercise autonomous decision making fully, it is usually desirable to help them understand their condition and obtain their assent to the care plan.

An important goal of ethics consultation is to help the family and care team arrive at consensus on a care plan that promotes the best interest of the patient and addresses the concerns, values, and preferences of all parties. The dying child needs palliation of symptoms and reassurance. The grieving parents need clinicians to share the burden of difficult decisions and provide emotional support and access to additional resources. Barriers to consensus include family history and conflict, information imbalance, and cultural background. Through effective communication and mediation, the parties may be able to reach agreement on mutually acceptable goals and plan of care.

Mrs. Ewing is an 86-year-old widow with dementia and severe heart disease. She lives in a nursing home, where she has been bedridden for a year. She occasionally speaks and follows some commands, but does not communicate in a consistent fashion. It is uncertain if she recognizes any of her family members or the people who care for her.

Mrs. Ewing was transferred to the local hospital, where she is being treated for congestive heart failure. Despite aggressive medical treatment, her condition has remained grave. Fluid has been removed from her lungs via a needle in the chest wall (thoracentesis), only to reaccumulate in two days. Recognizing that the prognosis is poor, her physician has addressed the treatment plan with her family. Her daughter has become extremely upset and insists that "everything should be done" for her mother. Mrs. Ewing's son, a dermatologist who does not live in town, has been in telephone contact and says, "Do whatever you have to do to keep her alive." He insists that his mother be transferred to the intensive care unit and that a second thoracentesis be performed.

The attending physician has explained that the available interventions would be painful and possibly unsafe, and would not likely alter the disease course. A permanent chest tube would need to be placed to continue withdrawing fluid, and Mrs. Ewing might require mechanical restraints to prevent her from pulling out the tube or the intravenous lines. If she has a cardiac or respiratory arrest, which is almost certain to occur soon, attempted resuscitation would likely be unsuccessful. If she were revived, she might face uncomfortable days on a respirator before her death. He advocates for a palliative care plan. The family remains adamant, however, stating that "nothing is worse than death."

Like parents of dying children, the adult children of dying parents often issue instructions to "do everything" or ask for specific interventions judged to be therapeutically ineffective or otherwise inappropriate. How these requests are handled can determine not only the effectiveness of the care plan, but also the residue of family comfort or guilt after the patient has died. If Mrs. Ewing's children believe that she was deprived of life-saving treatment because they were not good advocates, her death may be seen as their preventable failure. As an initial matter, then, ethics consultation should seek to defuse any sense of a power struggle with the family on one side demanding treatment and the professionals on the other side withholding it. The focus should begin and remain on the shared goal of identifying and promoting the patient's best interest.

Requests to "do everything" are a signal that the parties may not share the same understanding of the patient's condition and prognosis, the goals of care, the available treatment options, and the expected outcomes of the interventions being requested. The fact that Mrs. Ewing's son is a physician does not mean that he can be entirely objective in assessing the clinical situation. He may be experiencing the same unrealistic hopes for improvement as his sister and the same need to advocate for all available treatments. Indeed, as the family's in-house medical professional, he may feel additional pressure to effectively manage his mother's care.

Among the first things to determine are what "do everything" means to the family and what the interventions in question are expected to accomplish. Discussion should focus on clarifying the goals of care, the likely effectiveness of the proposed treatments in achieving those goals, the obligation to prevent suffering without benefit, and further explanation of the recommended plan of care. The family should be reassured that, while improvement is no longer feasible, comfort is an achievable priority that will receive the full attention of the team. The notion of aggressive palliative care as active intervention should be reinforced.

Ethics consultation can also reaffirm the special moral standing of the family. Mrs. Ewing's children may have intimate knowledge of her wishes that could inform the goals of care. Engaging in a benefit-burden assessment of the treatment options, including what is known about the patient's values and preferences, would be useful in decision making. If her wishes are unknown, the analysis should be based on the best interest standard. Discussion can emphasize their critical role in protecting Mrs. Ewing from interventions that will increase her suffering without providing benefit. In the event they disagree about care, the focus should be on their shared concern for their mother's well-being.

Physicians' concerns about honoring family requests may also need attention. Physicians are not obligated to follow every family demand, some of which are for medically inappropriate or futile treatment. Problematic requests should trigger discussion, clarification, and mediation where appropriate. Guided by their professional judgment and personal moral codes, physicians may legitimately refuse some requests. Their position, rationale, and commitment to the patient, as well as their offer to transfer the patient's care to another doctor, should be made clear to the family.

Limitation, either scarcity or expense, of resources introduces an additional and uncomfortable ethical element into the decision-making mix. If the decision is made to "do everything" for Mrs. Ewing, should she be given access to expensive resources, including a bed in the ICU? What if a critically ill 32-year-old also needed the bed? What makes sense clinically may not be the most appropriate course of action, all things considered. Even if the decision is made to treat Mrs. Ewing aggressively, it is still ethically appropriate to weigh her medical needs against the needs of others, when resources are limited.

FORGOING LIFE-SUSTAINING TREATMENT

Mrs. Martel is a 61-year-old hospital employee admitted for total abdominal hysterectomy (bilateral removal of uterus, tubes, and ovaries) and debulking for stage IV ovarian cancer. In the recovery room, she was without heartbeat for five minutes and suffered significant anoxic brain damage, although she retains brainstem function. She has been comatose but responsive to pain for one month and her care team believes that there is no chance for improvement.

The family has consented to a DNR order and has presented letters attesting to the fact that Mrs. Martel "would never want to live connected to tubes." Her husband and children have requested that she receive only comfort care and that artificial nutrition and hydration be stopped. Legal counsel and risk management are comfortable with the family's decisions, but the nursing staff is very troubled by this course of action. Since surgery, Mrs. Martel has been on an acute care floor where the notion of limiting life-sustaining treatment is disquieting. The nurses feel that they are doing nothing but turning the patient and, because she is receiving IM Dilantin to prevent seizures, they are causing her additional pain with the injections. They think that she is becoming congested and might be having difficulty breathing. Above all, they are distressed by the notion of discontinuing nutrition and hydration and "starving the patient to death."

In contrast to the family that wants everything done, the family that wants to forgo treatment can also present an ethical challenge for care professionals. Despite family consensus and caregiver understanding of the legal and ethical principles, limiting treatment at the end of life can be counterintuitive and disturbing to those whose mission is to preserve life. An ethics consultation can be very useful in helping care providers and families articulate their concerns and in reassuring them about the validity of the care plan.

A capable adult patient has a well-settled right to make an informed decision consenting to or refusing treatment, even if the decision leads to her death. These wishes can be expressed contemporaneously or prospectively. An appointed health care proxy agent can make these decisions on behalf of the incapacitated patient, based on wishes expressed in an advance directive, substituted judgment, or the best interest standard.

Absent an advance directive, the family is often best suited to represent the patient because of their long-standing and intimate relationship. The family is usually accorded a significant degree of discretion in making decisions for the incapacitated patient, although some states restrict the authority to limit treatment. Ethically, there should be a presumption that the family's knowledge of and concern for the patient is the best guide in making decisions about end-of-life care. While Mrs. Martel had not executed an advance directive or appointed a proxy agent, her family is agreed on what she would want in her current situation.

Legally, as well as ethically, there is no distinction between withholding and withdrawing life-sustaining treatment (LST). The key issues are (1) whether the interventions are benefiting the patient or contributing to suffering and prolonging the dying process, and (2) whether the patient or the surrogate believes they should be forgone. Yet, withdrawing artificial nutrition and hydration (ANH) feels different because of its association with nurturing. The notion that forgoing ANH at the end of life is starving the patient to death needs correction. Palliative care professionals should clarify for family and staff that withholding or withdrawing ANH from patients near death does not create hunger or thirst and, in fact, has been shown to often relieve discomfort during the dying process. Some religions and cultures stress the symbolic meaning of food and water and do not permit withdrawing or withholding ANH. Both ethical analyses and legal rulings, however, discuss ANH as a medical treatment like other interventions whose benefits and risks should be assessed in care planning.

The concerns of caregiving staff should always be considered in care planning but, in this situation, they deserve heightened attention. These acute care nurses are unaccustomed to limiting life-sustaining treatment, which they find clinically counterintuitive and ethically troubling. In addition, they are caring for a colleague with whom they cannot help but identify. The nurses need reassurance that they are doing a great deal for Mrs. Martel and her family by keeping her comfortable and treating her with professionalism, concern, and respect. The focus should be that, when cure or improvement is no longer feasible, the goals of care shift to maximizing comfort, minimizing suffering, and not prolonging the dying process. Involving the palliative care service in the planning and delivery of care should be educational and supportive for the nursing staff.

One important function of bioethics consultation is working with staff, including medicine, nursing, social work, and administration, to clarify and analyze difficult ethical issues. Sometimes more than one meeting is indicated to address multiple sets of issues. Here, bioethics might meet with the nurses to address their concerns and meet again with the family and care team to discuss the goals and plan of care, with particular attention to the most effective clinical setting. In this case, the palliative care or hospice unit is probably better equipped to attend to the patient's end-of-life needs, including identifying alternative methods for administering Dilantin and easing respirations. A bioethics consultation that includes palliative care professionals can reassure the family that, rather than a lower or less attentive level of care, the palliative care service provides expertise in symptom management at the end of life.

GOALS OF CARE

Frankie Abruzzi is a 31-year-old man, currently in the ICU in grave condition. He has a history of IV drug abuse, which he stopped seven years ago when he tested positive for HIV. For the past five years he has been on antiretroviral therapy. Also significant in his medical history is a heart valve replacement due to endocarditis contracted as a result of his drug use. According to his parents and immunologist, Dr. Stern, who has known him for several years, Frankie has coped fairly well emotionally with his condition and has been very conscientious about taking care of himself. Recently, Frankie and his wife divorced, but he has maintained contact with his young daughter.

Frankie was referred by Dr. Stern to Dr. Heiken, an oncologist, because of an elevated white blood count. He was admitted to the hospital for a bone marrow biopsy, which revealed a very early stage of leukemia. Interferon was started but discontinued shortly thereafter because Frankie continued to spike fevers, one of the side effects of interferon. According to Dr. Heiken, Frankie's leukemia is definitely treatable.

While in the hospital, Frankie developed abdominal swelling due to fluid buildup. He also developed an acute retroperitoneal bleed coming from his right kidney, which was removed. During surgery, Frankie became hypotensive for a protracted period and he has not regained consciousness. He is intubated and attempts to wean him from the ventilator have proved unsuccessful. He has developed left kidney failure, for which he has received dialysis on three occasions. Because of low blood pressure, however, dialysis has had to be discontinued, at least temporarily.

Frankie has no health care proxy or living will. His family consists of his two parents and a sister, all of whom seem genuinely concerned about doing what is best for Frankie and sparing him any unnecessary suffering. Yet their approaches to his care are very different. Mrs. Abruzzi and her daughter, who want to spare Frankie further needless suffering, have requested a DNR order and the withholding of dialysis and other cure-oriented treatment. In contrast, Mr. Abruzzi contests the DNR order and argues for continuing all other aggressive treatment because "Frankie is a fighter and he wouldn't give up." Dr. Stern advocates a palliative care plan that focuses on Frankie's comfort. Dr. Heiken explains that he cannot agree with forgoing resuscitation, dialysis, and other treatments because Frankie's condition is potentially reversible and he might be "salvageable." He says that, if the family decides to withdraw treatment, it will be difficult for him to be Frankie's physician and he will ask Dr. Stern to assume care of the patient.

The concept of autonomous decision making is based on the notion that capable patients are in the best position to make care decisions consistent with their own values and interests. The concept of surrogate decision making is based on the notion that people who know and care about the incapacitated patient will make the decisions he would make if he were able to do so. These insights into what matters to the patient inform the goals of care.

The difficulty arises when trusted and well-meaning surrogates have differing ideas of what the patient would want or what would be in his best interest. Frankie's devoted family members are advocating for the goals they each believe are best for him. His two doctors also have differing goals for Frankie based on their respective assessments of his clinical condition and prognosis. These well-intentioned but conflicting perspectives threaten to create a stalemate in care planning, interpersonal tension, and residual family conflict following Frankie's death.

Achieving consensus on a plan of care requires that the family and care professionals agree on the goals of care. A bioethics consultation would promote a review of what is known about Frankie's interests and values in light of what is known about his medical condition. Expectations of what continued treatment can accomplish should be clarified in light of Frankie's condition. Through discussion of the diagnosis, prognosis, treatment options, and patient wishes, the parties can reach a mutually acceptable plan of care with clearly defined goals (such as time-limited trial of specific critical care interventions).

The consultation should also consider Dr. Heiken's motivation to continue aggressive curative care in light of the clinical realities and his possible concerns about liability. Withdrawing life-sustaining measures, thereby allowing death, is sometimes confused with euthanasia or physician-assisted suicide. In other instances, physicians may act on strongly and deeply held convictions that prevent them from acceding to patient or family wishes. An available option, suggested by Dr. Heiken, is to transfer the patient's care to another physician.

Mrs. Pelz is a 105-year-old woman who was admitted from home with pneumonia. She lives with her daughter, Mrs. Dean, who is her health care proxy agent. For four years prior to admission, she was alert but noncommunicative, able to go from bed to chair and eat a little.

In the ER, Mrs. Pelz was intubated with her daughter's consent. Since admission, she has suffered multiple complications, including vaginal infections, pneumothorax, infections around the chest tube, and malnourishment because of poor intake. She is receiving nutrition and hydration through a nasogastric tube and antibiotics intravenously. She is currently not responsive, although her pulmonary function is improving enough that she may be able to be weaned from the ventilator.

Mrs. Pelz's prognosis is very poor and it is almost certain that, even with aggressive measures, she will never return to baseline. Her condition and prognosis have been explained to her family, including the likelihood that continued aggressive interventions will increase her suffering without providing benefit. According to Mrs. Dean, her mother had never expressed care wishes, except to say that she never wanted to be in a nursing home.

Mrs. Dean has authorized a DNR and stipulated that, if her mother is able to be weaned from the vent, she should not be reintubated and, if the nasogastric feeding tube is removed, it should not be replaced. She has based these decisions on her mother's irreversible condition and her belief that they will promote her mother's best interest by sparing her further needless suffering. Mrs. Pelz's granddaughter and great-granddaughters strenuously object to Mrs. Dean's decisions and want all supportive and curative measures continued. Their maturity and understanding of the clinical realities appear very limited, however, creating unrealistic expectations and resistance to information that is inconsistent with what they want to hear. The situation is complicated by dysfunctional family dynamics that create a passive-aggressive pattern of interaction between them and Mrs. Dean, who seems very isolated and anxious.

Even in the best circumstances, it is difficult for families to make decisions for critically ill patients. While the Abruzzi family members differed in their goals for Frankie's care, they were mutually supportive in their search for consensus on a way to promote his best interest. In contrast, decision making for Mrs. Pelz is complicated by family anger, guilt, denial, dysfunctional history, and conflicting interests, all of which are barriers to decision making.

An ethics consultation should begin by acknowledging the difficulty of the decision process and commending the family for struggling to do the right thing for the patient. Physician clarification of the clinical situation may help them recognize that the patient is dying and that care goals must accommodate that reality. When cure or improvement is no longer feasible, the goals of care become maximizing comfort, minimizing suffering, and not prolonging the dying process.

Bioethics mediation should be attempted in an effort to help the family resolve conflicts that are impeding care planning. Mrs. Dean needs special support in advocating for her mother's best interest in the face of overwhelming resistance and antagonism from her children and grandchildren. As the appointed proxy agent, she is empowered to make care decisions without family consensus and even without the guidance of her mother's explicit wishes. While family consensus is desirable, the care team's primary duty is to the patient and her best interest.

All parties should recognize that mediation is not family therapy. This family brings long-standing conflicts that will not be resolved in the clinical setting. What bioethics consultation can do, however, is emphasize the importance of leaving their interpersonal problems aside and focusing on their shared concern for Mrs. Pelz. The objective is to help family members give themselves permission to protect the patient from the burden of interventions that are no longer benefiting her.

Sample chart note
Re: Abigail Pelz
Reason for consultation: Clarification of patient's condition, prognosis, goals, and plan of care.

Mrs. Pelz is a 105-year-old woman with multiple health problems related to a recent respiratory insult and her generally debilitated condition. Despite aggressive interventions, she continues to deteriorate and will almost certainly not return to baseline. According to her attending and consulting physicians, she is dying. Her daughter, who is her health care proxy agent, has accepted the inevitability of her mother's death and requests no further cure-oriented interventions, but her granddaughter and two great-grandchildren appear to have unrealistic expectations, are reluctant to let go, and insist on pursuing aggressive treatment.

An ethics analysis considers the goals of care in the light of the patient's diagnosis and prognosis, the treatment options, and what is known about the patient's wishes. The benefits, burdens, and risks of therapeutic options are evaluated in terms of the patient's well-being. These considerations receive heightened scrutiny when, as here, the patient's condition is grave and irreversible, her prognosis is very poor, the treatments likely to benefit her are limited, she is unable to participate in decisions, and she has not communicated her health care wishes.

Under these circumstances, the goals of care focus on providing treatment that will benefit the patient without increasing her suffering or prolonging the dying process. To prevent unrealistic family expectations, it is especially important to distinguish why interventions are contemplated and what they are likely to accomplish. These issues were addressed during a meeting that included the patient's daughter, granddaughter and her husband, two great-grandchildren, the attending physician, resident, clinical care coordinator, rabbi, and bioethics consultant.

According to the care team, this patient will almost certainly not recover, despite aggressive treatment. For this reason, it would be clinically counterproductive and ethically unsupportable to burden her with additional cure-oriented interventions that would contribute to her suffering without providing benefit. Here, it is appropriate to help the family protect the dying patient from unnecessary and ineffective treatment. Accordingly, the team encouraged the family to recognize the limits of the patient's endurance, as well as the limits of what medicine can accomplish, and to focus on the goal of promoting her comfort and peace during the dying process.

The agreed-on plan is that the patient will remain on the vent, finish the current course of antibiotics, and continue to receive nutrition and hydration, but that no additional curative treatments will be started. All measures to enhance her comfort will be pursued. It will be important to help the granddaughter and great-grandchildren to support the patient's daughter and each other by recognizing their shared concern for the patient and the importance of acting together in her best interest.

INFORMED CONSENT AND REFUSAL

Mrs. Daws is a 57-year-old woman presenting to the ER in respiratory distress and hypoxia. She has a history of stage IV breast cancer, diagnosed five years ago, chronic schizophrenia, and mild retardation. She was treated briefly with chemotherapy, which was discontinued because she found the side effects so distressing. The cancer has metastasized to her ovaries and, following surgery three months ago, she was transferred to the medical center's long-term care facility for palliative chemotherapy. When she experienced shortness of breath today, she was brought to the ER. She is refusing intubation.

Her appointed health care agent is her husband, who is moderately mentally retarded. He is devoted to her and wants to be involved in her care. He is unable to understand her clinical condition or accept her terminal prognosis, however, and his anxiety is steadily increasing his agitation.

Mrs. Daws's level of cognitive function appears to be adequate for participation in care discussions and decisions. She seems to understand, certainly better than her husband, that she has breast cancer and that she will not recover from it. She understands, with appropriate apprehension and sadness, that there is no treatment that will make her better. The most compelling evidence of her decisional capacity is reflected in her long, close, and trusting relationship with her primary care physician and oncologist, Dr. Meyer. According to Dr. Meyer, she and the patient have engaged in many long discussions about her condition and care. In her opinion, Mrs. Daws appreciates the gravity and irreversibility of her condition.

The professionals caring for Mrs. Daws are very uneasy about whether to honor her refusal of intubation if her respiratory distress increases. The care team, including Dr. Meyer and clinicians in the ER, critical care, and pulmonary, all agree that intubation will not benefit her in the long term and that, once intubated, she will not be weanable. In the past, Mrs. Daws has been consistent, as she is today, that she does not want to die and wants treatment continued so that she can live as long as possible. She is also consistent in her refusal of intubation but it was not initially clear whether she would agree to intubation if it were the only way to remain alive.

For several reasons, Mrs. Daws is a patient who should be considered especially vulnerable to the risks of uninformed decisions with grave consequences. Her uncertain baseline capacity (compromised cognitive function and emotional instability), plus the current lack of clarity about her wishes and possible hypoxia, raise troubling questions about her ability to assume responsibility for refusing life-sustaining treatment. Further, her only family is her husband, whose cognitive deficits prevent him from functioning as an informed surrogate or even a stable support. Indeed, his emotional distress is distracting him from focusing on her situation. Under most circumstances, this patient would not be considered to have the ability to provide informed refusal of intubation.

Two factors alter the usual analysis. First, Mrs. Daws has a long and trusting relationship with Dr. Meyer, who has known and cared for her during the past several years. She is very familiar with the patient's level of understanding, wishes, values, and fears. She knows, for example, that Mrs. Daws is afraid of suffering and does not want to subject her husband to watching her distress. She has consistently asked Dr. Meyer to promise that she will not be in pain. Second, Dr. Meyer and the rest of the care team are convinced that intubation would contribute to the patient's suffering without benefiting her. A considerably higher degree of capacity would likely have been required for the patient to refuse life-sustaining interventions that the team considered to be in her best interest.

Dr. Meyers thus provides a combination of supported autonomy, substituted judgment, and best interest analysis. Her personal and medical knowledge enables her to support the patient and her husband, and refocus the goals of care toward the palliation that is needed.

MEDICAL FUTILITY

Bobby, a 6-month-old boy, was brought to the ER in full cardiac arrest by Ms. Clark, his 18-year-old mother. While bathing the infant, Ms. Clark had told her 2-year-old to watch the baby while she went to the kitchen for a moment. When she returned, Bobby was face down in the bathtub and not breathing. In the ER, he was successfully resuscitated and then transferred to the Pediatric Critical Care Unit (PCCU). At first, although he required oxygen support, he was able to breathe on his own. He also demonstrated reflexive responses to noxious stimuli. Within about 12 hours, however, he experienced respiratory failure and was intubated. At the time, all other outward indications of brainstem activity ceased. Although repeated neurological tests failed to confirm brain death, the consensus was that the baby would not regain responsiveness or any other meaningful brain function.

In conversations with Ms. Clark, the PCCU attending has attempted to explain Bobby's condition and prognosis, but she is unwilling or unable to entertain the possibility that her child will not recover. She has great trouble understanding and remembering what the physicians have told her and has some very unrealistic ideas about possible treatments. She has asked whether a brain transplant would be possible using her own brain and wanted to know whether the baby could be cloned. She is preoccupied with her responsibility for Bobby's near drowning and is unable to focus on discussions about end-of-life care, a DNR order, or transfer to a long-term care facility. She visits daily and, despite occasional glimmers of understanding, she continues to insist that her baby will make a full recovery. Although several tests now have confirmed brain death, she adamantly refuses to accept the determination or consider removal of mechanical supports.

The definition of medical futility has physiologic, qualitative, and quantitative components. The concept may be unhelpful except for the narrowest definition—failure of an intervention to achieve its therapeutic goal—which was applicable in this situation. Given Bobby's profound and irreversible neurological condition, interventions aimed at cure or improvement would be futile. Measures aimed at keeping him alive, however, might have been effective, although they would never lead to reversal of his brain damage. Now that brain death has been confirmed, mechanical supports are merely perfusing his organs, but will not return him to life. Helping his mother accept the reality of these distinctions is an essential but difficult part of the therapeutic interaction.

Ms. Clark's insistence on continued aggressive curative treatment is based on her poor understanding of medical information, compounded by her denial, guilt, and anger. The unimaginable pain of a parent unable to rescue her child is infinitely worse when she is responsible for the harm. The result is unrealistic expectations of and demands on staff, as well inability to begin the grieving process. These factors need to be addressed by the care team, including psychosocial support and counseling.

The controversial nature of futility, including where to draw lines limiting care, is inherently value-laden and subject to dispute. A critical judgment is who should make these assessments and decisions. While clinicians should not be the sole decision makers, it is unfair to ask families desperate for signs of improvement to recognize on their own when those hopes are unrealistic. Acknowledging the limits of medicine can begin the process of shared planning for what *can* be done in the patient's best interest.

Although the death of a child is always a tragedy, the determination of brain death is appropriate when supported by clinical and laboratory findings. Determination of brain death in a young child, especially one under a year old, is clinically and emotionally challenging for the care team and the family. Bobby's mother needs to be reassured that he is not suffering and that the care team will attend to his needs in a compassionate and dignified manner. Given her emotional fragility and protective denial, reasonable accommodations, discussed in chapter 9, are certainly appropriate for a specified time before mechanical supports are removed.

A final issue raised by this case is the relationship between futility and resource allocation. ICU care and life-sustaining treatment are scarce and expensive. The health care organization has a duty to be a judicious steward of community resources. A challenging question for the institution is whether parents' inability to accept their child's brain death because of psychological, philosophical, or religious barriers justifies continuing expensive medical care that ultimately drains community resources. The term "futility"—the failure of an intervention to be physiologically effective—is sometimes incorrectly used to justify not providing a scarce resource. Application of a scarce resource may work, but may be ruled out by the competing need of other patients. Grappling with this issue is the ongoing obligation of responsible health care organizations as they craft ethically principled policies and procedures.

PARENTAL DECISION MAKING

Luke is a 14-year-old boy and a long-term survivor of congenitally acquired HIV infection. His father, Mr. Bradley, is a physician's assistant, and makes all decisions regarding family medical care. Luke's mother died of AIDS and was cared for by Mr. Bradley during her illness. Nevertheless, Luke was not tested for HIV infection until he was 12 years old, at which time he tested positive. His father has been very resistant to the notion of telling Luke his diagnosis.

The medical center became involved in Luke's care shortly after his diagnosis. At that time, PCP prophylaxis and antiretroviral therapy were recommended. Mr. Bradley initially refused both, but finally was persuaded to start PCP prophylaxis with Bactrim. After his son had been on Bactrim for three weeks, Mr. Bradley discontinued medication without notifying the care professionals. The interruption in treatment was discovered during the next clinic visit, at which time Mr. Bradley explained that Luke had developed a fever and headaches, potential side effects of Bactrim. PCP prophylaxis was reinitiated with Dapsone instead of Bactrim. Again, he developed a fever and headaches and his father discontinued both the antibiotic and PCP prophylaxis.

During the summer, Luke developed neurological symptoms, including sleepiness, acting out, hypersexuality, and gait problems. In the fall, the cause of the symptoms was identified as HIV-related encephalopathy, an incurable condition that is AIDS-defining. Luke's symptoms currently are causing him a great deal of suffering. He is aware of what is happening to him, although the consensus is that he does not have decision-making capacity. He cries out that he is dying and believes that he is crazy. He is difficult to control and care for, creating disruption and distress at home. His 10-year-old sister has threatened to run away from home because of his behavior and its effects on family life. Psychotropic medications have been used to treat the effects of the encephalopathy but, because of adverse side effects, his father has discontinued all medications other than Ativan.

Care professionals have recommended that Luke receive D4T, an antiretroviral drug that will not produce a cure, but could ease his dementia and other neurological symptoms. Mr. Bradley has been considering this course of treatment, but has not made a decision to reinitiate antiretroviral treatment. Currently, Luke is (1) suffering severe symptoms caused by his encephalopathy; (2) receiving only Ativan, which is not providing significant symptom relief; and (3) not receiving medication, namely D4T, that might improve his symptoms.

Parents are typically accorded the responsibility for making health care decisions for their minor children, based on their presumed knowledge of and concern for them. The theory is that parents' mature judgment will enable them to act in ways that promote their children's best interest. Especially when the child's life is at stake, parents are usually not permitted to withhold beneficial treatment.

In this case, Mr. Bradley is indecisive about the treatment plan for many possible reasons. He may be experiencing some or all of the following emotions: denial that his child is dying, fear of losing his child, emotional stress of caring for a critically ill child, and a desire to protect his child from the distressing side effects of treatment. These barriers will have to be addressed by the care professionals in order to promote an effective care plan for Luke. Psychosocial support for the father may include involving additional support persons (other family members, friends, spiritual advisors), providing information in a comprehensible way, and allowing time for him to grasp the information and reach a comfortable decision.

Palliation of suffering must be the focus of the care plan. The effort should be to encourage Mr. Bradley to support the provision of medication that, while not curing Luke, will manage his symptoms. He should know, however, that his son's palliative needs will be met, even over his objections, and that clinicians will not withhold appropriate treatment because of his indecisiveness, beliefs, or values, however well intended. The crucial task is to empower the father and collaborate with him in ensuring that his child's best interests can be met.

Every medical intervention comes with potential benefits and side effects, some predictable, some unpredictable. The benefits of antiretroviral therapy are uncertain, as is the exact trajectory of Luke's disease. Decision making in the face of uncertainty is difficult, for patients, families, and clinicians. It is especially painful for the parents of sick and dying children, who feel powerless to make them better. Parents need consistent help from the care team, including regular consultation, counseling, and support.

Whether and how to involve the adolescent in the decision making is an individualized judgment that depends on numerous factors. The timing, manner, and content of the disclosure about his condition depends on what he knows, what he wants to know, the level of his maturity, and his ability to grasp and process the information and appreciate its implications. Here, although Luke has not been told explicitly that he has HIV/AIDS, his recollections of his mother's illness and his awareness of other sources of information make it likely that he suspects his diagnosis. The fear and isolation that he may be experiencing should be explained to his father in an effort to help him understand why Luke needs more open communication about his disease and treatment, and support and comfort during the dying process.

SURROGATE DECISION MAKING

Mrs. Charles is a 47-year-old woman without significant medical history. She is employed as a watch and clock repairer, and came to the ER with a swollen right thumb several days after sustaining an injury to that thumb at work. She was admitted and underwent surgical incision, drainage, and evacuation of suspected compartment syndrome. Following surgery, her condition deteriorated and she developed overwhelming sepsis and multi-organ system failure. The following day she underwent repeat surgery for necrotizing faciitis. Her condition continued to decline and, despite aggressive treatment, she remained dependent on ventilatory support, pressors, and hemodialysis. She required heavy sedation to manage her agitation. Several days after admission, she exhibited peripheral vascular compromise and developed dry gangrene of all extremities. Orthopedic evaluation established that bilateral amputation of both hands and both feet would be necessary to preserve her life.

The care team met with Mrs. Charles's family to explain her grave condition and the fatal prognosis without amputation. Although the patient had not appointed a health care proxy agent or executed a living will, her family was certain about what her decision would be under the circumstances. Her husband, father, and two siblings were united in their opinion that Mrs. Charles would not want to live without her hands and feet. They related numerous examples of her fierce independence. In addition to the delicate nature of her work, they cited her hobbies, which include playing guitar, skiing, and sailing. They repeated that, even if her life could be saved, the loss of her hands and feet would deprive her of the ability to do the things that bring her pleasure and the self-sufficiency so important to her. Knowing her preferences and values, they agreed that she would reject the surgery, even if death were the result.

The gravity of the decision's consequences prompted the care team to attempt lightening Mrs. Charles' sedation in an effort to engage her in a discussion of her options. When the sedation was decreased, however, the patient became very agitated and hypertensive, and the plan was abandoned. It looked as though the decision about amputation would have to be made by her family, and the consensus was that she would not be able to tolerate life as a multiple amputee.

The following day, as plans were being made for surgery, the care team tried once more to lighten the sedation and, this time, Mrs. Charles responded well. When she was alert and interactive, the care team and her family engaged her in discussion about her condition and options. To everyone's surprise, she insisted vehemently and repeatedly, "If the only way to keep me alive is to take off my hands and feet, then go ahead. Do whatever you have to do, just don't let me die."

Decision making on behalf of patients without capacity uses the following standards in order of preference: the patient's wishes as expressed directly through discussions with others or in advance directives; substituted judgment when the patient's wishes are not expressed but can be inferred; or, absent information about what the patient would choose, what is determined by others to be in the patient's best interest.

All states permit decisions about care, including end-of-life care, to be made by surrogates, based on the patient's explicitly expressed or documented wishes. Depending on the laws in the state where the patient is receiving treatment, these decisions may also be based on substituted judgment or the best interest standard.

An advance directive would have provided clear information about Mrs. Charles's wishes regarding some circumstances but perhaps not a situation as unanticipated as her current condition. Even without explicit instructions, however, her family had the benefit of knowing her values, preferences, decision-making history, and reaction to disability and dependence. Ideally, those insights could be confirmed contemporaneously by lightening her sedation enough to engage her in a discussion of her condition, prognosis, and options. Because that strategy did not appear to be feasible and time was running out, the decision fell to those who know her best. They were prepared to make the decision they genuinely believed she would make if she knew what they knew about her situation.

Given the gravity of the decision, the care team has a heightened obligation to ensure that the family clearly understands all the options, alternatives, and their implications. Efforts should also be made to confirm that the surrogate decision is grounded in promoting the patient's wishes and interests, rather than other considerations. In short, the team's obligation is to build in as many safeguards as possible to prevent a life-threatening mistake.

The unexpected twist to this case—Mrs. Charles's decision to proceed with the amputations—provides a cautionary postscript. Even when family or other surrogates are well-intended, convinced, and unanimous about what they believe the patient would choose, they may still be wrong. Like Mrs. Charles, patients who are suddenly faced with their own mortality may surprise even themselves by making choices they would not have anticipated. A critical take-away message is that, whenever possible, all efforts should be made to elicit and act on the patient's current wishes about current circumstances.

Mr. Feder is a 79-year-old man with end-stage dementia who was transferred to the hospital from the nursing home for treatment of pneumonia. He also has advanced metastatic prostate cancer. In the course of the diagnostic work-up, he was found to be suffering from a leaking aortic aneurysm, bilateral muscle abscesses, and an impacted bowel. The abscesses were drained and the impaction was relieved. He was started on a course of antibiotics and given a blood transfusion. The only remaining clinical issue is the aneurysm and the question is whether to perform a surgical repair.

This patient's profound dementia has left him with little responsiveness to his surroundings. He does not interact verbally, although he sometimes responds to simple commands and indicates discomfort by withdrawing from painful stimuli. His attending, Dr. Allen, says that Mr. Feder usually appears comfortable, although his recent medical problems caused him discomfort, which was evident in his behavior and reactions to clinical interventions.

According to Dr. Allen and the consultants from neurology and vascular surgery, repairing Mr. Feder's aneurysm will reduce the likelihood of a fatal rupture, but it will not improve his cognition or responsiveness. His pain will be increased postoperatively and the surgical mortality can be as high as 30%. Mr. Feder cannot understand his medical condition or the treatment options, and he is unable to participate in discussions or decisions about his care. He has no family or friends who might be involved in treatment planning.

Mr. Feder is an example of what has been described as the patient alone—an individual without decisional capacity, family, or other surrogates to participate in decisions about care. Patients alone are especially vulnerable because neither they nor anyone else who knows them can advocate for their interests. Without explicit information about Mr. Feder's wishes from recollected statements or advance directives, or inferences about his preferences based on knowledge of his values and decision patterns, the care team must rely on the best interest standard in determining the most appropriate course. This analysis requires others, in this case the care professionals, to consider what they believe will promote his best interest.

One criterion that is typically assessed, especially in the face of irreversible illness, is what effect the proposed intervention will have on the quality of the patient's remaining time. While quality-of-life judgments are usually reserved for the patient or those close to him, in this case that evaluation falls to his care providers. This analysis, assessing the relative benefits, burdens, and risks to the patient that would be expected as a result of the surgery, is reflected in the chart note following a bioethics consultation.

Sample chart note
Re: Kevin Feder
Reason for consultation: Question of the appropriateness of surgery for this patient.

This patient is a 79-year-old deeply demented man, admitted with pneumonia, metastatic prostate cancer, bilateral muscle abscesses, and bowel impaction. The pneumonia, abscesses, and impaction have been treated. A CT scan revealed a leaking aortic aneurysm and the question is whether it should be surgically repaired. I have discussed this case with the house staff, Dr. Allen, the attending, and Dr. Owen, the vascular surgeon. Following these discussions, I reviewed the case with Dr. Masters, the director of medicine.

This is a patient with little or no responsiveness to the world. He is reported to be generally comfortable, except during his recent medical problems. His cognitive status and ability to respond or interact will not be improved by surgery and his pain and discomfort will certainly increase. He has no ability to comprehend his medical situation, consider his options, or participate in making treatment decisions. The consensus of the treating team is that surgery will not substantially improve his condition.

This is a patient for whom the goal is comfort rather than cure. The appropriate plan is palliative care to ensure that he is as comfortable as possible, while avoiding aggressive curative measures, such as a surgical intervention that will only increase his pain and will not provide him with any improved quality of life. For this reason, both Dr. Allen and Dr. Owen expressed reluctance to intervene surgically. They both expressed concerns about his pain and suffering, as well as the surgical mortality, which could be as high as 30% in a patient with these characteristics. They both stated that, if the patient had family to participate in medical decision making, they would be comfortable with a decision not to intervene. Because this patient is alone with no family and no friends, he should not be automatically consigned to aggressive intervention that will not benefit him.

Dr. Masters, in a bioethics consultation on this case, stated that, if both treating physicians agreed, he would concur with medical management and aggressive palliative care.

CHAPTER 17

Sample Policies and Procedures

General Policies

    Access to bioethics consultation

    Advance directives

    Do-not-resuscitate (DNR) and do-not-intubate (DNI) orders

    Forgoing life-sustaining treatment

    Surrogate decision making for patients who lack decisional capacity

        The following general policies can be found at www.press.jhu.edu:

        Declaration of brain death

        Donation after cardiac death

        Managing requests for treatment judged to be medically futile
           or harmful

Specialized Policies

    These policies can be found at www.press.jhu.edu:

    Advance directives and POLST in psychiatric facility

    Ethics case consultation in hospice

    Informed consent in psychiatric facility

    Responding to a patient's desire to voluntarily stop eating and
       drinking (VSED) in hospice

    Restraint and seclusion in psychiatric facility

    Sexual activity in psychiatric facility

The review of institutional policies and procedures is one of the ethics committee's most important functions. Because of its interdisciplinary membership and focus, the committee brings a critical perspective to the analysis of the templates for clinical and organizational action. Of particular ethics concern is whether the policies and procedures effectively implement the values and mission of the institution, while maintaining the accepted standards of health care and business endeavor.

Policy and procedure documents can function in different ways, depending on their objectives, the needs of the institution, and the laws and regulations of the state in which the institution is located. All are intended to provide guidance for the staff in responding consistently to specific situations. Some are sets of instructions about what steps should be taken. Others list the forms that should be used in implementing a process. Still others identify the health care professionals responsible for certain activities. The most useful provide both education and direction, explaining the purpose and underlying principles of the policy, as well as the institutionally agreed-on plan of action. Policies often begin with an abstract or statement of purpose that summarizes their function, and some may also include the principles that they rely on for their rationale.

The following policies are presented as samples with the permission of several health care institutions around the country. No attempt has been made to survey care-providing organizations about their policies or to collect data on how they are drafted or implemented. Rather, the general policies were selected because they address clinical issues that have ethical implications and because most health care organizations have adopted some version of them, allowing for comparison of how different institutions address the same situations. However, no attempt has been made to annotate these policies to indicate their noteworthy features or to compare them to similar policies from other institutions. As noted elsewhere in this book, health care delivery is regulated by each state's law, and these differences are reflected in the policies that govern institutional procedures. The group of specialized policies represents those whose provisions are specific to institutions that provide specialized care, such as psychiatric centers, hospices, or long-term care facilities.

There is no one ideal way to draft a policy. However, as your ethics committee considers drafting a policy for your institution, or is asked to review an already existing policy, the following general guidelines may prove useful:

- The purpose of the policy. What is the policy designed to do? What issue does it address? This would usually go at the beginning of the policy.
- The scope of the policy. To whom does the policy apply? Which categories of patients or health care providers are covered by the policy? This may be a short statement, followed later in the policy by a more extensive discussion.
- Definitions. Have key terms used in the policy—such as advance directive, brain death, and so on—been defined? This might be included in the section on scope or would most usefully follow right after it.
- Basic principles. What ethical principles or principles of professional or organizational ethics undergird the policy? Not all policies contain this, but a statement of the policy's ethical foundations may be useful as an educational tool.
- Procedures for implementation. Does the policy outline the various procedures that should be performed in order to execute the policy and identify the persons who are responsible for doing so? This is often the longest section of the document.
- Ethics follow-up. Does the policy state how ethical issues that remain unresolved can be referred to an "ethics mechanism" (in the words of the Joint Commission accreditation requirements) such as an ethics committee or consult service? (Your institution may have a separate policy for this or it may be included as a section of another policy.)

General Policies

ACCESS TO BIOETHICS CONSULTATION
(general; see online for an access policy for hospice)

Purpose

1. To ensure that patients, their families and designated representatives, and the caregiving staff are provided the opportunity to participate in the deliberation of the bioethics consultation service and bioethics committee on issues that affect patient care.
2. To establish a process for timely access to the bioethics consultation service for the analysis and resolution of ethical problems and conflicts in patient care.
3. To establish a process for access to the full bioethics committee when, in the judgment of the bioethics consultation service, patient care issues would benefit from wider deliberation.
4. To establish a process whereby the bioethics committee is available to the medical center caregiving and administrative staff for education and review of policies related to bioethical issues.

Scope

This policy extends to all medical center caregiving and administrative staff, patients, families, and designated representatives throughout the integrated delivery system.

Function

1. All ethical issues in the clinical setting are appropriately addressed by the bioethics consultation service, composed of members of the Division of Bioethics at the medical center. Members of the consultation service are available whenever a consult is requested to provide timely and continued assistance in clarifying and resolving ethical dilemmas. A summary of the consult is documented in the patient's chart.

   Ethical issues for which consultation might be sought include, but are not limited to

   - developing, signing, and honoring of advance directives
   - participation in the health care decision-making process
   - withholding and withdrawing life-sustaining treatment
   - do-not-resuscitate orders
   - informed consent to and refusal of treatment
   - patient dignity, confidentiality, and privacy
   - patient rights and responsibilities

2. The bioethics committee is available when a wider ethical analysis would be helpful. The interdisciplinary committee meets on a regular and ad hoc basis to

- provide advisory and nonbinding recommendations for resolution of conflicts in care decisions;
- participate in developing and reviewing medical center policy when matters of ethics are involved; and
- provide educational programs in bioethical issues, both within the medical center and for the wider community.

Access

Anyone involved in patient care associated with the medical center—patient, family member or designated representative, or staff member, regardless of site—with an ethical concern or problem can access the bioethics consultation service by contacting the Division of Bioethics. After hours, request for ethics consultations requiring immediate attention will be handled by the appropriate administrative nursing coordinator.

Caregiving and administrative staff members who wish to present bioethical issues, policies, and educational matters to the bioethics committee should directly contact the committee chair or co-chair through the Division of Bioethics.

Notification of Patient, Family, or Designated Representative

When the request for bioethics consultation comes from a patient, family member, or designated representative and the case will be presented to the full bioethics committee as part of the clinical consultation, those requesting will be notified and invited to participate in deliberations.

Permission of the patient, family, or designated representative is not required for either a consultation or full committee review.

Confidentiality

All deliberations of the bioethics consultation service and the bioethics committee are confidential, and all records and documentation are protected.

ADVANCE DIRECTIVES

Purpose

This policy informs associates and medical staff about federal and state laws that govern patients' rights to make advance health care decisions, including consent to or refusal of medical, surgical, or diagnostic interventions. Staff members are required to provide patients with (1) information about advance directives, (2) the opportunity to formulate advance directives, and (3) the offer of assistance in doing so. Care providers are required to be aware of and respect patient care wishes expressed in advance directives. Patients will not be discriminated against based on whether they have advance directives.

Scope

This policy applies to all medical center associates in the network and affiliated physicians and their staffs in other clinical settings.

Definitions

Advance directive: A written or oral expression of a capacitated individual's health care instructions, including general preferences and consent to or refusal of specified treatments or interventions. These instructions, including living wills and health care proxy appointments, are recognized by state law as constituting evidence of a person's health care wishes, stated in advance of decisional incapacity. They take effect only when the individual is deemed to have lost the capacity to make health care decisions. (Do-not-resuscitate [DNR] orders are considered a specific type of advance directive and are covered in a separate medical center policy.)

Living will: A list of instructions, written by a capacitated individual, about therapeutic interventions that he does or does not want under specified conditions, usually at the end of life. A living will is used as guidance in making health care decisions for an incapacitated patient and is especially useful for those without other persons who can make decisions for them. It may constitute clear and convincing evidence of a patient's wishes.

Health care proxy: A document in which a capacitated individual delegates health care decision-making authority to another person (a health care agent), in accordance with the Health Care Proxy Law.

Health care agent: An adult, 18 years of age or older, who has been authorized through a health care proxy appointment to make health care decisions on behalf of a temporarily or permanently incapacitated patient, with exceptions listed below (see section II on provisions of the health care proxy law). An alternate agent is also appointed by the patient to assume decision-making responsibilities in the event the primary agent is unable or unwilling to do so.

Family members, even next of kin, do not automatically assume the responsibility or authority of a health care proxy agent. *Only the appointment by a capable individual authorizes a person to be an agent and only a valid proxy document provides evidence of that appointment.*

Decision-making capacity: The ability to understand and appreciate the nature and consequences of health care decisions, including the benefits, burdens, and risks of therapeutic and diagnostic interventions; the alternatives to proposed health care; and the ability to make and communicate an informed decision about treatment.

Reasonably available agent: A health care agent who can be contacted with diligent efforts by the attending physician or someone acting on behalf of the attending or the medical center.

I. Policy Implementation

Health care providers are responsible for the close scrutiny and interpretation of the provisions of their patients' advance directives. Patients who are currently incapable of making their own decisions and have left explicit written or verbal instructions, in a living will or in a health care proxy, depend on their care providers to be aware of and respect their treatment wishes. The provisions of advance directives are activated only when patients have lost decisional capacity and are in specified conditions. For this reason, it is essential to determine whether the incapacitated patient meets those criteria before treatment decisions by others are based on the patient's advance directive.

Medical Center Physicians' Responsibilities

1. Attending physicians and other licensed independent practitioners should routinely discuss advance directives with capacitated patients and encourage them to appoint health care agents or, if they have no one to appoint, to complete living wills. (When clinically indicated, the risks, benefits, and burdens of a do not resuscitate [DNR] order, another form of advance directive, should also be discussed.)

2. The house staff should include discussion of advance directives in the history and physical completed for all in-patient admissions.

3. When clinically indicated, the attending physician makes a capacity determination and documents the determination in the patient's medical record.

4. Whenever a decision requiring informed consent is needed, the attending physician must reevaluate the patient's capacity to make that specific decision.

5. If the attending physician determines that the patient lacks the capacity to make health care decisions but has sufficient capacity to appoint a health care agent, she should encourage the patient to do so.

6. If the attending has determined that the patient lacks decisional capacity and the patient has a health care agent, the attending will discuss with the health care agent the benefits, burdens, risks, and the alternatives to any proposed procedure. The agent has the right to receive any and all medical information that the patient would have received if capacitated.

7. The physician is required to honor in good faith the health care agent's decisions as if made by the patient. If, however, the physician has concerns about the health care agent's understanding of the patient's wishes, the agent's capacity to make decisions on the patient's behalf, or other questions about the health care proxy decision process, the bioethics committee or the medical director's office should be consulted.

8. When a physician becomes aware that the patient has revoked the proxy appointment, the physician must document the revocation in the patient's medical record and, if appropriate, discuss this action with the agent.

9. If a physician is unable to honor a health care agent's decision(s) based on the physician's sincerely held religious or moral beliefs, the physician must contact the medical director or designee, to transfer the patient to a physician willing to abide by the agent's decision(s), and so advise the agent.

10. Care providers are encouraged to contact either or both of the following available resources with questions or concerns about advance directives:
    a. bioethics committee
    b. office of the medical director

During evenings, weekends, and holidays, the associate director of nursing (ADN) should be contacted via the page operator.

II. Legal Authority

A. The Patient Self-Determination Act is a federal law that requires all medical center staff to determine whether patients have advance directives, inform them of their right to execute advance directives, and provide them with assistance in doing so.

B. The Health Care Proxy Law is a state law that allows a capable patient to appoint a health care agent with legal authority to make health care decisions for the patient after capacity has lapsed. A health care agent's decision-making authority has priority over that of any other surrogate.

The Health Care Proxy Law permits a patient to delegate to another person (health care agent) all or part of the patient's authority to make health care decisions in the event he loses decisional capacity. Unless specifically limited in the appointment document, the agent is authorized to make all decisions the patient would make, including decisions about life-sustaining treatment. The agent is required to make determinations consistent with what the patient would have chosen if he had decision-making capacity or, when the patient's wishes are unknown, with what is in the patient's best interest.

Decisions about artificial nutrition and hydration may be made by the agent, but *only* if she knows or can ascertain the patient's wishes about these interventions.

An agent may not make decisions about autopsy or organ donation, unless she is otherwise authorized to do so.

A living will can be used in conjunction with a health care proxy to provide the agent with additional guidance about the patient's wishes. In the event that the agent's decisions are inconsistent with the terms of the living will, the bioethics committee or the medical director's office should be consulted.

If a patient has specified health care instructions in an advance directive and neither the agent nor the alternate agent is available, the bioethics committee or the medical director's office should be contacted for assistance in reviewing the patient's instructions.

A copy of the health care proxy should be placed in the patient's medical record upon admission / new patient registration or as soon thereafter as possible.

III. Health Care Proxies and Agents

A. Who May Appoint a Health Care Agent?

Any competent person 18 years old or older, any married person, or any parent may appoint a health care agent. Adults are presumed competent to appoint a health care agent, unless they have been deemed incompetent by a court.

B. Who May Be Appointed a Health Care Agent?

Any competent adult (18 years of age or older) may serve as a health care agent, with the following exceptions: a hospital employee may not serve as agent for any patient at the hospital, unless he is related to the patient, or the patient appointed the agent before admission to the hospital. Physicians are the only exception to this rule.

A patient may appoint her physician as agent, but the physician may not serve as both agent and attending physician once the agent's decision-making authority begins.

A physician who has been appointed as a patient's agent may not determine the patient's capacity to make health care decisions.

A person not related to the patient may not be appointed as agent if, at the time of the appointment, she is serving as health care agent for 10 or more other people.

C. Lack-of-Capacity Determinations

A patient may have the capacity to appoint an agent to make decisions on his behalf, yet lack the capacity to make the more complex treatment decisions the agent will make. The decision-making authority of the health care agent is activated *only* when it is determined that the patient is temporarily or permanently incapacitated and ends when capacity is regained.

A determination that the patient lacks the capacity to make specific health care decisions must be made by the *attending* physician, with a reasonable degree of medical certainty.

When the attending physician is also the patient's proxy, another attending physician must make the determination of capacity.

a. For a health care decision that *does not require forgoing life-sustaining treatment*, the *determination of incapacity need only be made by one attending physician.*

b. If the agent is to make a decision about forgoing (withholding or withdrawing) life-sustaining treatment, the attending physician must *consult with another physician to confirm the patient's lack of capacity.* The consultation must be recorded in the patient's medical record.

Notice of a determination of incapacity must be given verbally to the agent. If the patient is able to comprehend, verbal and written notice of an incapacity determination must also be given to the patient. If family members or significant others object to the determination of incapacity, or the health care decision(s) made by the agent, but the patient does not object, the person objecting must obtain a court order to overturn the incapacity determination or health care decision. Unless or until a court order is obtained, the health care agent's decisions prevail.

If and when the patient regains decision-making capacity, the agent's authority ceases. The physician should notify the agent and document the change in the chart.

The attending physician's determination of incapacity must be documented in the patient's medical record.

Mentally Ill Patients

Mental illness does not by itself constitute or indicate decisional incapacity. However, if lack of capacity is due to mental illness, the attending physician making the incapacity determination must be (or must consult with) a board-certified psychiatrist. The consultation must be documented in the patient's medical record.

Mental illness (under the Health Care Proxy Law) does not include dementia, such as Alzheimer's disease.

Mentally Disabled Patients

If lack of capacity is due to mental retardation or developmental disability, the attending physician making the incapacity determination must be (or must consult with) a physician or clinical psychologist who is employed at a school for the developmentally disabled; or has been employed for at least two years and is qualified to render care in an Office of Mental Retardation and Developmental Disabilities (OMRDD) facility; or has had special training or at least three years' experience in treating developmental disabilities and meets other criteria to be established in ORMDD regulations.

D. The Health Care Agent's Decision-Making Authority

When the patient is not capable, the decisions of an appointed agent take precedence over the decisions of any other person (e.g., a surrogate appointed under the DNR law), unless the health care proxy document indicates that the patient limited the agent's authority at the time of appointment, or the court appoints a guardian to make decisions about the patient's health care. Unless otherwise limited, the agent is authorized to make any and all health care decisions that the patient would make if capacitated. If, however, forgoing of nutrition or hydration is contemplated, the agent must have specific knowledge of the patient's previously expressed wishes regarding nutrition or hydration.

Before making any decisions on behalf of an incapacitated patient, the agent must consult with a physician, registered nurse, licensed psychologist, or certified social worker, as indicated by the nature of the decision to be made.

The agent must carry out the patient's previously expressed specific wishes and act in accordance with the patient's religious or moral beliefs to the extent that they are known or can reasonably be determined. If the patient's previously expressed instructions are inconsistent with the plan of care considered by the treating team to be clinically appropriate for her current medical condition, the agent should confer with the attending physician and make decisions consistent with what the patient would likely decide under the unanticipated circumstances. If the patient's wishes, religious beliefs, or moral beliefs cannot be ascertained, the agent must act in the patient's best interest.

To make informed decisions on behalf of an incapacitated patient, the agent should be provided with all information about diagnosis, prognosis, and therapeutic alternatives that would normally be provided to the patient if capacitated. The attending physician may share with the agent any relevant communications he previously had with the patient.

E. Dispute Management

Disputes, such as those regarding determinations of capacity, between or among the agent, family/surrogate, and doctor require consultation. The bioethics committee or the office of the medical director or risk management should be contacted. They will contact the Legal Department if a legal opinion from a medical center counsel is required.

F. Health Care Proxy and Do-Not-Resuscitate (DNR) Orders

When the patient lacks decisional capacity, the health care agent's decision(s) takes precedence over the decisions of any other person (e.g., a surrogate under the DNR law). The existence of a health care proxy document does not negate the need for a DNR order or for DNR attending physician documentation and consent forms.

Before consulting a health care agent about DNR decisions, two physicians must confirm and document the patient's lack of capacity, utilizing the attending physician's DNR documentation form. Thereafter, the agent may be asked to consent to a DNR order in accordance with the do-not-resuscitate (DNR) policy.

If the agent agrees to consent to a DNR order, the oral or written consent to DNR form should also be completed and the DNR order (either electronic or written) should be entered.

If conflict exists between a DNR form previously signed by the patient and the agent's current instructions, the bioethics committee or the office of the medical director should be consulted.

DO-NOT-RESUSCITATE (DNR) AND DO-NOT-INTUBATE (DNI) ORDERS

Purpose

To set forth policies and procedures for deciding to forgo cardiopulmonary resuscitation (CPR) in the event of a cardiac or respiratory arrest and entering a DNR order. A DNR order does not limit any other care and can be consistent with aggressive treatment. If there is no DNR order, the law assumes the patient wants and consents to CPR, and a code must be called. (The extent and duration of the code are based on the medical judgment of the physician(s) present.)

This DNR policy meets medical, legal, ethical, and accreditation standards to help medical center physicians and other associates provide optimal patient care and protect patients' rights. Any questions concerning this policy should be directed to the office of the medical director or the bioethics committee. Attached to this policy are forms that must be completed before a DNR order is issued.

Note: Do-not-intubate (DNI) orders are closely associated with but distinct from do-not-resuscitate (DNR) orders. (See discussion of do-not-intubate orders as appendix to this policy.) In summary:

In a cardiopulmonary *arrest*, a DNR order permits withholding both intubation and other components of CPR. A separate DNI order is not needed.

In situations *other than an arrest*, a separate DNI order is needed to forgo intubation since a DNR order *only* applies to cardiopulmonary arrest. A DNI order is appropriate when a patient/surrogate chooses to forgo intubation or reintubation for present or future moderate to severe respiratory distress or when a patient has requested not to be intubated under *any* future circumstance.

Clear and convincing evidence of the patient's wishes regarding resuscitation is required if the patient lacks decisional capacity. DNI orders in nonarrest situations are fully covered in the do-not-intubate (DNI) policy.

*Not discussed in text.

X. Dispute Mediation and Judicial Review
   A. Dispute Mediation Process and Judicial Review
   B. Dispute Mediation Committee Membership
   C. Mandatory Mediation
XI. Other Issues/Concerns about DNR Orders or DNR Policies and Procedures (P&P)

I. Definitions

Adult: Any person who is 18 years of age or older, has custody of a child, or has married.

Attending physician: The physician with primary responsibility for the patient's treatment and care. More than one physician, sharing responsibility, may be the attending physician.

Capacity: Capacity to make a DNR decision means the ability to understand and appreciate the nature and consequences of a DNR order, including the benefits, burdens, and risks of CPR, and to reach an informed decision regarding a DNR order. Every adult is presumed to have decisional capacity unless there has been a *clinical determination of incapacity* or a *legal determination of incompetence.*

Cardiopulmonary resuscitation (CPR): Measures to restore cardiac function or to support ventilation in the event of a cardiac or respiratory arrest. These measures include manual chest compression, intubation, artificial respirations, direct cardiac injection, intravenous medications, electrical defibrillation, and open-chest cardiac massage. CPR excludes measures taken in the absence of an arrest, such as intubation to improve ventilation and cardiac function.

Close friend acting as surrogate: Any adult who knows the patient and presents a completed affidavit to the attending physician.

Concurring physician: An attending physician, selected by the patient's attending physician, to provide a concurring opinion about the patient's diagnosis, prognosis, or decisional capacity.

Dispute mediation process: A mechanism for resolving conflicts arising between or among health care professional(s), the patient, or patient's family or surrogates. Any disagreement about entering a DNR order must be referred to mediation, during which time the order may not be written and an existing DNR order must be suspended. If the patient (or someone purporting to speak on the patient's behalf) objects to the DNR order, the staff member hearing the objection should document the objection in the patient's medical record. The order should not be written without consulting with the medical director or designee.

DNR based on medical futility: The DNR law defines CPR medical futility as follows: (1) CPR will be unsuccessful in restoring cardiac and respiratory function, or (2) the patient will experience repeated arrests in a short period of time before death occurs.

DNR surrogate: An adult, other than a health care agent, selected in accordance with the State Public Health Law, to make decisions about a DNR order on behalf of an incapacitated patient. The list of potential surrogates and order of priority is found on both the oral DNR consent form, appendix B, and the written DNR consent form, appendix C.

Do-not-resuscitate (DNR) order: An order not to attempt CPR in the event of a cardiac or respiratory arrest. Such an order may include all CPR measures or may be limited to specific procedures. A DNR order for an outpatient requires a separate order.

Emergency medical services personnel: The personnel of an agency providing initial emergency medical assistance, including but not limited to first responders, emergency medical technicians, and advanced emergency technicians. These personnel are legally required to honor nonhospital DNR orders when called to attend a patient who has experienced a cardiopulmonary arrest in the field.

Extraordinary burden: In determining whether CPR would be an extraordinary burden, factors to be considered include but are not limited to whether CPR would cause more harm than benefit because of a patient's frailty, debility, or illness.

Health care agent: An adult to whom health care decision-making authority has been delegated through a health care proxy. The agent's powers are only activated by a determination that the patient lacks decisional capacity. The decisions of the agent supersede those of any other person. If, however, the agent's decision seems contrary to the patient's previously expressed wishes, the agent must indicate what changed wishes of the patient support the agent's decision. A copy of the Health Care Proxy Form should be placed in the patient's medical record.

Hospital emergency service personnel: The personnel of the Emergency Department of the medical center, including but not limited to, attending physicians, registered professional nurses, other nursing staff, and registered physicians assistants assigned to the medical center's Emergency Department.

Mental illness: An affliction manifested by a disorder or disturbance in behavior, feeling, thinking, or judgment to such an extent that the patient requires care, treatment, and rehabilitation. Mental illness does not include delirium or dementia, such as Alzheimer's disease, or other disorders related to delirium or dementia.

Minor: Any person under 18 years of age except one who has custody of a child or who has married or is serving in the armed services.

Nonhospital DNR order: An order that directs emergency medical services personnel and medical center Emergency Department staff not to attempt CPR if the patient suffers a cardiac or respiratory arrest in the field or in the Emergency Department or other ambulatory area.

Permanently unconscious: Irreversibly unconscious, without thought, sensation, or awareness of self or environment, including an irreversible coma, persistent vegetative state, or the end stage of certain degenerative neurological conditions.

Terminal condition: An illness or injury from which there is no recovery and which reasonably can be expected to cause death within three months to two years, depending on the underlying diagnosis.

Witness: Any capacitated adult who attests to the validity of a verbal consent or written signature.

II. General Guidelines
    A. Overview

The DNR law established rules under which capacitated patients and, in appropriate circumstances, others speaking on behalf of the incapacitated patient, may consent to issuing a DNR order. This policy describes the circumstances under which DNR orders should be entered and reviewed.

Every patient is presumed to consent to the administration of CPR in the event of cardiac or respiratory arrest, unless a DNR order is written.

To forgo *other* life-sustaining treatments, see the forgoing life-sustaining treatment policy. All patients, even those with DNR orders, should receive care that is appropriate to their medical conditions. A DNR order refers only to cardiopulmonary resuscitation (CPR) and does not limit any other care or treatment for the patient or authorize denial or withdrawal of treatments other than CPR.

    B. Summary of Steps for Attending Physicians for Obtaining a DNR Consent and Entering a DNR Order. There are separate procedures for patients (a) with capacity, (b) without capacity and with a surrogate, and (c) without patient and with no surrogate.

Objection by Patient, Agent, or Other DNR Surrogate to a DNR Order Based on Medical Futility

If the patient, the patient's health care agent, or other potential DNR surrogate objects to the attending physician's entering a DNR order based on medical futility, the matter must be submitted to dispute mediation, and the order may not be entered until the mediation is completed. (See "Dispute Mediation and Judicial Review," section X.) If the dispute mediation committee agrees that a DNR order based on medical futility may be written, the steps in section II above should be followed.

    C. Role of House Staff in Obtaining Consent to and Entering DNR Orders

As described in section II-B above, obtaining consent to and entering a DNR order is primarily an attending physician responsibility. However, the house staff, in conjunction with the attending physician, may perform the following steps in the policy and procedure.

    E. Health Care Providers Objecting to a DNR Order

        1. *Attending Physicians*: An attending physician who becomes aware of a patient or family request for a DNR order and who objects to a DNR should promptly make known to the person requesting the DNR order her objection to the issuance of such an order and the reason(s) for this objection. The physician should either submit the matter to dispute mediation or make all reasonable efforts to arrange to transfer the patient to another attending physician.

III. Consent for DNR Orders
    A. Elements of Informed Consent to a DNR Order

Before a DNR order may be entered, the attending physician or other responsible physician must obtain either oral or written consent to a DNR order from the patient or a legally authorized agent or other surrogate. The person consenting should be provided with information about the patient's diagnosis and prognosis, the reasonably foreseeable risks and benefits of CPR for the patient, and the consequences of a DNR order. Oral consent should be documented on the Oral Consent to DNR Form.

B. DNR Consent for Adults with Capacity

Consent to a DNR order must be obtained from the capacitated patient. Oral consent requires the signatures of two witnesses, one of whom must be a physician affiliated with the medical center.

If the attending physician determines that the patient would suffer significant and imminent harm from a discussion of CPR ("therapeutic exception" to the disclosure requirement), he should contact the bioethics committee or the medical director's office for further direction before entering the DNR order. *The signature of the medical director or designee is required for a "therapeutic exception" to discussing a DNR order with a capacitated patient.*

C. Determination of Incapacity

a. An attending physician and a concurring physician must determine that a patient lacks capacity and must document this opinion on the Attending Physician's DNR Documentation Form. While house staff may not act in place of the attending physician, fellows and senior house staff licensed in this state may act as concurring physicians on evenings, weekends, or holidays when delaying the DNR order to wait for a concurring attending physician would be harmful in light of the patient's condition.

"Capacity" to make a DNR decision means the ability to understand and appreciate the nature and consequences of a DNR order, including the risks and benefits of CPR, and to reach an informed decision. Every adult patient is presumed to have decisional capacity unless there has been a clinical determination of incapacity in accordance with this section or a court determination of incompetence. A finding that a patient lacks capacity to make a decision about DNR does *not* necessarily mean that the patient lacks capacity for other decisions since capacity is decision-specific.

b. *Criteria for Surrogate Consent to DNR*

A DNR order based on a surrogate's consent may not be issued unless an attending physician and concurring physician determine and document in the DNR order that the patient has at least *one* of the following medical conditions (terms defined in section I):

(1) the patient has a terminal condition; *or*

(2) the patient is permanently unconscious; *or*

(3) CPR would be medically futile; *or*

(4) CPR would impose an extraordinary burden on the patient in light of the patient's medical condition and the expected outcome of the CPR (e.g., the patient is so frail, debilitated, or ill that CPR would

cause more harm than benefit; however, advanced age and infirmity alone do not constitute sufficient basis for this determination).

    c. Concerns about Surrogate Decision Making

    The office of the medical director or the bioethics committee should be contacted immediately if:

      (1) There is a question about whether a surrogate is available, willing, and competent to act.

      (2) There is any reason to question whether the surrogate's decision is based on the patient's wishes, including a consideration of the patient's religious or moral beliefs.

      (3) There is any reason to question whether the surrogate is making the decision based on the patient's best interests if the patient's wishes are not known and cannot be ascertained.

      (4) There is any reason to believe that there is anyone higher on the surrogate list who is available, willing, and competent to act on behalf of the patient.

      (5) The surrogate consents to a DNR order and the patient objects, in which case a DNR order should not be written and the office of the medical director or the bioethics committee should be contacted.

      (6) There is conflict about the DNR consent between or among the following individuals: the patient, anyone on the surrogate list, or the care providers. (See "Dispute Mediation and Judicial Review," section X.)

      (7) If a patient, health care agent, or DNR surrogate objects to a DNR order, the order may not be written and the office of the medical director or the bioethics committee or risk management committee should be contacted. (See "Dispute Mediation and Judicial Review," section X.)

I. Patients Who Are Minors

    1. In order to write a DNR order for a patient who is a minor a parent or legal guardian of the patient must consent to a DNR order before the order may be issued. Consent may be *either* oral *or* written.

    2. The parent or legal guardian of a minor shall consider the minor's wishes and religious and moral beliefs in making a decision about consenting to a DNR order.

    3. If the minor patient is able to understand the consequences of a DNR order and expresses a preference, the assent of the patient should be obtained before a DNR order is written. If it appears that the minor patient has capacity sufficient to provide consent, the determination of capacity must be made by the attending physician in consultation with the parent or guardian and must be documented in the patient's medical record. The parent(s) of a minor patient must also consent if the minor is under 18 years of age. Written consent must be witnessed by two adults, using the Written Consent to DNR Form.

    4. If either parent or the minor objects to entering a DNR order, or the attending physician has questions about a parent or guardian's authority to consent to a DNR order, the order must not be written, and the office

of the medical director, the bioethics committee, or the risk management committee should be called. (See "Dispute Mediation and Judicial Review," section X.)

V. Renewing DNR Orders

The attending physician should review the DNR order whenever the patient's medical condition materially changes to determine if the order is still appropriate in light of the patient's condition. Such review, however, does *not* require the physician to obtain consent each time the order is renewed.

If there is concern about a possible delay in renewing the DNR order, the physician in charge of the patient care unit/service should be consulted to expedite the matter.

VI. Revoking Consent to a DNR Order

A capacitated patient, a health care agent, or a DNR surrogate who has consented to a DNR order may revoke the consent at any time by notifying the attending physician or a member of the clinical staff orally or in writing or by *any* act evidencing a specific intent to revoke the consent.

Any health care professional who becomes aware of a revocation must notify the attending physician of the revocation.

However, if a health care agent or DNR surrogate for an incapacitated patient wishes to revoke a DNR order to which the patient (when capacitated) had consented, the bioethics committee or the office of the medical director should be consulted.

VII. Canceling DNR Orders

A. General Rule

The attending physician is responsible for canceling any DNR order that should no longer be in effect, whether because consent was revoked or the patient's condition changed.

B. Patient Who Regains Decisional Capacity after a Surrogate Consented for the Patient to a DNR Order

Medical center associates who believe that a patient (who had previously been determined to be without capacity) has regained capacity should immediately contact that patient's attending physician. The attending physician should review the patient's condition and document any change in the patient's decisional capacity in the progress notes. If the patient has indeed regained capacity, the attending physician should cancel the DNR order. If the patient's medical condition is such that a DNR order is still indicated, the attending physician should seek consent to a DNR order from the now-capacitated patient.

VIII. Nonhospital DNR Orders

A. Honoring a Nonhospital DNR Order

A nonhospital DNR order is an order that directs emergency medical services personnel and Emergency Department staff *not to attempt CPR if the patient suffers a cardiac or respiratory arrest* in the community, in the hospital's ambulatory departments, including the Emergency Department, or in a nonhospital health care facility.

A nonhospital DNR order should be honored as if it were a hospital-initiated DNR or a DNR order for a patient transferred from another hospital or health care facility. The Emergency Department attending or the inpatient attending physician should evaluate the patient's suitability for a DNR order. The attending physician should honor the patient's DNR decision unless "other significant and exceptional medical circumstances warrant disregarding the order."

X. Dispute Mediation and Judicial Review
  A. Dispute Mediation Process

A dispute mediation process will be employed to resolve any conflict concerning a DNR order. Any interested person may submit a DNR issue to dispute mediation. To submit a case to an ad hoc dispute mediation committee the person requesting the dispute mediation should notify the office of the medical director, who must then notify the attending physician and the bioethics committee. Once notified, the attending physician must ensure that no DNR is written or, if written, the DNR is suspended, until: (1) the issue is resolved, (2) the mediation process has concluded its efforts to resolve the dispute, or (3) 72 hours have elapsed from the time the dispute is submitted, whichever occurs first. When the dispute mediation process has been concluded, the decision should be implemented in accordance with this policy.

A representative of the committee should enter in the progress notes: (1) when and by whom the request for dispute mediation was received; (2) when dispute mediation occurred; and (3) the outcome of the dispute mediation process.

Persons participating in dispute mediation must be informed of their right to judicial review at the conclusion of the process. If disagreements persist after the above time frame, the Legal Department must be contacted to bring the matter to resolution.

  B. Dispute Mediation Committee Membership

    1. The ad hoc dispute mediation committee should include representatives from the bioethics committee, the medical director's office, the risk management committee, and other resources, as indicated. If required, the medical center's dispute mediation committee will be convened and will be composed of members of the medical center's bioethics committee selected by the medical center president or her designee, and must include an administrative representative, a physician, and a registered nurse. Special membership requirements obtain when the case involves lack of capacity due to mental illness, mental retardation, or developmental disability.

    2. In situations involving patients with mental illness, mental retardation, or developmental disability, the committee must also include a board-certified psychiatrist.

  C. Mandatory Dispute Mediation

The following are situations in which the attending physician must submit the matter to dispute mediation:

    1. When the attending physician has actual notice that any persons on the surrogate list (or, if the patient is from an office of mental hygiene–regulated facility, the facility director) opposes a DNR decision by

another surrogate, even if the person objecting is lower on the surrogate list.

2. A physician or the medical center administration opposes a patient's or surrogate's DNR consent, and the physician has chosen not to transfer care of the patient before dispute mediation.

3. One parent objects to a DNR order for a minor.

4. When the patient resides in a facility regulated by the office of mental hygiene (OMH).

Appendix

Do-Not-Intubate (DNI) and Do-Not-Resuscitate (DNR) Orders

A do-not-intubate (DNI) order should be used to forgo intubation in circumstances *other* than cardiopulmonary arrest.

I. Procedure for Entering a DNI Order

DNI orders are *separate* from DNR orders.

In a cardiac or pulmonary *arrest* a DNR order *includes not intubating* the patient.

However, in *nonarrest* conditions requiring intubation, including moderate to severe respiratory distress, a *separate DNI order* is required to forgo intubation. Nonarrest situations are *not* covered by the DNR law.

A. DNI Order for a Capacitated Patient

A patient *with* decisional capacity may choose not to be intubated at any time in the future *or* only under certain specified conditions after full discussion with the attending physician.

1. If the patient *wants to be intubated* in *all circumstances except a cardiopulmonary arrest, no separate* DNI order is needed, and a DNR order will suffice.

2. If the patient has consented to a do-not-resuscitate (DNR) order and also requests not to be intubated or reintubated for respiratory distress, a *do-not-intubate order should also be entered.*

3. In the rarer circumstance that a patient does not wish to have a do-not-resuscitate (DNR) order but requests not to be intubated under any circumstance, the patient should be advised that having a DNI order without an accompanying DNR order would severely limit the physicians' ability to provide effective resuscitation if CPR were required.

B. DNI Order for an Incapacitated Patient with a Health Care Agent

If the patient has an appointed health care agent, the agent may request that the patient not be intubated for significant respiratory distress or other noncardiac or pulmonary arrest condition, just as the patient would if the patient had decisional capacity.

C. DNI Order for Patient without Capacity, with Surrogate

When an incapacitated patient has a surrogate who is not an appointed health care agent, the attending may *only* enter a do-not-intubate (DNI) order to forgo intubation for significant respiratory distress or in another *nonarrest* situation under the following conditions:

1. A *DNR order has been entered*, based on one of the *four medical conditions* stipulated in the DNR policy (*i.e., terminal condition,*

permanent unconsciousness, medical futility, or extraordinary burden) and

2. The patient's family or other surrogate are in agreement about the patient's wishes and are able to clearly *describe to the attending physician* the patient's prior wishes. (This constitutes clear and convincing evidence of the patient's prior wishes not to be intubated in the present circumstances.)
3. A second attending physician enters a concurring opinion about the patient's lack of decisional capacity and the patient's medical condition.
4. The attending physician should complete the required documentation and enter either a written or an electronic DNI order.

(*Note*: If the above conditions for a DNI order have been met, there is no need to obtain written evidence from family/surrogate or review by the Legal Department and the medical director.)

II. Review, Modification, or Revocation of a Do-not-Intubate (DNI) Order

A. The attending physician should review the DNI order every 7 days for inpatients and every 60 days for altered level of consciousness (ALOC) patients and whenever the patient's condition materially changes, to determine if the order is still appropriate in light of the patient's condition. The review, however, does not require the physician to obtain consent each time the order is renewed.
B. If a patient *regains decisional capacity,* the DNI order authorized by the agent or other surrogate *must be revoked* and the attending must discuss treatment options with the *patient.*
C. If the *patient's condition improves,* the attending physician must *reassess* the patient's prior declared choices in light of the patient's changed condition to determine whether forgoing intubation is still indicated. The attending should discuss this assessment with the patient/agent or other surrogate, as medically indicated.
D. If the *patient, agent, or other surrogate revokes or otherwise modifies her consent* to a do-not-intubate order, any health professional who becomes aware of this change must contact the attending physician immediately. The attending *must cancel the order.* Thereafter, if indicated, dispute mediation may be initiated by contacting the bioethics committee or the medical director's office.

FORGOING LIFE-SUSTAINING TREATMENT
Purpose

To assist patients, patient representatives, and staff when making a decision to forgo (withdraw or withhold) life-sustaining treatment.

Policy

The patient has a legal and ethical right and primary responsibility for self-determination, including the right to forgo treatment. There is no legal or ethical distinction between withholding and withdrawing treatment. Decision making at the medical center reflects legal and ethical standards when life-sustaining treatment is forgone; specifically,

- When a patient lacks the necessary decisional capacity to participate in treatment decisions, the patient's representative will make such decisions on behalf of the patient. The patient will be included in these decisions whenever possible. Decisions made by the patient's representative will reflect the patient's wishes. If the patient's wishes are unknown, the decision will reflect the patient's best interests.
- Whenever the decision to forgo life-sustaining treatment is made, the patient will receive care that maintains dignity and comfort.
- The patient's condition will be reviewed periodically to assure that the decision, the plan of care, and implementation of that plan continues to be appropriate.
- When there is a decision to forgo life-sustaining treatment, the patient, patient representative, or staff may have concerns regarding the appropriateness of a course of action. When this occurs, the medical center will provide mechanisms to address these concerns.
- The attending staff physician or other health care providers are not obligated to comply with the patient's decision if the treatment would be contrary to accepted standards of clinical practice or the law.
- In cases where implementing the patient's decision would be contrary to the deeply held personal or professional beliefs of the attending physician or other health care provider, that individual has the right to withdraw from the patient's case. Should such a conflict occur, the patient will not be abandoned, but will be assisted by the physician and medical center staff in obtaining care that is consistent with the patient's wishes.

Procedure

1. Determining the Decision Maker:
   a. Patient with Decisional Capacity: If the patient has the necessary decisional capacity, the patient will make all treatment decisions. A patient has decisional capacity if the patient has the ability to understand, reflect on, and reiterate the medical situation, including the consequences of the decision to forgo treatment. Decisional capacity may be presumed in the absence of any impairment of judgment. The attending physician usually determines decisional capacity. The physician may consult other health care providers, family members, or others who know the patient to determine the current level of decisional capacity.
   b. Patient without Decisional Capacity: In those instances in which the patient lacks decisional capacity, the patient's representative will make the

decision regarding forgoing life-sustaining treatment. In the usual order of priority, the following individuals may act as the patient's representative:

1) In the case of a minor, the child's parents or legal guardian.
2) In the case of an adult,
   a) the individual designated by the patient in a health care directive as her agent or a legal guardian appointed by a court;
   b) the spouse;
   c) an adult son or daughter;
   d) either parent;
   e) an adult brother or sister;
   f) other close family members; and
   g) in some circumstances a close personal friend of the patient.
3) If a patient does not have a representative to make decisions on the patient's behalf, does not have an advance directive, and there is no other reliable evidence of the patient's wishes, the attending physician may contact the ethics committee.

2. The Decision-Making Process
   a. The attending physician shall ensure that the patient or the patient's representative making the decision understands the following before the decision to forgo life-sustaining treatment is made:
      1) the patient's current medical status, including the likely course of the condition if treatment is withheld or withdrawn;
      2) interventions that might be helpful to the patient, including a description of the treatment options, their risks, and anticipated benefits and burdens; and
      3) the attending physician's professional opinion regarding the available alternatives.
   b. in the case of the patient without decisional capacity, the decision regarding treatment will be consistent with the stated directives of the patient as expressed in an advance directive or, if there is no advance directive, the decision will be consistent with other reliable expression of the patient's wishes. If there is no advance directive or other reliable expression of the patient's wishes, the decision will be in the best interests of the patient, taking into consideration the patient's values, life philosophy, or spiritual beliefs.
   c. Throughout the decision-making process, the attending physician is encouraged to consult with her colleagues and other members of the health care team.
   d. When a decision to forgo treatment has been made, the attending physician will communicate the decision to the other members of the health care team and document the decision in the medical record.

3. Documentation: When the participants have reached a decision to forgo life-sustaining treatment, the attending physician will document the decision in the patient's medical record. Documentation should include
   a. participants in the discussion;
   b. who the decision maker is;

c. if the patient is determined to lack adequate decisional capacity, the rationale for determining decisional capacity;

d. summary of the information presented and the discussion that led to the decisions; and

e. specific decisions reached, including treatment to be continued and treatment to be withheld; considerations should include but not necessarily be limited to ventilation, blood products, medication, hydration and nutrition, dialysis, and other interventional procedures.

4. Development and Implementation of the Care Plan: The care plan will particularly address ongoing assessment and management of pain and psychological stress. In addition, the plan will be documented in the medical record and will include

a. the patient's resuscitation status and an order if the patient is to be DNR/DNI;

b. orders for what specific treatments will be withheld or discontinued;

c. maintenance of dignity, comfort, and hygiene and mechanisms to ensure that patient and family members are not abandoned, but have access to ongoing communication with the staff; and

d. orders for medication.

1) The goal of treatment is to relieve pain and suffering to the fullest extent possible consistent with the patient's wishes.

2) Health care professionals must make every effort to relieve the pain and suffering of the dying patient. Relief of pain and suffering may require either intermittent or continued administration of large doses of analgesics and sedatives which, in circumstances other than anticipated death, would be considered inappropriate. Dying patients should be assured the maximal possible comfort, even in the face of impending death as heralded by falling blood pressure, declining rate of respirations, or altered level of consciousness. Vital signs may be obtained to assess the patient's status in the dying process, but should not influence decisions about administering medications in the presence of continued pain or other distressing symptoms for which the medication is an accepted treatment. The attending staff physician will clearly document in the patient's chart all clinical indications for administration of medication, including all dosage changes.

SURROGATE DECISION MAKING FOR PATIENTS WHO LACK DECISIONAL CAPACITY

General

Typically, health care decisions are made by capable patients based on their goals, values, preferences, and appreciation of the clinical realities. The legal and ethical presumption of decisional capacity creates an obligation to respect the consent or refusal of treatment by adult patients absent evidence that capacity is lacking. When patients lack the ability to make care decisions for themselves, this responsibility is assumed by surrogates who are charged with acting in accordance with incapacitated patients' known preferences or to promote patients' best interest.

Purpose

The purpose of this policy is to clarify the clinical and ethical issues raised when care decisions must be made on behalf of patients who lack the capacity to make these decisions for themselves, and outline the procedures for capacity assessment and surrogate decision making. Because these decisions are presumed to reflect the incapacitated patients' known preferences or to promote patients' best interest, the surrogates charged with this responsibility should be the persons who know the patients best and are most concerned with their welfare. This presumption is reflected in the governing hierarchy of surrogates. Accordingly, this policy outlines the situations in and the criteria by which decisional capacity is assessed; and the governing legal hierarchy of surrogates appropriate to make care decisions on behalf of incapacitated patients.

Procedure for Assessing Decisional Capacity

When, in the judgment of one or more members of the care team, a patient appears to lack the capacity to make care decisions, that concern will be communicated to the attending physician / treating practitioner, who will conduct a capacity assessment. Decisional capacity is considered to include the ability to

- understand the basic facts of one's diagnosis, prognosis, and the relevant treatment options;
- weigh the benefits, burdens, and risks of the treatment options;
- apply a set of personal values;
- arrive at a decision that is consistent over time; and
- communicate the decision.

Decisional capacity is a clinical determination best made by a physician/practitioner caring for the patient. The assessment may benefit from but does not require a psychiatric evaluation unless there is evidence to suggest psychiatric illness, clinical depression, substance abuse, or other psychiatric condition. Because capacity is decision specific rather than global, the assessment should focus on the patient's capacity to make the specific decision at hand, leaving open the possibility that capacity may be sufficient for other decisions.

Procedure for Determining Decision-Making Capacity

The attending physician / treating practitioner's assessment of the patient's decisional capacity will be documented in the medical record. If the patient is determined to *have sufficient capacity* to make the necessary decisions about care, the patient's consent or refusal will be honored. If the patient is determined to *lack sufficient capacity* to make the necessary decisions, the care team will turn to surrogates in the following order to assume decision-making responsibility:

- court-appointed guardian with authority to make health care decisions for the patient;
- health care agent or alternate agent, pursuant to the patient's appointment in an advance directive;
- surviving spouse or civil union partner;
- domestic partner, as defined in section 3 of P.L.2003, c.246 (C.26:8A-3);
- adult children, according to age;
- parents;
- adult siblings, according to age;
- grandparents;
- adult grandchildren;
- uncles or aunts;
- adult nephews or nieces;
- adult cousins;
- adult stepchildren;
- adult relatives or next of kin of previously deceased spouse;
- any other relative or friend.

To gain as much insight as possible into the patient's goals, values and preferences, and approximate as closely as possible the decisions he would make if capable, the ethical imperative is to engage the decision-making efforts of individuals who know the patient best before moving to those with a less vested relationship to him. For that reason, a good faith effort will be made to contact members in each level of the hierarchy in turn, moving to a lower level only when it has been determined that no one in a higher level is able or willing to assume decision-making responsibilities.

Standards for Surrogate Decision Making

Surrogate decision making is based on the following standards:

- direct evidence of the wishes of a formerly capable patient, specifically in an advance directive;
- substituted judgment, which draws on what is known of the formerly capable patient's wishes, values, and history of decision making;
- best interest standard, which reflects what the surrogate(s) judge to be in the best interest of an incapacitated patient whose wishes and values are either unknown or unformed.

Duration of Decision-Making Responsibility

Surrogate decision-making authority lasts only for the duration of the patient's incapacity. If and when the patient regains decisional capacity, he resumes making independent care decisions.

The decisions of a capable patient survive the loss of capacity. For example, the decision of a capable patient to consent to a DNR order must be honored if and when the patient arrests and loses decision-making capacity. This decision is validly documented in the DNR order and *may not be revoked by anyone else, including next of kin.*

Delegation of Decision-Making Responsibility by Capable Patients

Capable patients may also elect to delegate decision-making responsibility to another person, especially if this has been a settled pattern prior to hospitalization. The patient's preference for a surrogate will be noted in the medical record and the patient will be kept informed of care decisions and other clinical developments to the extent that this information is desired. Patients with sufficient capacity to delegate decision-making responsibility should be encouraged to do so by means of an advance directive, appointing the chosen party as a legal health care agent for this and subsequent hospitalizations when decisional capacity may have lapsed.

PART III

ORGANIZATIONAL CODES OF ETHICS

As discussed in chapter 12, organizational ethics is grounded in the notion that organizations, not just the individuals who work in them, are moral agents with ethical obligations. Accepting that designation means that, like other moral agents, organizations should be expected to have an articulated set of values, standards, and goals that animate the decisions they make and the actions they take. One such statement is an organizational code of ethics, an expression of the norms that govern behavior and set the organization apart from other entities. These codes can be perceived as a form of self-identification, proclaiming what the organization believes in and strives to achieve.

Codes of ethics are distinguished from compliance codes by their normative reach beyond the minimum demands for adherence to legal and regulatory requirements. While codes of compliance specify expectations in terms of such requirements, and are relatively clear-cut in what they require, codes of ethics set the bar at a higher level—the ethical obligations of the organization—and address matters that typically resist neat and easy solutions. To be sure, corporate compliance is an aspect of ethical corporate behavior. But, ethical organizational practices encompass far more than compliance with law and regulation. Certain issues will be addressed by both sorts of codes; others are only addressed by ethics codes and have no counterpart in compliance codes.

The chapters in part I provide the rationale for the moral obligations that health care organizations and providers are expected to discharge. The fiduciary relationship that characterizes the therapeutic interaction binds care providers—individuals and organizations—to a heightened level of ethical expectation and accountability. Accordingly, codes of ethics for care providers and care-providing organizations set out the values, norms, and goals that govern behavior and decision making in the clinical, administrative, research, and educational settings.

Developing a code of ethics is an endeavor unlike any others in which your committee is likely to engage. Rather than simply gathering information and setting out a preamble, process, and procedure, this is an exercise in organizational introspection and consensus building that reflects clinical, administrative, research, and academic perspectives. For that reason, the first step is bringing the concept of an organizational code of ethics to senior leadership and the board of governors for endorsement. In making this pitch, it is important to emphasize the difference between a code of ethics and other documents that describe the organization or establish its standards of conduct or compliance. Explain that the code targets populations both internal (senior and mid-level leaders, clinical and administrative staff) and external (the larger professional and lay communities). As such, it provides a unique opportunity to define the organization and shape the way others perceive it.

Because the code is grounded in ethics, it is useful to develop the early drafts—and there will be more than a few—in your ethics committee or a dedicated working group of the committee. Begin by reviewing relevant foundational documents, such as the organizational mission and vision statements. Next, identify the ethical principles and values that define the organization's moral agency, and describe the behaviors and activities that demonstrate a shared commitment to the ideals articulated in the mission and vision statements. Institutional policies and guidelines should be reviewed to ensure that they are consistent with the code as it develops.

The working draft should now be circulated with requests for comments and suggestions from all the organization's constituent perspectives. Rather than soliciting general feedback, you might target the vice presidents, directors, or chief officers responsible for the different services and departments, such as academic affairs, clinical services, compliance, employee relations, finance, human resources, information and technology, legal, marketing, patient care, public relations, quality and safety improvement, research, and risk management. When these perspectives are incorporated into the draft code, the revised document should be reviewed again by your ethics committee and then returned for final approval of executive leadership and board of governors. This is a time- and labor-intensive undertaking but one that is well worth the effort.

The sample codes of ethics presented below reflect how the respective organizations define themselves, their mission, and their obligations. As you read through them, see which elements might resonate with your organization.

We begin with the following code, which is fairly typical of codes of ethics that are called "organizational" or "institutional."

Regional Medical Center Code of Conduct

PREAMBLE

The Regional Medical Center (RMC) has a code of conduct "to define personal and professional standards of conduct and acceptable behavior for all people while carrying out assigned responsibilities at RMC, including its regulated sites." It is the responsibility of individuals to act in a manner consistent with this code of conduct and to support the code of conduct by holding others accountable to these standards. Code of conduct violations need to be reported to a supervisor, either directly, or via Patient Safety Net, RMC's online event and service concern reporting system.

When reported, violations of this code of conduct will be addressed through appropriate administrative, departmental, and human resource policies related to inappropriate behavior and conduct. RMC will not tolerate acts of retribution or consequence to any employee who carries out the standards of or reports violations to this code of conduct.

The standards of conduct summarized below will help to ensure a positive environment for staff, patients, visitors, and a culture that optimizes patient care and safety.

Standards of Conduct and Professionalism

1. Treat all persons, including patients, families, visitors, employees, trainees, students, volunteers, and health care professionals with respect, courtesy, caring, dignity, and a sense of fairness and with recognition of and sensitivity to the needs of individuals from diverse backgrounds (including gender, race, age, disability, nationality, sexual orientation, and religion).
2. Communicate openly, respectfully, and directly with team members, referring providers, patients, and families in order to optimize health services and to promote mutual trust and understanding.
3. Encourage support and respect the right and responsibility of all individuals to assert themselves to ensure patient safety and the quality of care.
4. Resolve conflicts and counsel colleagues in a non-threatening, constructive, and private manner.
5. Teach, conduct research, and care for patients with professional competence, intellectual honesty, and high ethical standards.
6. Promptly report to your supervisor, any individual who may be impaired in his ability to perform assigned responsibilities due to any cause (e.g., emotional issues, substance abuse).
7. Promptly report adverse events and potential safety hazards and encourage colleagues to do the same.
8. Willingly participate in, cooperate with, and contribute to briefings and investigations of adverse events.
9. Respect the privacy and confidentiality of all individuals. Adhere to all RMC policies and HIPAA regulations regarding personal health information.
10. Uphold the policies of RMC.
11. Utilize all RMC facilities and property, including telecommunication networks and computing facilities, responsibly and appropriately.
12. Participate in education and training required to perform job duties.
13. Be fit for duty during work time, including on-call responsibilities.

There are two observations to make about this and similar codes. First, these are codes of organizational *ethics* and not, or not only, codes of *compliance*. The standards of conduct enumerated above express central ethical values in the practice of medicine and are important elements of the professionalism that is essential to a climate that promotes the ethical delivery of health care.

Although they can be classified as ethics codes, however, they are minimalist in the sense that the standards are not explicitly anchored in ethical imperatives that give them moral weight and explain why they are obligatory. For example, the first and ninth standards require that all persons be treated with fairness, dignity, and compassion, but is silent about the core ethical principle of respect for persons. The third standard would be strengthened by invoking the foundational principle of respecting autonomous decisions. The seventh and eighth standards speak to the need for disclosure of information without reference to the notion of truth telling, which is the basis of trust-based relationships. While not explicitly stated, standards 6 and 7 are grounded in the moral imperatives of protecting vulnerable patients and preventing actions likely to cause harm. In reviewing or helping to formulate a code of ethics for your institution, you need to decide what you want from a code. Will it be a set of directives for ethical professional conduct, or will it also attempt to provide some justificatory framework for them?

The second and perhaps more important observation is that this and similar codes are not really codes of *organizational* ethics at all, in the sense in which we are using the term. These codes set out directives for all professional staff working in the institution. They articulate how *individual* clinicians and administrators should act; they do not address what the *organization* itself should do. But, as was argued in chapter 12, the organization is not just an entity that is the place where professionals practice. It is a moral agent in its own right and, accordingly, it has a set of rights and responsibilities. An organizational code of ethics will articulate these and, perhaps, their moral basis, as well.

The following two codes, by contrast to the one above, adopt the organizational perspective. The various provisions of both, for example, all state what "Metropolitan Medical Center" or "University Medical Center" does, what *it* creates, pursues, engages in, supports, and strives to achieve. Such codes are still rather rare by comparison with codes of professional ethical conduct. But, as changes in the practice of medicine are increasingly looking at the organizational context in which health care is delivered, such codes fill a vital need.

Metropolitan Medical Center Code of Ethics

Metropolitan Medical Center strives to abide by the ethical principles embodied in this code of ethics in all aspects of patient care, medical education, clinical research, and community service, and in all aspects of administrative functions related to those services. These ethical principles describe guidelines for honorable behavior for health care providers, managers, and all other associates and volunteers. Metropolitan strives to realize these standards in all its clinical and organizational activities.

ORGANIZATIONAL PRINCIPLES

Metropolitan Medical Center recognizes that managers and associates have ethical obligations to patients, staff, and the community. Therefore,

1. Metropolitan creates an ethical organizational environment by
   - promoting ethical decision making through mechanisms that integrate ethical analysis into clinical and administrative deliberation and policy development;

- protecting the rights of human subjects and promoting the welfare of animals in research protocols;
- developing mechanisms for implementing the ethical principles in the code and establishing a process for resolving ethical disputes;
- involving staff in ethical decision making on the organizational and clinical levels by promoting discussion of ethical issues, expression of ethical concerns without fear of reprisal, and consideration of whether behavior is ethical;
- listening and attending to the concerns of patients and families;
- reducing institutional barriers to patients and families receiving information and guidance from providers and making informed health care decisions; and

- creating effective, efficient, and confidential dispute resolution mechanisms to address ethical conflicts and concerns on the organizational, administrative, and clinical decision-making levels.

2. Metropolitan pursues a socially responsible agenda by
   - addressing the health of the community by working with individuals and groups to identify public health care needs, establish priorities, and provide adequate notice of available services;
   - promoting accessible, affordable, and convenient primary care;
   - building community alliances that work with community organizations and individuals to promote public health and safety, and coordinate health care delivery; and
   - supporting teaching and research as important parts of its responsibility to the community and the larger society.

3. Metropolitan engages in responsible stewardship by
   - conserving limited health care resources by using them efficiently and responsibly, and distributing them beneficially and cost-effectively;
   - promoting cost-effective care through cooperative clinical decision making that uses resources wisely, by avoiding both under- and overtreatment, and encouraging patients to assume responsibility for monitoring and improving their health;
   - maintaining continuous quality review to assess the effectiveness of resource utilization and clinical outcomes;
   - incorporating ethical principles and reasoning into resource planning and utilization review in order to promote financial accountability at all organizational levels;
   - promoting measures, including incentive plans, to increase provider productivity, motivate effective resource utilization, provide high-quality patient care, and enhance the work ethic;
   - providing the same standard of care, regardless of payment source, by enforcing policies that define equity and prohibit discriminatory provision of care;
   - identifying and cultivating potential sources of public and private funding for patient care, medical education, and research; and
   - devoting a portion of its institutional budget to funding uncompensated care for the uninsured and underserved.

4. Metropolitan supports fair marketing and communication practices by
   - promoting realistic consumer expectations by accurately reflecting the institution's health care delivery record and capabilities, and limiting promises to what the institution can actually provide;
   - promoting informed consumer choice by providing the public with accurate and balanced information about existing and planned institutional resources, treatment capabilities, and areas of specialization; and
   - disclosing information to patients about institutional relationships that create actual, potential, or apparent conflicts of interest.

CLINICAL PRINCIPLES

Metropolitan Medical Center recognizes that its primary mission is to ensure the provision of high-quality, ethically based patient care. Therefore:

1. Metropolitan monitors quality of care by
   - promoting best clinical practice by using measures of quality that reflect the current research on clinical outcomes and practice guidelines;
   - including all departments and disciplines in system-wide continuous quality improvement to improve the quality of care and promote clinical skills;
   - monitoring and reducing adverse clinical events by focusing on patient safety, and identifying and eliminating practice patterns and systems that deviate from accepted standards of care;
   - promoting continuity of care by sharing appropriate medical information, coordinating services among providers, and developing discharge plans that monitor the transition from hospital to the community or other care facilities; and
   - abiding by the principle of truth telling and requiring appropriate personnel to disclose health-impairing mistakes to patients and, where indicated, their families, in order to respect autonomy and prevent or mitigate harm.

2. Metropolitan supports ethical clinical decision making by
   - stressing the importance of ethically based and informed health care decision making by requiring that providers confirm the patient's decisional capacity and, if the patient lacks capacity, identifying the appropriate surrogate;
   - supporting informed choice by clearly informing patients, proxies, or other surrogates about treatment options and their benefits, burdens, and risks, with special attention to decision making for patients incapable of making health care choices;
   - respecting the rights of all concerned parties by protecting patient and family interests, providing clinical information for informed consent and refusal, enhancing patient and family voice in clinical decision making, and addressing patient and family concerns and complaints;
   - supporting a principled dispute resolution system that addresses treatment and interpersonal conflicts, strives for consensus, and is based on ethical, medical, and legal principles; and

- recognizing that mediator neutrality is essential in addressing and resolving clinical disputes between and among staff, patients, families, and other surrogates.

3. Metropolitan promotes multidisciplinary clinical consultation by
   - promoting collaborative clinical management and supporting the authority of specific multidisciplinary teams;
   - supporting attending physicians' professional judgment and authority, while requiring institutional oversight and joint clinical management and implementing a plan of care that reflects the patient's best interest, regardless of financial compensation; and
   - continuing its long-standing commitment to readily accessible comprehensive primary care services through its network of ambulatory care clinics, supplemented by specialty care services.

4. Metropolitan protects patient privacy and confidentiality by
   - making the protection of patient information central to patient care and related services;
   - creating mechanisms that provide authorized persons easy and timely access to computerized patient information, while safeguarding patient privacy and confidentiality;
   - restricting access to medical records and other health information, including billing information, to those with a "need to know" in order to provide direct patient care, review the quality of care, and pursue other legitimate clinical or organizational goals;
   - educating staff about their obligations regarding access to and disclosure of patient information;
   - advising patients that medical information will not be disclosed to others, including family and friends, without patient permission, except as permitted by law; and
   - establishing policies and practices that protect against breaches of confidentiality and punish illegitimate access, use, or disclosure of patient information.

University Health Network Code of Ethics

PURPOSE OF THE UNIVERSITY HEALTH NETWORK CODE OF ETHICS

Ethics is the study of how decisions are made about actions, especially when facing conflicting choices. While ethics may concern decisions about actions that are right or wrong, more often ethics is about decisions when two or more worthy options are available and only one can be implemented. These analyses are informed by values, ethical principles, and theories of reasoning.

A code of ethics sets out the standards that inspire efforts to surpass what is required by laws and regulations and achieve a higher level of performance. To do that, a code of ethics expresses the values and principles that guide ethical decision making and the standards used to evaluate decisions, policies, and actions. In addition to defining the principle-based foundations of what University Health Network (UHN) *does*, this code is aspirational and articulates what the organization *strives to achieve*. Accordingly, this code of ethics identifies the values that define UHN and the ethical principles and obligations that guide decisions and actions in its organizational, clinical, educational, research, and business settings.

Ethics has special relevance in the health care setting because the moral core of caregiving creates ethical imperatives unique to health care organizations. Organizational ethics is grounded in the notion that organizations, not just the people who work in them, are moral agents with ethical obligations. The decisions organizations make and the actions they take have ethical implications and consequences. Just as the ethical obligations of each profession hold its members to elevated standards of conduct, so do equally high standards bind the organizations in which professionals practice.

These expected standards are heightened even more for organizations, such as medical centers, whose practitioners assume direct responsibility for the welfare of others with whom they have a fiduciary relationship. The fiduciary obligation imposes on UHN, its staff, and its practitioners the duty to put the interests of those who rely on them—patients, students, research subjects—before their own individual or corporate interests. It is this special relationship that establishes the trust-based bond between those who provide and those who receive care, and sets the healing professions apart from all other service enterprises. Because the fiduciary commitment goes beyond hierarchy, the organization is able to fulfill its moral obligations only through the actions of every team member at every level in every discipline, department, or capacity.

The UHN code of ethics embodies the mission of offering the highest-quality health care, wellness, teaching, and research, and the vision of achieving leadership in excellence. The foundation established at the organizational level creates the ethical environment for health care delivery, teaching, research, and business practice. Because its defining principles and values ground activity throughout UHN, all policies, practices, and standards of professional conduct are consistent with this code of ethics.

OBJECTIVES AND PRINCIPLES

- UHN creates an ethical organizational environment by
  - ensuring that all clinical, administrative, academic, and research activity throughout UHN reflects the organization's guiding principles and values of quality, integrity, professionalism, teamwork, and communication;
  - articulating to internal and external audiences what UHN stands for, what animates and ethically justifies its decisions and actions, and what patients, staff, and the public can expect;
  - modeling at the leadership, management, and staff levels the attitudes and behaviors that
    - fulfill UHN's charitable mission by providing high-quality care to all patients without regard to race, creed, gender, sexual orientation, or ability to pay;

- promote the dignity, security, and professionalism of all team members, including clinical and non-clinical staff, administrators, researchers, and educators;
- put the welfare of patients and research subjects before the interests of any individual, group, or organization;
- foster ethical research that strives to add to generalized knowledge while protecting human subjects;
- foster education and mentorship of care professionals;
- provide ample time and resources for the delivery of high-quality care;

- promote integrity and professionalism in all clinical, academic, research, and business interactions;
- identify and manage conflicts of interest;
- promote responsible stewardship of limited resources;
- monitor and enhance the quality of patient care;
- foster justice in access to healthcare
- recognizing and valuing staff efforts to provide exceptional service;
- ensuring that all members of the UHN community know the desired standards, are accountable for their actions, and feel safe sharing their questions, concerns, insights, and suggestions;
- ensuring that principle-based policies that guide actions are transparent and accessible for review by
  - sharing with management and staff the evolution of short- and long-range plans and goals;
  - sharing with management and staff the results of surveys and changes in financial incentives, management structure, and staffing
- partnering with other health care organizations to achieve common goals of improving patient experience, promoting population health, and creating more affordable health care;
- creating mechanisms for effective, efficient, and confidential dispute resolution;
- encouraging the identification, reporting, and study of untoward occurrences;
- fostering the fiduciary relationship between and among governance, leadership, and the wider community;
- promoting responsible stewardship of health care resources by
  - conserving health care resources in the clinical, administrative, research, educational, and research settings by using them efficiently and appropriately;
  - distinguishing between scarce and expensive resources in organizational planning and decision making;
  - modeling responsible stewardship of resources in all settings
- UHN creates an ethical clinical environment by
  - fostering the fiduciary relationship between care professionals and patients by
    - placing the interests of patients before those of health care professionals or the organization;

- distinguishing between what patients and surrogates request and what patients need;
- providing medically necessary care in which the anticipated benefits to the patient outweigh the anticipated burdens and risks
- o promoting the dignity, security, and professionalism of caregiving staff by
  - modeling attitudes and behavior that demonstrate respect for caregiving staff;
  - ensuring that caregiving staff are neither unfairly advantaged nor disadvantaged in their work because of race, religion, ethnicity, gender, or sexual orientation;
  - protecting caregiving staff from harm based on discriminatory or other malicious criteria;
  - protecting staff from harassment, verbal or physical threat, or other forms of intimidation by patients, visitors, or other staff;
  - mentoring staff so that roles and responsibilities are commensurate with experience and skills;
  - conferring on staff the authority to make and take responsibility for clinical decisions commensurate with each caregiver's role and skill set;
  - teaching and mentoring new health care professionals by
    - modeling the highest standards of professionalism;
    - modeling the integration of ethical principles and standards in all areas of clinical work
- o promoting respect for the autonomy of capable patients by
  - ensuring that patients' care goals and preferences are elicited and, when clinically indicated, integrated into the plan of care;
  - determining what patients know and want to know about their medical condition and how involved they want to be in care planning and decision making;
  - ensuring that the decisions of capable patients are communicated and honored, before and after capacity has lapsed;
  - offering information and assistance in creating advance directives or Practitioner Orders for Life-Sustaining Treatment (POLST), as appropriate;
  - ensuring that advance directives and POLST are available and accessible during current hospitalizations and maintaining these documents for use in future patient encounters;
  - identifying the appointed agents or informal surrogates who will make decisions in the event that patients' decisional capacity is temporarily or permanently lost;
  - providing patients and surrogates sufficient accurate, relevant, and timely information about diagnosis, prognosis, and treatment options in a manner that is understandable and culturally sensitive, and ensuring that the information has been understood by the patient and surrogate;
  - engaging certified interpreters, rather than family or other surrogates, when patients or surrogates prefer to use a language other than English

- o collaborating with patients and surrogates in shared decision making about the goals and plan of care by
  - meeting regularly with patients and surrogates to review the patient's evolving condition and its implications for revising goals and plan of care;
  - providing information, options, and recommendations regarding care planning;
  - distinguishing the responsibilities of patients, surrogates, and practitioners in developing and implementing goals and plans of care;
  - interacting with patients and families with respect, honesty, and empathy

- o protecting vulnerable patients who lack decisional capacity by
  - identifying patients whose decisional capacity is diminished, fluctuating, or lapsed;
  - determining whether patients with diminished capacity still have sufficient capacity to appoint others to make decisions for them;
  - identifying the appointed agents or informal surrogates who will make decisions on behalf of incapacitated patients;
  - providing agents or surrogates with information, guidance, and support in the process of decision making on behalf of incapacitated patients
- o promoting patient best interest and protecting patients from harm by
  - ensuring that only interventions likely to benefit patients are offered for consideration;
  - ensuring that care is provided only by qualified professionals;
  - ensuring that the anticipated benefits to patients of proposed interventions outweigh the anticipated burdens and risks;
  - explaining to patients and surrogates why interventions they have requested are or are not clinically indicated and why interventions that will not benefit patients or risk causing them harm will not be provided;
  - ensuring that untoward clinical events are responded to with procedures for determining the cause, preventing reoccurrence, and disclosing to patients or surrogates information necessary to understand and mitigate harm;
- o protecting patient confidentiality and privacy by
  - protecting personal health information learned in the diagnostic and therapeutic encounters with patients;
  - disclosing personal health information only to health care professionals providing direct patient care or other services;
  - assuring patients that personal health information will only be disclosed to family and friends consistent with their expressed preferences;
  - helping family and other surrogates understand why withholding health information from capable patients is ethically and clinically problematic, and would be considered only if a clinical assessment determined that disclosure would put the patient at risk of imminent and significant harm

- UHN creates an ethical research environment by
  - fostering the fiduciary relationship between research investigators and subjects by
    - placing the interests and safety of subjects before the interests of investigators or sponsors;
    - ensuring that subjects understand the distinction between research and treatment in the research setting;
    - promoting research that minimizes risk to subjects and maximizes benefit to society
  - promoting respect for the autonomy of research subjects by
    - confirming that potential subjects have sufficient decisional capacity to provide informed and voluntary consent to participate in research;
    - confirming that consent for incapacitated patients to participate in research does not put them at more than minimal risk;
    - ensuring that subjects receive and understand sufficient information about the purpose, conduct, risks, and benefits of proposed research;
    - ensuring that subjects understand that their initial consent and continuing participation in research is voluntary and may be withdrawn at any time;
    - ensuring that subjects understand that their decision about participating in research will not affect the health care that they receive
- UHN creates an ethical business environment by
  - supporting fair marketing practices by
    - offering only those services, resources, and outcomes that UHN can deliver;
    - disseminating accurate information to facilitate patient choice and decisions by vendors or others who do business with the organization;
    - making publicly available information about organizational relationships that create actual, potential, or apparent conflicts of interest
  - engaging in ethical business decision making by
    - balancing the need for clinical, research, and educational resources with the need for organizational growth and development;
    - providing and billing only for services that are medically indicated;
    - ensuring transparency so that stakeholders understand the organization's short- and long-term planning;
    - ensuring that organizational leadership is accountable to stakeholders;
    - entering into contracts that have clear business justification, are commercially reasonable, and whose terms reflect fair market value;
    - ensuring that the impact of business decisions takes into account their effect on the larger community
- UHN creates an ethical academic environment by
  - integrating ethics into all stages of academic pursuit;
  - requiring that students demonstrate understanding of ethical theory and conduct in clinical and non-clinical settings;
  - fostering intellectual honesty, transparency, discovery, and innovation;
  - requiring that students and faculty demonstrate accountability for ethical behavior in their academic activities;

- developing curricula and clinical training that focus on patient-centered and interdisciplinary care;
- developing and presenting educational material and clinical training in ways that are sensitive to and respectful of culture, religion, and ethnicity, with recognition of and respect for personal creed;
- providing an exceptional educational experience that prepares outstanding clinicians and academicians, and contributes to the body of health care knowledge;
- fostering community engagement and social justice

Drafting a code of ethics sets up an immediate and difficult balance between comprehensiveness and accessibility. In an effort to include all the organization's constituent parts, responsibilities, and activities, as well as their ethical reach, the resulting statement can become long, dense, and inaccessible to all but the most dedicated reader. The risk is that a code whose core values and commitments should resonate with every member of the organization, from CEO to part-time employee, becomes so self-consciously intellectual that its essence is lost in the verbiage. For that reason, in addition to simplifying and clarifying the text in your code, you might consider adding an abbreviated and streamlined version, a summary code that captures the salient points in easily understood language.

PART IV

KEY LEGAL
CASES

By including this section in the handbook, we are not suggesting that, in addition to its other responsibilities, your ethics committee should assume the functions of your institution's Legal Department. As emphasized throughout this handbook, the unique contribution of ethics committees is the application of ethical analysis to clinical and organizational issues. Nevertheless, it is important to recognize that the provision and assessment of health care takes place in a context shaped partly by the constraints of statutory and case law. This legal landscape, in turn, reflects the evolution of societal norms, judicial philosophies, governmental pragmatics, and, sometimes, political agendas. As noted in part I, almost all law governing health care is state-specific, and your committee will benefit from familiarity with how the relevant laws and regulations in your state affect the care provided in your institution. Perhaps the simplest way to do this is to review your institution's policies, all of which must be consistent with your state's laws. Examples of health care institutional policies are discussed in chapter 17.

This section, then, is intended not to teach law, but to provide an overview of key legal developments that inform your work. Rather than an exhaustive catalogue of bioethics-related case and statutory law, the following cases and statutes have been selected because they represent important legal milestones that have affected and, in some cases, profoundly altered health care and bioethics. In some instances, they illustrate the ways different courts or legislatures address similar issues. In others, it is possible to see the disconnect between law and ethics that creates tensions addressed in ethics committee deliberation. Because of their historical significance, several of these cases are also referred to in the relevant chapters of part I.

The cases have been summarized to highlight the ethical issues they raise, keeping the legalese to a minimum. For those wishing to consult the original text, each case is presented with its legal citation and web link, as well as a brief parenthetical statement of the holding, the legal principle derived from the court's opinion or decision. Further information about these and other pertinent cases and statutes can be found in the references at the end of this section. For example, a brief but very informative and accessible explanation of the American constitutional structure, including the relationship between federal and state courts, appears in *Law and Bioethics: An Introduction* by Jerry Menikoff.

The authors gratefully acknowledge the help of Georgina Campelia as co-author of this section.

Informed Consent

The doctrine of informed consent and refusal has its roots in the law of battery, which holds that unconsented-to touching, even treatment intended to be beneficial, is unlawful. The earliest, most well-known, and widely quoted expression of this philosophy was by Justice Benjamin N. Cardozo, who said, "Every human being of adult years and sound mind has a right to determine what shall be done with his own body; and a surgeon who performs an operation without his patient's consent commits an assault for which he is liable in damages" (*Schloendorff v. Society of New York Hospital*, 105 N.E. 92, 93 (N.Y. 1914)).

The signal case establishing the principle of informed consent was *Canterbury v. Spence*, 464 F.2d 772 (D.C. 1969) (http://biotech.law.lsu.edu/cases/consent/canterbury_v_spence.htm) (holding that the physician is obliged to provide sufficient information about a procedure's risks so that a reasonable patient can make an informed decision). The case concerned a patient who underwent surgery for back pain, fell out of bed during recovery, and suffered paralysis. Among the plaintiff's claims was that he had not been informed before surgery of the risk of paralysis. The court held that, not only consent, but *informed* consent is necessary before medical treatment is undertaken.

The issue before the court was the kind of risks that must be disclosed and here two opposing philosophies were articulated. One camp believed that the doctor should disclose risks considered standard by the medical community, a view that would require expert medical testimony during trial. The other camp held that the standard should be what the reasonable patient would consider a significant risk, requiring disclosure of a far greater range of risks. The *Canterbury* court held that the reasonable patient standard was more appropriate because it shaped the disclosure duty according to what the patient needed to know. Controversy remains about whether the nature and content of disclosure should be determined by the doctor's duty to inform or the patient's understanding of the disclosure. Although states are still about evenly split on which approach to follow, the medical community standard is the majority view.

More recently, two California cases further developed the doctrine of informed consent. *Moore v. Regents of the University of California*, 793 P.2d 479 (Cal. 1990) (http://online.ceb.com/CalCases/C3/51C3d120.htm) (holding that informed consent requires physician disclosure of "personal interests unrelated to the patient's health" but potentially affecting medical judgment), examined the doctor's conflict of interest. The case concerned the deliberate withholding from the patient of his doctors' plans to use tissue removed from his body for likely profitable research. Having made the diagnosis of hairy-cell leukemia and realizing the unique properties of Mr. Moore's tissue, the doctors applied for a patent on the cell line from the tissue before removing his spleen. On appeal, the court found that, even if the treatment had a therapeutic purpose, the patient's ignorance of the doctors' research and financial interest in his tissue, which may have affected their medical judgment, impaired his ability to give truly informed consent.

Arato v. Avedon, 858 P.2d 598 (Cal. 1993), (http://law.justia.com/cases/california/cal4th/5/1172.html) (holding that the duty to obtain informed consent does not require a physician to disclose a patient's statistical life expectancy), concerned the nature of the patient's health-related information that is necessary for informed decision making. After being diagnosed with a virulent form of cancer, the patient consented to chemotherapy and radiation treatment. The doctors explained to the patient and his family the poor prognosis for this type of cancer and the experimental but promising nature of the chemotherapy; they did not, however, provide statistical information on his life expectancy. The suit brought following the patient's death claimed that, had he known the short life expectancy and the small chance of successful cure, he would not have undergone the treatment, and thus he had not given fully informed consent. The suit further claimed that his ignorance of his situation prevented him from adequately ordering his affairs, resulting in his family suffering financial hardship.

The *Arato* court found that the physicians had provided the patient with what was required to give an informed consent—sufficient information material to the treatment decision to enable the patient to make a knowledgeable choice. The unreliability of statistical morbidity data, plus the patient's apparent reluctance to learn his life expectancy, removed the physicians' burden to disclose the information. Because of its emphasis on not imposing unwanted, potentially distressing information, it has been suggested that *Arato* represents an expansion of the therapeutic exception to the disclosure obligation.

Grimes v. Kennedy Krieger Institute, 366 Md 29, 782 A2nd 807 (2001) (www.courts .state.md.us/opinions/coa/2001/128a00.pdf) (holding that children may not be used as research subjects in nontherapeutic studies that expose them to risk of injury or damage to their health), reaffirmed children as a class deserving heightened protection in research. In 1993, the Kennedy Krieger Institute (KKI) launched research to determine the effects of various lead paint abatement interventions on homes in urban Baltimore. The study was undertaken in response to the increasing number of landlords abandoning properties in low-income areas rather than meet the cost of mandatory full lead paint abatement. Endeavoring to find less costly abatement methods and stem the property abandonment, the local government recruited landlords and reimbursed them according to a sliding scale based on five levels of intervention. Groups I, II, and III received increasingly comprehensive repair and maintenance. No additional repairs were done to Group IV homes, which had already been abated of lead paint, or Group V homes, which were presumed to be lead paint free because they were built after 1980.

To enroll study subjects, KKI recruited families with young children already living in these homes and paid them to allow periodic sampling of dust, water, soil, and blood. Assessment of the effectiveness of the different abatement procedures consisted of "measuring the extent to which the . . . healthy children's blood became contaminated with lead, and comparing that contamination with levels of lead dust in the houses over the same periods of time" (Morse R. 2003). Two children who were part of the study subsequently sued KKI, claiming that KKI had breached its duty to research subjects by failing to fully disclose the known hazard of lead paint to children and its presence in the homes where they continued to live. Both plaintiffs claimed in their negligence suits that the KKI study increased rather than decreased the children's exposure to a known hazard, thereby putting them at foreseeable risk of harm. The circuit court granted KKI's motion for summary judgment (prompt disposition of a controversy without trial when the facts are undisputed or only one question of law is involved) on the grounds that it did not owe a duty to the plaintiffs and that no contract or "special relationship" existed between the researchers and the study subjects. The court of appeals of Maryland, however, ruled that the circuit court had erred in granting KKI's motion and vacated (annulled) the rulings, sending the cases back to the lower court for retrial.

In its analysis, the court of appeals found that, given the parties' interests and the nature of the nontherapeutic enterprise, the consent forms signed by KKI and the children's parents did create a valid contract and a "special relationship" between the researcher and research subjects. The court distinguished the physician-patient and researcher-subject relationships, noting that, especially in nontherapeutic research studies, the parties may have conflicting interests and, as in these cases, the research may involve foreseeable risks. The court took special notice of the requirements of true informed consent, including the disclosure and understanding of "all material facts," necessary for risk-benefit assessment, especially in health-related research. Finally, the court held that even with their consent, parents may not expose their vulnerable children to health risks without therapeutic benefit, even to generate knowledge that will benefit society.

The ethical importance of *Grimes v. Kennedy Krieger Institute* lies in the court of appeals ruling that the interests of society in new research are potentially in conflict with the interests of research subjects. The ruling sets out three ways in which a "special relationship" between researcher and subject can be created, a flexible framework for injured subjects to seek redress, and a clear prohibition against exposing vulnerable children to risks that are more appropriately undertaken by informed and capable adult subjects.

The well-settled right of capable persons to consent to or refuse medical treatment has been invoked periodically in an effort to broaden the scope of self-determination in health care decision making—see, for example, *Washington v. Glucksberg*, 521 U.S. 702 (1997) (www.law.cornell.edu/supct/html/96-110.ZC2.html) (holding that the U.S. Constitution does not encompass a right to physician assistance in ending one's life). *Abigail Alliance for Better Access to Developmental Drugs v. Eschenbach*, 495 F. 3d 695 (D.C. Cir. 2007) (www.abigail-alliance.org/WLF_FDA .pdf) (holding that there is no constitutional right to unapproved drugs by terminally ill patients), presented the Court of Appeals for the District of Columbia with another opportunity to find a new fundamental right under the due process clause of the Fifth Amendment.

Abigail Alliance, an advocacy group of terminally ill persons and their supporters, claimed that competent, terminally ill patients who had exhausted all other approved treatment options have a fundamental right to access experimental drugs that have passed Phase I clinical testing but have not received the FDA approval necessary for clinical use as therapy. The Alliance argued that, with knowledge of the relative risks and benefits, these patients have the right to assume the risks of potentially life-saving experimental drugs without FDA interference. The DC district court held that the Constitution does not protect such a right. A three-judge panel of the DC court of appeals reversed that decision, but the full court of appeals declined to further expand the scope of fundamental rights and held that there is no constitutionally protected right to experimental drugs.

Privacy

Historical and religious prohibitions against interfering with procreation were at the root of some states' statutory criminalization of contraception. These statutes were struck down in 1965 when the U.S. Supreme Court, in *Griswold v. Connecticut*, 381 U.S. 479 (1965), (www.law.cornell.edu/supremecourt/text/381/479) (holding that the constitutionally protected right to privacy of married persons was violated by laws restricting the use of or dissemination of information about contraception). The executive director and a physician at a Connecticut Planned Parenthood clinic were convicted under a state law that made it a criminal offense to provide counseling on contraception to married couples.

Griswold was a landmark case because it (1) legalized the use of contraception by married couples and the freedom of their doctors to counsel them regarding its use; and (2) found in the Constitution a "penumbra" (or implication) of rights not specifically articulated in the text, but emanating from fundamental constitutional guarantees. These guarantees, according to the Court, included the very important zone of privacy in marital relations. This reasoning gave rise to the concept of privacy as autonomy, the protectable right to personal decision making. The far-reaching importance of this approach is that it allowed the *Griswold* Court, and subsequent Courts, to find a generalized right to privacy capable of accommodating a broadened scope of protected personal interests. The interests found to be protectable under the expanding right to privacy included those intimate areas of life related to personal decisions, such as marriage, procreation, child rearing, family definition, and abortion.

Griswold thus created a zone of privacy, which it accorded a high degree of protection. According to constitutional interpretation, fundamental rights are those that are so central to individual liberty that they can be abridged only when the state can demonstrate a compelling interest in doing so. The difficulty of overcoming this very high standard is the constitutional safeguard against arbitrary state intrusion in the lives of individuals. The *Griswold* line of reasoning, however, lost much of its vitality in *Bowers v. Hardwick*, 478 U.S.186 (1986) (www.law.cornell.edu /supremecourt/text/478/186) (holding that the right to privacy does not include a fundamental right to engage in consensual sodomy, even within the privacy of one's home), a decision considered to restrict privacy as autonomy. Based on homosexual activities, Hardwick was charged with violating the provisions of a Georgia state sodomy law. When the district attorney chose not to pursue the matter, Hardwick sued, challenging the constitutionality of a law that criminalized private, consensual sexual behavior. The Court distinguished consensual sodomy from any constitutionally protected right and clearly signaled its reluctance to expand further the definition of fundamental rights.

Nineteen years later, however, the Court overturned *Bowers* in *Lawrence and Garner v. Texas*, 539 U.S. 558 (2003) (http://supreme.justia.com/cases/federal/us/539/558 /case.html) (holding that the Texas statute that criminalized sexual intimacy by same-sex couples, while not criminalizing the same behavior by different-sex couples, violates the due process clause of the Fourteenth Amendment). The Court upheld the privacy and liberty rights of adults, ruling, "The Texas statute furthers no legitimate state interest which can justify its intrusion into the personal and private life of the individual." Nevertheless, in recent years, the Supreme Court has declined to expand the scope of individual privacy rights.

The Defense of Marriage Act (DOMA) (www.gpo.gov/fdsys/pkg/BILLS-104 hr3396enr/pdf/BILLS-104hr3396enr.pdf), enacted by the U.S. Congress and signed into law by President Bill Clinton in 1996, singled out same-sex couples for unequal treatment under federal law. Section 2 permits states to refuse recognition of valid same-sex marriages performed and recognized in other states. Section 3, which was declared unconstitutional in 2013, eliminates all same-sex couples, regardless of marital status, from all federal laws and regulations, thereby denying them all the federal benefits and protections available to heterosexual couples.

President Clinton and other legislators ultimately responded to growing public pressure and called for DOMA's repeal. In 2011, Attorney General Holder, at the direction of the president, announced that the Department of Justice would stop defending DOMA in court. Given the increasing number of states recognizing same-sex marriage (at the time of this writing, 19 plus the District of Columbia and 8 Indian tribes), it seems likely that DOMA will eventually be repealed and replaced with the Respect for Marriage Act, which guarantees every married couple the certainty of recognition, protection, and benefits under federal law in all states.

Confidentiality

The need to protect the public health has been invoked to justify breaching the professional duty of confidentiality, as in state laws requiring health care providers to report suspected cases of child abuse and neglect; wounds that are the result of gun shots, knives, or other pointed instruments; burn injuries of specified severity; and cases of reportable communicable diseases.

More recently, courts have recognized a professional obligation to disclose information that will protect identified third persons put at specific risk by patients' ability and intention to do harm. The legal duty to protect identified persons endangered by a foreseeable harm was first recognized in a negligence suit brought by the parents of a young woman murdered by her boyfriend. The case was *Tarasoff v. Regents of University of California*, 551 P.2d 334 (Cal. 1976) (http://scholar.google .com/scholar_case?case=10716111142563485073) (holding that a therapist who concludes that a patient poses a foreseeable danger to a third person is under a duty to notify the potential victim). Even though Prosenjit Poddar had confided during his psychotherapy session his intention to kill Tatiana Tarasoff and the psychologist subsequently alerted the police, the therapist did nothing to warn the potential victim directly. The court reasoned that "the public policy favoring protection of the confidential character of patient-psychotherapist communications must yield to the extent to which disclosure is essential to avert danger to others. The protective privilege ends where the public peril begins."

The *Tarasoff* reasoning has been incorporated into the partner notification laws of most states, which now require that sexual and needle-sharing contacts of HIV-positive patients be informed that they have been exposed to the virus and should be tested. *Tarasoff* is also noteworthy because it significantly broadened the scope of professional duty to include not only the immediate patient, but also an identified third party at risk who had no direct clinical connection to the care provider.

The exponential increase in ability to capture, store, interpret, and make diagnostic and therapeutic use of genetic information has presented myriad foreseen and unforeseen challenges. Decoding the human genome represents, in many ways, the quintessential Pandora's box, revealing unimagined potential for benefit and harm. Among the threshold questions are, now that we know how to access this information, what can we do with it, what should we do with it, how shall we protect it, how shall we protect ourselves from it? An especially chilling theme, envisioned in the 1997 film *Gattaca*, is the dystopian society where individuals' genetic destiny is determined prenatally and controls their entire future. The Genetic Information Nondiscrimination Act (GINA) was written and signed into law in 2008 in response to concerns about how genetic information might be misused to discriminate against people based on their genetic predisposition to certain limiting health conditions. The scope of the law is limited to employment and health insurance, access to which profoundly affects the life quality of individuals and populations. While the ultimate goal of creating genetic profiles is personalized medicine—a lifetime plan of care that is safer, more effective, more accessible, and affordable because it is suited to one's genetic profile—the possibilities for misuse of the information are equally compelling. The law's potential effectiveness in protecting individual rights is still unknown, but is likely to be highly scrutinized as an indicator of science as a societal benefactor.

Health Care Decision Making

FORGOING LIFE-SUSTAINING TREATMENT

Among the most difficult bioethical dilemmas are decisions to refuse or terminate life-sustaining treatment, made either by capable patients or on behalf of patients without capacity. In 1975, what became known as the "right to die," but is really the right to refuse unwanted treatment, was brought to national attention when 21-year-old Karen Ann Quinlan lapsed into a persistent vegetative state (PVS). Although doctors determined that her condition was irreversible, they were reluctant to accede to her family's wishes and discontinue life support measures. In a unanimous landmark decision, *In re Quinlan*, 355 A.2d 647 (N.J. 1976) (www.uta.edu/philosophy/faculty/burgess-jackson/In%20re%20Quinlan,%2070%20N.J.%2010,%20 355%20A.2d%20647%20(1976).pdf) (recognizing a constitutionally protected right to refuse life-sustaining treatment and upholding the exercise of that right by the family of a patient in PVS), the New Jersey Supreme Court held that removal of the respirator necessary to keep Ms. Quinlan alive would not constitute criminal homicide because death would result from existing natural causes.

In an analysis that weighed the interests of the state against the benefits and burdens to the patient, the *Quinlan* court noted that "the State's interest [in maintaining] life weakens and the individual's right to privacy grows as the degree of bodily invasion increases and the prognosis dims." The court based its protection of the right to refuse treatment on the constitutionally protected right to privacy, what some commentators have called "privacy as autonomy."

Courts that have found persuasive evidence of terminal illness or unbearable suffering plus decision-making capacity have held that patients' decisions to terminate life-sustaining treatment are reasonable and supportable. *Satz v. Perlmutter*, 362 S.2d 160 (Fla.App. 1978) *aff'd* 379 S.2d 359 (Fla. 1980) (www.leagle.com/decision/197852 2362So2d160_2448) (upholding a competent individual's right to refuse unwanted life-sustaining treatment) concerned a 73-year-old patient with amyotrophic lateral sclerosis, also known as Lou Gehrig's disease, a progressively debilitating and incurable disease. Although generally paralyzed and dependent on mechanical breathing assistance, he was alert, fully competent, and able to speak. He understood that his condition was terminal and he wanted to have the breathing tube removed from his trachea, knowing that this would cause almost immediate death. Indeed, he had attempted, unsuccessfully, to remove the tube himself. He was supported in this decision by his family.

The hospital, fearing both civil and criminal liability, refused to honor his request. The patient petitioned for a court order preventing the hospital from interfering with his decision. The state intervened, citing four state interests in keeping a patient alive, which had been articulated in an earlier case, *Superintendent of Belchertown State School v. Saikewicz*, 373 Mass. 728 (1977) (http://masscases.com /cases/sjc/373/373mass728.html) (holding that the probate judge acted appropriately in enforcing the patient's decision to decline life-prolonging treatment in light of no sufficient state interest to counterbalance that decision). These four justifications were the state's (1) interest in the preservation of life; (2) duty to prevent suicide; (3) need to protect innocent third parties; and (4) need to maintain the ethical integrity of the medical profession. The court found that "the condition is terminal, the patient's situation wretched, and the continuation of his life temporary and artificial." Accordingly, despite the state's four interests in maintaining life, the court held that the plaintiff's decision to terminate his life-supporting treatment was reasonable.

Refusal of life-sustaining treatment by a capable patient on religious grounds is illustrated by *Fosmire v. Nicoleau*, 551 N.Y.S.2d 876 (1990) (http://scholar.google.com /scholar_case?case=13093476897919645004&hl=en&as_sdt=6&as_vis=1&oi =scholarr) (holding that the Supreme Court should not have authorized the requested blood transfusions without consent or discussion with the patient, who was competent at the time of treatment), in which a Jehovah's Witness refused the blood transfusions necessary to save her life during childbirth. The court held that, at the time of treatment, this patient was competent to express her wishes and make a health care decision. The court considered the four state interests in keeping a patient alive, especially the claim that preserving her life was for the benefit of her children, and found that the state had failed to show paramount interest in preventing the patient from exercising her right to refuse treatment.

A patient's right to refuse nutrition and hydration was addressed in *Bouvia v. Superior Court of Los Angeles County*, 225 Cal. Rptr. 297 (Cal.Ct.App. 1986) (http:// people.brandeis.edu/~teuber/bouvia.html) (holding that a decisionally capable person may refuse artificial feeding enforced to sustain life, even if the person is not terminally ill). Cerebral palsy and arthritis had slowly robbed the 28-year-old patient of the use of her limbs and she was completely dependent financially as well as physically. Nevertheless, she was intelligent and competent, and had graduated from college. When she tried to starve herself to death by refusing food, a nasogastric tube was inserted through which she was force fed. Her request to have the tube removed was denied by the lower court, which found that, because she was incurably but not terminally ill, she could potentially live for years.

The appellate court, however, held that a competent person's right to refuse unwanted life-sustaining treatment encompasses forced tube feedings, and that the absence of a terminal prognosis does not affect that right. The court emphasized that the right to refuse treatment belongs to the competent patient and is not to be limited or denied by physicians or courts. It is interesting that the concurring opinion foreshadowed the assisted dying debate by saying that, rather than having to starve herself, Ms. Bouvia should have been able to call on her doctors to help her achieve a painless death.

SURROGATE DECISIONS TO FORGO
LIFE-SUSTAINING TREATMENT

The substituted judgment standard of decision making for an incapacitated patient was first articulated in *Superintendent of Belchertown State School v. Saikewicz*, 370 N.E.2d 417 (1977) (http://masscases.com/cases/sjc/373/373mass728.html) (holding that an individual incompetent from birth has the same right as competent individuals to refuse medical treatment and is not required to undergo unwanted life-sustaining treatment). The case concerned Joseph Saikewicz, a profoundly retarded 67-year-old man with the mental age of less than 3 years. The issue before the court was whether to treat his leukemia with chemotherapy, which would cause him considerable discomfort and had a 30% to 50% chance of extending his life for 2 to 13 months, or forgo therapy, in which case he would die within weeks.

In reaching its ruling, the *Saikewicz* court began by recognizing the patient's lifelong incapacity to make decisions and using an objective standard to consider what would be in his best interest. But then the court proposed an alternative method of decision making for this patient—substituted judgment—suggesting that the incompetent individual's choices could be inferred by a surrogate decision maker based on what is known about his wishes and values. The court's somewhat strained reasoning was that those who are and have always been legally incompetent still have the same right as others to refuse life-sustaining treatment, and to deny them that right just because they are incompetent devalues their worth.

Despite the utility of the substituted judgment standard in surrogate decision making, the way it was used by the *Saikewicz* court has been largely discredited by subsequent courts and commentators. Substituted judgment is typically reserved for those situations in which previously capable patients have a known history of preferences that can guide decision making on their behalf. Precisely because persons who are profoundly retarded have no such history, decisions for them must rely on the best interest standard, drawing on what *others* believe will promote their well-being. The *Saikewicz* court blurred this distinction and relied on the fiction that the always-incompetent patient has values and wishes that can be divined by surrogate decision makers, explaining that "the decision . . . should be that which would be made by the incompetent person, if that person were competent, but taking into account the present and future incompetency of the individual." The risks of applying this contrived reasoning in the clinical setting are discussed in chapter 2 and were pointed out later by the *Storar* court considering a similar case.

The standards for making decisions on behalf of the never-competent and the formerly competent were more clearly distinguished in a pair of 1981 cases. *In re Storar*, 52 N.Y.2d 363 (N.Y. 1981) (https://mywebspace.wisc.edu/rstreiffer/web/Course Folders/BioandLawF99Folder/Readings/In_re_Storar.pdf) (holding that the guardian of a lifelong incompetent person may not withhold medical treatment in a belief that such withholding is in the incompetent person's best interest), concerned a profoundly retarded 52-year-old man with terminal bladder cancer whose mother petitioned for an order discontinuing the blood transfusions necessary to keep him alive. The patient had been from birth incapable of making a reasoned determination about his health care and his mother rejected the recommended transfusions because they caused him discomfort and would extend his life by only three to six months. Here, the question was whether the patient's best interests were served by allowing his mother or the hospital to have decision-making authority.

In its ruling, the court analogized the patient to a child incapable of exercising his autonomy, even though he was chronologically an adult. Note that, in contrast to the earlier *Saikewicz* court, the *Storar* court relied on the notion of best interest, rather than engaging in the fiction that the wishes of a never-competent person could be used to guide decision making. In explaining why it declined to use substituted judgment, the court said of the *Saikewicz* reasoning that asking what an incompetent person would decide if competent "would be similar to asking whether if it snowed all summer would it then be winter?" Relying on what it considered to be the patient's best interest, the *Storar* court held that, while a parent may consent to or refuse treatment on behalf of a child, the parent may not deprive a child of life-sustaining treatment.

The companion case to *Storar* was *Matter of Eichner*, 52 N.Y.2d 363 (N.Y. 1981) (http://wings.buffalo.edu/bioethics/eich1.html) (holding that the agent of an incompetent person may authorize the termination of life-sustaining measures if such termination is consistent with the prior wishes of the patient when competent). Also known as the Brother Fox case, the matter concerned an elderly priest who suffered brain damage and lapsed into a coma as a result of postoperative cardiac arrest. Brother Fox's guardian, Father Eichner, petitioned for an order discontinuing life support in accordance with Brother Fox's previously expressed wishes not to be kept alive artificially if he were in a vegetative state. Finding that Brother Fox's numerous statements at the time of the *Quinlan* case constituted clear and convincing evidence of his care preferences, the court held that the patient's wishes to have life-sustaining measures removed, as expressed through his representative, should be honored.

A pivotal case addressing both surrogate decision making and the right to refuse life-sustaining treatment was *In re Conroy*, 486 A.2d 1209 (N.J. 1985) (http://law.justia.com/cases/california/calapp2d/117/194.html) (holding that an incompetent person's life support may be removed if doing so is demonstrably in the incompetent person's best interest). The case concerned an 83-year-old nursing home resident with multiple, serious, and irreversible physical and cognitive impairments that left her unable to do anything for herself and minimally responsive to her surroundings. Regardless of treatment, she was expected to live less than a year.

The court permitted removal of her feeding tube, articulating a range of surrogate decision-making standards for terminally ill patients. The court established three tests for determining when life-sustaining treatment may legitimately be withheld or withdrawn from an incapacitated patient: (1) *subjective test*—what is known about what the patient wanted, based on her prior explicit verbal or written statements; (2) *limited objective test*—"trustworthy evidence" about what the patient would have wanted plus clear indications that the treatment would only prolong suffering; and (3) *pure objective test*—without knowledge of what the patient would have wanted, but with clear indications that the burdens of the treatment "markedly outweigh" the benefits *and* that continuing treatment would be "inhumane."

Perhaps the most famous and precedentially important case of this kind was *Cruzan v. Director, Missouri Department of Health*, 497 U.S. 261(1990) (http://supreme .justia.com/cases/federal/us/497/261/case.html) (holding that the Constitution is not violated by a state statute requiring "clear and convincing evidence" of the prior consent of a comatose patient before terminating life-sustaining measures). The case concerned Nancy Beth Cruzan, a 25-year-old woman in PVS for 7 years, whose parents petitioned for an order to discontinue artificial nutrition and hydration. The U.S. Supreme Court, in its only such decision, upheld Missouri's right to insist on the demanding "clear and convincing evidence" standard for determining the wishes of an incompetent patient regarding the termination of life support. Because it is the only Supreme Court decision regarding refusal of life-sustaining treatment, the *Cruzan* holding remains binding on all lower courts addressing these matters.

In a ruling with far-reaching implications, the *Cruzan* Court recognized the liberty interest of a competent individual to refuse unwanted treatment, but found insufficient evidence of the prior wishes of *this* patient. The Court noted that the grave and irreversible consequences of a decision to withdraw life-sustaining treatment justified refusing such a request without certainty about the patient's wishes when competent. The Court held that imposing the stringent clear and convincing evidence standard did not violate due process protections, partly because of the state's interest in preventing abuse when the family is unavailable, unable, or unwilling to act as surrogate decision maker. The Court noted that, because due process did not require the state to give decision-making authority for termination of life support to anyone but the patient, the state was not required to give family members the right of substituted judgment. The ruling *permits but does not require* states to insist that evidence of prior competent wishes to end life support meet the demanding clear and convincing standard of proof. Presently, Missouri and New York require application of this standard in the clinical setting, significantly limiting the ability of nonappointed surrogates in those states to make end-of-life decisions for incapacitated patients.

Finally, it is worth noting Justice O'Connor's dissent, in which she said that the clear and convincing standard denies many people the opportunity to refuse treatment because so few leave explicit instructions or indicate their wishes in the event of incapacity. Therefore, she predicted, the *Cruzan* decision did not foreclose the possibility that the constitutionality of surrogate decision making might be considered in the future. Indeed, it has been suggested that some state statutes authorizing health care proxy appointments represented, in part, a response to the uncertainty created by the clear and convincing evidence standard articulated in *Cruzan*.

More recently, three cases captured national attention because of the struggles the patients' families endured as they attempted to make surrogate decisions for their loved ones. In 1990, Terri Schiavo suffered a cardiac arrest, leading to severe hypoxic-ischemic encephalopathy. During the ensuing several months, her condition led treating and consulting physicians to concur that she was in a persistent vegetative state (PVS). Her husband, Michael, was appointed her legal guardian and Ms. Schiavo was transferred to a long-term care facility where she was cared for and sustained by artificial nutrition and hydration (ANH) through a feeding tube. By the mid-1990s, Mr. Schiavo understood that his wife's condition was irreversible but Mr. and Mrs. Schindler, Terri's parents, were convinced that she was responding to treatment and would recover. In 1998, Mr. Schiavo petitioned the court for permission to remove the feeding tube he was certain his wife would have refused if she could do so. In 2005, the decision to remove ANH was upheld (http://abstractappeal.com/schiavo/trialctorder02-05.pdf).

As the U.S. Supreme Court ruled in *Cruzan*, states may set their own evidentiary standards for determining the wishes of now-incapacitated persons, and Florida law required "clear and convincing evidence that the decision would have been the one the patient would have chosen had the patient been competent or, if there is no indication of what the patient would have chosen, that the decision is in the patient's best interest" (Quill 2005). After six days of evidentiary hearings, including testimony that Terri Schiavo had expressed her wish not to have her life maintained by mechanical means, the trial court ruled that Mr. Schiavo's request should be honored and the feeding tube was removed. The Schindlers, however, supported by outside organizations and officials, continued to oppose forgoing life-sustaining treatment, igniting a series of court proceedings and feeding tube removals and reinsertions. In 2003, at the request of Governor Jeb Bush, the Florida legislature passed Terri's Law to override the court decision and the feeding tube was reinserted. Ultimately, the ruling of the trial court was upheld by the Florida Second District Court of Appeal and subsequent appeals to the Florida Supreme Court and the U.S. Supreme Court were denied. During the legal proceedings, the acrimony between Michael Schiavo and his in-laws, exacerbated by special interest groups, politicians, and elected officials, played out in public. Finally, on March 18, 2005, 15 years after her cardiac arrest, Terri Schiavo's feeding tube was removed for the last time and she died 13 days later.

More recently, two mirror-image cases—one in which the patient's family challenged the declaration of death and sought to keep her on life support, and one in which no one challenged the declaration of death but the hospital and the state sought to maintain the patient's body on mechanical supports until fetal viability—generated strong feelings across the country. In December 2013, in Oakland, California, 13-year-old Jahi McMath was found by multiple independent neurological exams to meet the criteria for brain death, following complications of surgery for sleep apnea. Her grieving family was unable to accept her death and sought judicial intervention to prevent physicians from discontinuing her ventilatory support. Three weeks after the initial determination of death, the court ordered her body released to the custody of her family. With continued ventilatory support and added nutritional support, Jahi's body was moved to a facility where her physiologic functions are reportedly being sustained.

In November 2013, in Fort Worth, Texas, 33-year-old Marliese Munoz was declared brain dead after collapsing with a pulmonary embolism. The diagnosis was final and uncontested by the care team or her family. Both Mrs. Munoz and her husband were EMTs and had had many discussions about the treatment they would and would not want under different clinical circumstances. So, Mr. Munoz and his wife's parents were stunned to learn that John Peter Smith Hospital would not comply with their instructions or honor the late Mrs. Munoz's wishes to have ventilatory support removed. The hospital said that Texas law forbade removing life support from a pregnant patient and Mrs. Munoz was 14 weeks pregnant. The hospital's intention was to maintain her body on mechanical supports until 20 weeks of gestation and then deliver the baby. After that, Mrs. Munoz could be declared dead and removed from the machines supporting her organs.

Mr. Munoz sought judicial intervention and the court ruled that the law invoked by the hospital had been misread and misapplied in this case. The Texas Advance Directives Act (TADA), discussed below, restricts physicians' ability to terminate unwanted life support at the request of a terminally ill pregnant woman, her advance directive or her surrogate(s).* The court ruled that, because TADA was intended to be applied to living pregnant women and Mrs. Munoz had been declared dead, the law had no bearing on this case and that the hospital had to comply with Mr. Munoz's instructions. More than a month after she had collapsed, Mrs. Munoz and her undelivered fetus were cremated.

MEDICAL FUTILITY

In the case of *Betancourt v. Trinitas Regional Medical Center* (2010) (Lower Court Ruling: http://thaddeuspope.com/images/Betancourt_v_trinitas_3-4_2_.pdf; Appellate Court: http://caselaw.findlaw.com/nj-superior-court-appellate-division/1535060.html) (case dismissed as moot by the Appellate Court based on the death of the patient), the court considered "whether a hospital . . . can be compelled to provide inappropriate treatment . . . contrary to recommended standards of care." Ruben Betancourt, a 73-year-old man, was admitted to Trinitas Regional Medical Center in January 2008 for surgical removal of a malignant tumor from his thymus gland. The operation went as planned but, in the surgical ICU, the tube connecting him to the ventilator became dislodged, depriving him of oxygen for an undetermined period of time. As a result, he suffered anoxic encephalopathy, irreversible brain damage that left him unconscious and non-communicative, with no neurological function above the brainstem level. When his neurological condition remained unchanged, the consensus on the treating team was that

---

* At least 31 states have laws with similar restrictions on the rights of pregnant women to refuse unwanted treatment, and the Texas law is among the 12 most restrictive.

Mr. Betancourt was in a persistent vegetative state (PVS) from which he would not recover. His family disputed the diagnosis, however, claiming that he exhibited signs of responsiveness.

Following discharge, Mr. Betancourt received care in several New Jersey rehab facilities. He was readmitted to Trinitas in July 2008, with end-stage renal disease (ESRD), chronic obstructive pulmonary disease (COPD), hypertensive cardiovascular disease, and congestive heart failure (CHF). His life depended on ventilatory support, tube feedings, and dialysis. During the next six months, the patient's condition continued to deteriorate. In addition to his other co-morbidities, his skin was crumbling, he had osteomyelitis, and his inability to digest food prevented healing of his open wounds. In the words of one treating physician, he was "an elderly moribund patient who was actively and palpably dying" (*Amicus* brief, Trinitas, 2009).

The Trinitas medical staff agreed that continued treatment would be futile in reversing or improving the patient's condition and was merely prolonging his dying. The physicians counseled the family to forgo further life-sustaining measures, including dialysis to manage the ESRD, and consent to a do-not-resuscitate (DNR) order, which would preclude attempted cardiopulmonary resuscitation (CPR) if his heart stopped. When consensus with the family could not be reached, physicians discontinued dialysis and entered a DNR order in the medical record. The Betancourt family commenced legal action, requesting that Trinitas be ordered to resume treatment and that the patient's daughter be named as his guardian. The district court issued a temporary restraining order (TRO), requiring the hospital to resume dialysis and continue treatment during the trial.

The issues before the court, which reflect the ethical and legal dilemma whenever medical futility is considered, are captured in the following excerpts from the court's decision (*Betancourt* 2009):

> Plaintiff Betancourt: "whether a medical provider on its own initiative can terminate life support services for a patient";
> Defendant Trinitas: "whether a medical provider may be required to provide medical care to a patient where the treatment is futile, against the standard of care and inhumane."

The district court, however, chose to answer neither of these questions, confining itself to the narrow issue of patient self-determination and surrogate decision making. Thus, the question the court answered in the affirmative was whether a guardian should be appointed to articulate the patient's wishes and approved the patient's daughter to assume that role. The ruling was explained by asserting that Trinitas had asked the court to "take the role of surrogate decision maker . . . [by] determining the proper course of treatment for Mr. Betancourt, a task which . . . is outside the role of the court" (*Betancourt* 2009). The issue left unaddressed was not whether the court should be deciding the appropriate course of treatment, but whether the court would affirm the authority of *care professionals* to use their clinical judgment and determine the appropriate course of treatment for a patient.

Mr. Betancourt continued receiving treatment at Trinitas, where he died in May 2009. Despite his death, the case was accepted for appellate review because of the importance of the issues, their public policy implications, and the likelihood of their repetition in similar situations. The court of appeals took 26 pages to rule that it would not address the questions before it, reasoning that matters of medical treatment should not come before a court and that matters of health care provider authority should be addressed by the legislature (Superior Court of New Jersey 2010). Because the only substantive ruling in *Betancourt* is by a trial court, it has no precedential value in New Jersey or any other state. Nevertheless, for the very reasons the appellate court granted review, *Betancourt* has attracted considerable attention and will likely be referenced as long as the question of professional responsibility in cases of medical futility remains unresolved.

STATE ACTION TO PROVIDE GUIDANCE IN CASES OF MEDICAL FUTILITY

Among the most difficult cases are those, like *Betancourt*, in which terminally ill or dying patients or, more often, their surrogates, request the initiation or continuation of treatment considered by the medical team to be medically futile or harmful. In 1999, the Texas legislature undertook a response to this challenge by creating the Texas Advance Directives Act (TADA), also known as the Texas Futile Care Law, described as "a new law [that] appears to be the first in the nation to provide a legally sanctioned, extrajudicial, due process mechanism for resolving disagreements about end-of-life care between patients and providers" (Fine 2001, p. 26).

The law takes as its foundation the principle that health care professionals are under no obligation to offer or provide treatment that will not benefit and may harm the patient. Recognizing that concerns about legal liability and the lack of consensus on a definition of "medical futility" discouraged physicians from refusing requests for non-indicated treatment, the TADA drafters made its standards entirely procedural. The law sets out a series of steps intended to confirm the medical futility of the requested treatment; ensure review and concurrence by clinical leadership, the ethics committee, and legal counsel; and offer assistance in transferring the patient to another facility willing to provide the requested treatment.

Throughout the process, the patient continues to receive the disputed treatment, as well as medically indicated care and the team meets with the patient or surrogate at each step in an effort to achieve consensus on a resolution. After 10 days, if consensus with the family is not achieved and no other hospital willing to provide the disputed treatment is found, the hospital may unilaterally withdraw the disputed treatment. The patient or surrogate may seek judicial extension to find another provider. If no extension is sought or granted, the disputed treatment is withdrawn. TADA has provided a model for state statutes and institutional policies, an example of which can be found in chapter 17.

PHYSICIAN-ASSISTED DYING

Note that, while the *Cruzan* Court found that the Constitution protects an individual's liberty interest in refusing unwanted medical treatment, it did not find a constitutionally protected "right to die." In 1997, the U.S. Supreme Court ruled in two cases that sought to turn the right to refuse treatment into a right to assisted death. The plaintiffs in *Washington v. Glucksberg*, 521 U.S. 702 (1997), claimed that the Fourteenth Amendment due process clause could encompass a protected right to determine the time and manner of one's death and to obtain physician assistance in doing so. The plaintiffs in *Vacco v. Quill*, 521 U.S. 793 (1997) (www.law.cornell.edu /supct/html/95-1858.ZO.html) (holding that New York's prohibition on assisting suicide violates the equal protection clause of the Fourteenth Amendment), claimed that, under the Fourteenth Amendment equal protection clause, terminally ill patients not maintained on life support are treated unequally compared to terminally ill patients who *can discontinue* life support.

The Supreme Court rejected both arguments in two rulings that have more to do with palliative care than assisted dying. The Court held that, while there is no constitutionally protected right to assisted suicide, there is a protected interest in pain relief. The Court reaffirmed the doctrine of double effect, saying that it is both legally and ethically appropriate to give terminally ill patients as much medication as necessary to relieve pain, even if the unintended effect is to hasten death. The Court also strongly reaffirmed the distinction between forgoing life-sustaining treatment and assisted suicide. Finally, the decisions indicated that, if states did not statutorily make it easier and less threatening for physicians to provide adequate analgesia to patients who need it, the Court would not rule out the possibility of revisiting the issue of assisted dying in a future case. These rulings have far-reaching implications for palliation throughout the therapeutic continuum, especially at the end of life.

Robert Baxter, marine veteran, long-haul truck driver, and passionate outdoorsman, was dying from lymphocytic leukemia when he joined the advocacy group Compassion & Choices and four Montana physicians in a case claiming that Montana's constitutional guarantees of privacy, dignity, and equal protection encompass the right to choose and access assistance in dying. Mr. Baxter died on December 5, 2008, just hours after the district court agreed with his claim, ruling that "the Montana constitutional rights of individual privacy and human dignity, taken together, encompass the right of a competent terminally ill patient to die with dignity." The Montana attorney general appealed the ruling but, on December 31, 2009, the Montana Supreme Court, in *Baxter v. Montana*, upheld the lower court ruling, making Montana the third state to legalize assistance in dying and the first to do so under case rather than statutory law.

Medical Decision Making for Minors

In general, the legal trend has traditionally favored the decisions of parents or guardians concerning a child's welfare. One landmark case illustrating this deference was *Parham v. J.R.*, 442 U.S. 584 (1979) (http://scholar.google.com/scholar_case?case =15981297995569250470&q=Parham+v.+J.R&hl=en&as_sdt=6,33&as_vis=1) (holding that a state may permit parents to have their child institutionalized without a formal hearing). A borderline retarded child manifesting aggressive and antisocial behavior petitioned the court through an appointed guardian, requesting that he be moved from Georgia's Central State Hospital to a less harshly restricted environment that would meet his needs. The court denied J.R.'s petition, holding that a minor's substantial liberty interest in avoiding unnecessary confinement is outweighed by the superior decision-making capacity of his parents who are presumed to act in their child's best interests.

In contrast was *Custody of a Minor*, 379 N.E.2d 1053 (Mass. 1979) (www.court listener.com/mass/boY3/custody-of-a-minor/) (holding that, when even well-intentioned parental conduct threatens the welfare of a child, the interests of the child and the state may compel intervention). The case concerned 3-year-old Chad Green, a child suffering from acute lymphocytic leukemia. His parents believed that his best chance of cure lay in discontinuing standard chemotherapy and substituting metabolic therapy, including massive doses of vitamins and the drug laetrile. A lower court found that the child's condition required conventional therapy and warranted removing him from the legal custody of his parents. The appellate court affirmed, finding that, despite the traditional legal presumption that parents are the best judges of what is in their child's best interest, the compelling evidence here showed that Chad's well-being was seriously threatened by his parents' refusal to comply with medically proven therapy. The court held that the health and safety of a child must be the primary interest of the state, even when that interest overrides the authority of parents to care for their child.

The continuum of ethical decisions related to endangered or severely handicapped newborns is illustrated by two cases that captured national attention. At one end was the 1982 case of Baby Doe, who was born in Bloomington, Indiana, with tracheoesophageal fistula, a defect preventing the oral ingestion of food. While the condition is fatal, it is also easily remedied with surgery. However, the defect is more common in infants with Down syndrome, as was true in this instance. Although Down syndrome children run the gamut from profoundly retarded to educable and self-sufficient, the referring obstetrician testified that the infant would have a "minimally acceptable quality of life." The Indiana Supreme Court upheld the parents' refusal to permit surgical repair of the esophageal opening and the infant died. In this instance, the court did not elect to override parental decision even though the infant's life was at stake. Moreover, the only acknowledged reason for withholding treatment was the Down syndrome. The resulting public outcry was based at least partly on the perception that, by withholding life-sustaining treatment, the parents were meeting their own needs to be relieved of the burden of a handicapped child.

The resulting Baby Doe regulations, issued in 1984, were intended to prevent seriously ill infants from being deprived of necessary medical attention. Drawing on existing law that made it illegal for agencies receiving federal funds to discriminate on the basis of handicap, these rules required hospitals to post notices stating that "nourishment and medically beneficial treatment (as determined with respect to reasonable medical judgments) should not be withheld from handicapped infants solely on the basis of their present or anticipated mental or physical impairments" (Furrow et al. 1991, p. 1184). The notices included a toll-free hotline number to facilitate reporting violations of the regulations, which would trigger intervention by "Baby Doe squads" of physicians, attorneys, and administrators. After several court challenges, the Baby Doe regulations were struck down by the U.S. Supreme Court, which ruled that parents had the right to refuse treatment for their children, regardless of handicap. Revised and less stringent regulations appeared in 1987 as amendments to the Child Abuse Prevention and Treatment Act.

At the other end of the spectrum was *In re Baby K*, 16 F.3rd 590 (4th Cir. 1994) (http://law.justia.com/cases/federal/appellate-courts/F3/16/590/492033/) (holding that life-sustaining treatment is required in an emergency setting, even if the treatment is medically futile). Baby K was an infant born with anencephaly, a condition that left her with a functioning brainstem that kept her body alive, but no upper brain function that would enable her to develop awareness or cognitive ability. In the opinion of treating physicians, providing ventilatory assistance was inappropriate, given the infant's limited life expectancy and dismal quality of existence. Nevertheless, the court upheld the mother's wishes for the infant to receive breathing assistance in the emergency room whenever she experienced respiratory distress. The court's reasoning was that, under the Emergency Medical Treatment and Active Labor Act (EMTALA), the Rehabilitation Act of 1973, and the Americans with Disabilities Act (ADA) of 1990, life-sustaining treatment is required in an emergency setting, even if that treatment is deemed medically futile. In this case, Baby K's breathing difficulty qualified as an emergency medical condition, the diagnosis of which triggered the hospital's duty to provide the infant with stabilizing treatment or transfer her to another facility in accordance with the provisions of EMTALA.

Reproductive Rights

ABORTION

The case that legalized abortion in the United States was *Roe v. Wade*, 410 U.S.113 (1973) (www.law.cornell.edu/supremecourt/text/410/113) (holding that a state anti-abortion statute that prohibits abortion except to save the life of the mother, regardless of the stage of pregnancy or other factors, violates the due process clause of the Fourteenth Amendment and denies a woman's right to privacy). The case was heard by the U.S. Supreme Court as the review of a challenge to a Texas law banning all abortions except those necessary to save the life of the mother. The Court held that the right of privacy "founded in" the Fourteenth Amendment's protection of "personal liberty and restriction of state action" was broad enough to encompass a woman's right to terminate her pregnancy under conditions limited only by the state's interest in her welfare and in the life of the unborn after viability. Moreover, the Court held these rights to be "fundamental" and "implicit in the concept of ordered liberty."

Roe represented a watershed in American legal, medical, and ethical thinking, and has had consequences far beyond the abortion issue. Considered by many to be the Court's most controversial ruling, the case was perceived as both a landmark for women's rights and an excessive level of judicial activism. To read the text of the remarkable Supreme Court opinion and concurrences is to read an encapsulation of the divisiveness and soul searching that marked—and still marks—this emotional issue.

Ultimately, the Court chose not to address the difficult issue of when life begins and declined to find that a fetus is a "person" within the meaning of the Fourteenth Amendment. To do so would have accorded the fetus due process protections that would have effectively invalidated the right to abortion. Instead, the Court referred throughout the opinion to "potential life," consistent with the trimester framework using viability as its standard.

The Court based its reasoning on the right to privacy in personal decisions it found in the Fourteenth Amendment and cited the inherent medical factors. Thus, the *Roe* Court held that a statute criminalizing abortion except as a life-saving measure regardless of other considerations violates the due process clause of the Fourteenth Amendment. More specifically, the Court devised a regulatory scheme based on fetal development and viability, holding that during the first trimester, the decision to abort was within the zone of private decision making between the pregnant woman and her doctor; during the second trimester, the state may regulate abortion only to protect the health of the mother; and, during the third trimester, the state's interest in promoting life enables it to regulate and even prohibit abortion except to save the life of the mother. The policy was that the state's interest in promoting life and its associated right to intervene increases as the development and viability of the fetus advances.

The sweeping scope of *Roe* was modified in two subsequent Supreme Court decisions, although both reaffirmed a woman's right to an abortion. *Webster v. Reproductive Health Services*, 492 U.S. 490 (1989) (www.law.cornell.edu/supremecourt /text/492/490) (upholding a state's right not to fund abortion and to require viability testing), relaxed the rigid trimester framework, allowing states to focus on fetal viability in regulating abortion. The case was heard as a review of an order invalidating a Missouri state scheme to prohibit state-funded abortion. Finding that states were under no obligation to subsidize health care of any kind, the U.S. Supreme Court held that a state could refuse to fund any particular type of health care, such as abortion. The Court also did not find unconstitutional a state requirement that life can be protected after viability, the determination of which may be required as a condition of permitting an abortion. Accordingly, the ruling upheld the right of a state to withhold funding for abortion as it might for any other health care and to require viability testing prior to terminating any pregnancy of more than 20 weeks' duration.

The second case was *Planned Parenthood of Southeastern Pennsylvania v. Casey*, 505 U.S. 833 (1992) (www.law.cornell.edu/supct/html/020794.ZR.html) (striking down state law provisions that unduly burden a woman's right to an abortion, discarding the trimester scheme entirely, and substituting the undue burden test to regulate abortion). Responding to the challenge of a Pennsylvania statute, the U.S. Supreme Court held that (1) it was necessary to reaffirm the essential holding of *Roe v. Wade* recognizing the right of a woman to have an abortion prior to the point of fetal viability; (2) the rigid trimester scheme adopted in *Roe* to regulate abortion should be replaced by a test to determine whether the restrictions on abortion placed an "undue burden" on a woman; (3) the medical emergency definition and the requirements for informed consent, 24-hour waiting period, parental notification, and reporting and record keeping did not impose an undue burden, and were thus not invalid; and (4) the spousal notification provision did impose an undue burden and was, therefore, invalid.

The U.S. Supreme Court next addressed reproductive rights in 2007 in *Gonzales, Attorney General v. Carhart et al.* 550 U.S. 124 (2007) (www.supremecourt.gov /opinions/06pdf/05-380.pdf) (upholding the federal Partial-Birth Abortion Ban

Act of 2003, prohibiting intact dilation and extraction [IDX, D&X, or intact D&E], an abortion procedure typically, albeit rarely, performed in the mid- to late second trimester). *Casey* had reaffirmed the constitutional right of a woman to terminate a pregnancy before fetal viability and prohibited states from creating obstacles that place an "undue burden" on the exercise of that right. *Casey* also required states to have a health exception to the ban, permitting pregnancy termination after fetal viability when necessary to preserve a woman's life or health, an exception not included in the Partial-Birth Abortion Ban Act.

Following the *Casey* ruling, anti-abortion groups endeavored to increase support for abortion restrictions by expanding the scope of their argument. Rather than framing the matter as a conflict between women's rights of self-determination and states' interest in protecting human life, abortion was presented as a threat to both women and their potential offspring, justifying certain restrictions as necessary to protect women from harmful choices to terminate their pregnancies. One of the allegedly harmful options from which women were said to need protection was intact dilation and extraction, and the Partial-Birth Abortion Ban Act authorized the punishment of physicians who perform this procedure. The law had been declared unconstitutional in California, New York, and Nebraska district courts, and the Nebraska ruling had been affirmed by the U.S. Court of Appeals for the Eighth Circuit. In *Carhart*, the Supreme Court affirmed the constitutionality of the Partial-Birth Abortion Ban Act, including its lack of an exception to protect a woman's life or health, and further limited the availability of pregnancy termination.

STATE ACTION TO REDEFINE "PERSON"

Rather than confining their efforts to overturning *Roe v. Wade*, anti-abortion advocates have enlisted conservative state legislatures in drafting or revising laws that either constrain how women and their physicians make and implement reproductive decisions (see below), or redefining child abuse and neglect laws to include protection before birth.

As an example, in 2011, Mississippi voters were asked to consider a "personhood" amendment (*A Life Begins at the Moment of Fertilization Amendment, also known as Initiative 26*) to the state constitution, stating that life begins at conception and extending to embryos and fetuses the full independent and protectable rights of persons in the United States. Voters rejected the amendment because of its overly broad scope, which would ban not only all abortion without exception, but also threaten the legality of some forms of contraception, stem cell research, and in vitro fertilization. After the defeat, the advocacy group Personhood Mississippi headed up an effort to revive the amendment for the 2013 ballot, which voters also rejected.

The issue of abortion remains not only highly controversial, but central to much of the legal and political activity in this country. Opponents of abortion rights have as their stated goal the overturning of *Roe v. Wade* and, toward that end, they lobby for or against candidates for political and judicial positions. Seemingly unrelated matters, such as child health regulations, drug enforcement policies, stem cell research restrictions, and protections against domestic violence, are perceived by many as efforts to chip away at the right to abortion without actually overturning *Roe*. Indeed, where one stands on the issue of abortion has become a litmus test of where one's social and political sympathies lie.

The U.S. Supreme Court addressed the collision of reproductive and religious rights in *Secretary of Health and Human Services, et al. v. Hobby Lobby Stores, Inc* (decided June 30, 2014), www.supremecourt.gov/opinions/13pdf/13-354_olpl.pdf (holding that some corporations can claim a religious exemption from a legal requirement that companies with 50 or more employees offer a health insurance plan that covers contraception for female employees or pay a fine). The Court considered arguments regarding a conflict between women's reproductive rights (specifically, contraception coverage) and employers' rights to religious freedom. Hobby Lobby is an arts and crafts company with approximately 21,000 employees (Forbes), founded by the current CEO David Green (Mears 2014). Green and his family claim to have founded the company based on Christian beliefs that conflict with regulations promulgated by the Department of Health and Human Services (HHS) under the Patient Protection and Affordable Care Act (PPACA), which mandates coverage of contraception in the health plans offered by specified employers for female employees. Religious employers, such as houses of worship, and religious nonprofit organizations are exempt from this requirement.

In September of 2012, Hobby Lobby filed a lawsuit in the U.S. District Court of the Western District of Oklahoma, requesting religious exemption from the contraception coverage requirement by appealing to the First Amendment and the Religious Freedom Restoration Act (RFRA). The RFRA requires the government to use the "least burdensome" means to enforce law that interferes with religious convictions (Mears 2014). The case was appealed to the Supreme Court, which heard argument in October 2013 and issued a 5–4 ruling in favor of Hobby Lobby in June 2014 (www.hobbylobbycase.com/the-case/case-timeline/). The Court found that the contraception requirement in the PPACA was in violation of the RFRA because it was not the "least burdensome" means of enforcement. While the ruling has been welcomed in some quarters, it has also generated considerable concern regarding the potential for increasing claims to religious exemption from laws that apply to the general public, and decreasing access to certain forms of health care (specifically, contraception) for women.

SURROGATE PARENTING

The most famous surrogacy case, and one that embodies all the potential risks and heartaches, was *In re Baby M*, 537 A.2d 1227 (N.J. 1988) (http://biotech.law.lsu.edu/cases/cloning/baby_m.htm) (holding surrogate motherhood contracts void as against public policy because they extract payment of money for the termination of parental rights). Mr. and Mrs. Stern contracted with Mary Beth Whitehead, a married woman already a mother, to be impregnated by artificial donor insemination using Mr. Stern's sperm. After delivery, Ms. Whitehead reluctantly surrendered the baby, but then changed her mind, regaining the child and leaving the state. Although the trial court upheld the agreement, the appellate court found the contract void as a matter of public policy because it required payment of money for the termination of parental rights, and because it severed the relationship between a child and her natural parents, which is not in the best interests of the child. Ultimately, the court looked to the best interest of the child, as it would in any adoption, and awarded custody to the Sterns, with visitation rights to Ms. Whitehead.

MATERNAL-FETAL CONFLICT

On occasion, a pregnant woman's assertion of autonomy brings her right to refuse unwanted treatment into conflict with the state's interest in protecting the unborn. Courts have generally opted to save the fetus where possible, as illustrated by the case *In re A.C.*, 573 A.2d 1235 (D.C. 1990) (http://academic.udayton.edu/lawrenceulrich /inreac.htm) (holding that a terminally ill woman must undergo a caesarean section to save her fetus). Although A.C. had agreed to a section at 28 weeks' gestation, the court approved the hospital's petition for surgery at 26.5 weeks. The baby died three hours after birth. The decision was subsequently vacated when it was shown that neither A.C.'s rights nor her decisional competence had been correctly evaluated because she had been so heavily medicated. Rather than offering the patient's dubious "informed consent" to authorize surgery, the treatment decision should have been based on substituted judgment, drawing on what was known of her prior wishes when she had unquestioned capacity.

Maternal-fetal conflict is also reflected in attempts to prosecute pregnant women for behavior that puts the fetus at risk. Some cases have argued that child abuse and neglect statutes include "fetus" within the meaning of the term *child* for purposes of finding liability for failure to protect the health and safety of the unborn. For example, *Jefferson v. Griffin Spalding County Hospital Authority*, 274 S.E.2d 457 (1981) (www.leagle.com/decision/1981333247Ga86_1288.xml/JEFFERSON%20v.%20 GRIFFIN%20&c.%20HOSPITAL%20AUTH.) (holding that rejection of necessary medical care, including a caesarean section, rendered a fetus a neglected unborn child). Likewise, *Whitner v. State*, 492 S.E.2d 777 (S.C.1997) (http://caselaw.findlaw .com/sc-supreme-court/1238430.html) (holding that a viable fetus is a "person" according to the Children's Code and, therefore, could be a victim of child neglect) found that the South Carolina state abuse statute included fetuses within the meaning of the term *child*. Although the ruling was subsequently reversed, this case represented the first time that a state's highest court upheld a woman's conviction for criminal neglect of her unborn child because she used cocaine while pregnant.

In *Samantha Burton v. State of Florida* (District Court of Appeal 2010) (http:// opinions.1dca.org/written/opinions2010/08-12-2010/09-1958.pdf) (reversing lower court order and upholding right to refuse medical treatment when the state cannot show compelling state interest for overcoming this right), the question of whether the state may compel a pregnant woman to engage in or refrain from engaging in activities, depending on their effect on her fetus was broadened considerably. The circuit court had found that Samantha Burton had failed to follow her doctor's instructions, thereby placing her pregnancy at high risk and placing her fetus at substantial and unacceptably high risk of severe injury or death. Basing its ruling on an earlier Florida case holding that "as between parent and child, the ultimate welfare of the child is the controlling factor" (*MN v. Southern Baptist Hosp. of*

Florida, 648 So.2d 769 (Fla. 1st DCA 1994)), the circuit court compelled Samantha Burton to "submit to any medical treatment deemed necessary by the attending obstetrician, including detention in the hospital for enforcement of bed rest, administration of intra-venous medications, and anticipated surgical delivery of the fetus" (*Burton* 2010).

In reversing the lower court order, the district court of appeal painstakingly reviewed the fundamental constitutional right to refuse medical treatment and the well-settled rule that the state must show a compelling state interest sufficient to overcome this or any fundamental right. Here, the standard established in *Roe v. Wade* and all succeeding rulings related to reproductive rights is that the state's interest in the potentiality of life becomes compelling at the point of fetal viability, a determination not required in the state statute or established in Samantha Burton's pregnancy. The court found that the rule "the ultimate welfare of the child is the controlling factor" was misapplied because it derived from the case of an eight-month-old child rather than a fetus. Finally, the court invoked the basic principle that, even when a compelling state interest has been shown, the means to pursue that interest must be "narrowly tailored in the least intrusive manner possible to safeguard the rights of the individual," a requirement not met by the lower court ruling.

PRE- AND POSTNATAL DECISION MAKING

The search for common ground is especially difficult in the contentious and highly polarized area of reproductive rights, where people of intelligence and good will often passionately disagree. In 2008, however, pro-choice, pro-life, and disability advocates came together with liberal and conservative legislators to support the Prenatally and Postnatally Diagnosed Awareness Act: Public Law 110-374, 122 Stat. 4051 (www.gpo.gov/fdsys/pkg/PLAW-110publ374/html/PLAW-110publ374.htm), co-sponsored by Senator Edward Kennedy (D-MA) and Senator Sam Brownback (R-KA). This federal legislation aimed to "amend the Public Health Service Act to increase the provision of scientifically sound information and support services to patients receiving a positive test diagnosis for Down syndrome or other prenatally and postnatally diagnosed conditions" (Summary of Act). The unusual alliance supporting the measure and its successful passage and signing by President Barack Obama have been attributed to its focus on disclosure of balanced information that had scientific validity and would be useful to those endeavoring to become knowledgeable and make informed decisions about bearing and raising children afflicted with certain conditions.

STERILIZATION

Perhaps the most egregious misuse of state power in the name of public protection was *Buck v. Bell*, 274 U.S. 200 (1927) (http://caselaw.lp.findlaw.com/scripts/getcase.pl?navby=CASE&court=US&vol=274&page=20) (upholding the state's right to authorize forced sterilization of institutionalized persons afflicted with hereditary forms of mental retardation, provided that safeguards exist to prevent abuse). Carrie Buck, an 18-year-old involuntary inmate of a state mental institution, was the first person to be sterilized under the 1924 Virginia compulsory sterilization law. She was selected because of a perceived familial pattern of mental deficiency: she, her mother, and her daughter were all determined to be "feeble-minded." The U.S. Supreme Court upheld the state's involuntary sterilization of institutionalized mental defectives to prevent a future drain on society's resources. Justice Holmes's chilling assessment that "three generations of imbeciles are enough" is especially tragic in view of the later-suggested possibility that both Carrie Buck and her daughter were, in fact, mentally normal.

State Action to Protect Public Health

The authority of the state to safeguard the public health has traditionally been considered so vital that, in exchange for state protection, citizens have been required to relinquish specific individual liberties. For example, *Jacobson v. Massachusetts*, 197 U.S. 11 (1905) (https://supreme.justia.com/cases/federal/us/197/11/case.html) (holding that a statute mandating vaccination was justified even though it infringed on individual rights), established that, by its authority to safeguard public welfare, the state may use its police power to compel vaccination. In its ruling, the U.S. Supreme Court also emphasized the state's reciprocal obligation to use its power discriminately, targeting its regulations to achieve only the identified state goal without unnecessary abridgment of individual liberties.

The Medical Device Amendments (MDA) of 1976 created a system of federal oversight of medical devices that would preempt state oversight systems and provide clear and consistent standards. Under the MDA, federal oversight of medical devices operated on a sliding scale, varying according to the type of device being considered. The most rigorous scrutiny is applied to Class III devices subjected to Food and Drug Administration (FDA) premarket approval. These devices are permitted to enter the market only if FDA review of their design, labeling, and manufacturing specifications concludes that these particulars provide reasonable assurance of safety and effectiveness. No modifications to the devices are permitted without FDA permission.

In *Riegel v. Medtronic, Inc.* (2008) (www.law.cornell.edu/supct/html/06-179.ZS .html) (holding that the MDA's preemption clause barred the claims of strict liability, breach of implied warranty, and negligent design, testing, marketing, and manufacturing because they claimed violation of New York common law rather than federal law), Donna Riegel brought suit against Medtronic after its catheter, a Class III device that had received FDA premarket approval, ruptured in her husband's coronary artery during cardiac surgery. The district court held that the MDA's preemption clause barred the claims of strict liability, breach of implied warranty, and negligent design, testing, marketing, and manufacturing because they claimed violation of New York common law rather than federal law. The Second Circuit Court of Appeals affirmed the district court ruling, as did the U.S. Supreme Court. The case is noteworthy in the ongoing effort to delineate the proper protective role of government in a well-regulated society.

State Action to Control What Practitioners Must or Must Not Discuss with Their Patients

The efforts of groups or individuals with special interest, religious, or political agendas to influence public policy have increased significantly. An equally concerning trend is state legislation that controls the therapeutic interaction. These actions are distinguished from the well-settled responsibility of states to establish standards of public health and safety, professional societies to establish standards of competence, or voter consensus on desired social objectives. Not surprisingly, these initiatives relate to controversial matters on which there is little or no societal agreement.

MANDATED DIAGNOSTIC INTERVENTIONS AND DISCUSSIONS PRIOR TO PREGNANCY TERMINATIONS

A growing number of states have standardized protocols that are required whenever a patient requests information about or implementation of pregnancy termination, all intended to enhance women's understanding of the significant step they are about to take. For example, 22 states regulate the provision of ultrasound by abortion providers; 12 states require verbal counseling or written materials to include information on accessing ultrasound services; 9 states require that a woman be provided with the opportunity to view an ultrasound image if her provider performs the procedure as part of the preparation for abortion; 7 states require that an abortion provider perform an ultrasound on a woman seeking an abortion and require that the provider offer the woman the opportunity to view the image; 5 states require that a woman be provided the opportunity to view an ultrasound image; 3 states mandate that an abortion provider perform an ultrasound on each woman seeking an abortion and require the provider to show and describe the image. In addition to mandating the disclosure of often unwanted information or images, several states' procedures require waiting periods or additional travel that impose the undue burdens on access to abortion services that are prohibited under *Casey*.

For example, in 2005, South Dakota passed the Informed Consent for Abortion law, requiring that women requesting pregnancy termination be given a written statement saying that "the abortion will terminate the life of a whole, separate, unique, living human being with whom she has an existing relationship" (S.D. Codified Laws, § 34-23A-10.1 [2006]) (http://legis.sd.gov/Statutes/Codified_Laws/Display Statute.aspx?Type=Statute&Statute=34-23A-10.1). The statement must also include a description of the "statistically significant risk factors to which the pregnant woman [who chooses abortion] would be subjected," including depression, psychological distress, and a heightened risk of "suicide ideation and suicide" (South Dakota Codified Laws secs. 34-23A1). Women were required to sign each page of the statement to verify their understanding of its contents and physicians were required to confirm their patients' understanding.

The constitutionality of the statute was challenged in Planned Parenthood Minnesota, North Dakota, South Dakota v. Mike Rounds, 375 F. Supp. 2d 881 (D.S.D.

2005) (http://media.ca8.uscourts.gov/opndir/11/09/093231P.pdf) (upholding the lower court's decision to allow the South Dakota law to take effect), with the assertion that the law required physicians to provide information that far exceeded the "truthful and nonmisleading information" permitted under *Casey*. Moreover, because the law did not provide for physicians to disagree with or depart from the required statements, it mandated "unconstitutional compelled speech, rather than reasonable regulations of the medical profession." The Eighth Circuit Court of Appeals affirmed the lower court decision, noting that the law mandated women to read and sign the state's moral and philosophical position rather than unbiased, evidence-based information that would assist independent, informed decision making.

West Virginia is one of several states requiring a vaginal ultrasound for women requesting pregnancy termination, even for women who have been raped. Similarly, Texas requires that a woman seeking an abortion undergo a sonogram at least 24 hours before the procedure and that the physician who will be performing the abortion display the sonogram image and make the fetal heartbeat audible.

GAG LAWS PREVENTING DISCUSSION OF HEALTH-RELATED MATTERS

In response to a Florida mother who claimed that her Second Amendment rights were violated when, during a routine examination, a physician asked her child about guns in the home, the Privacy of Firearms Owners Act (CS/CS/155) was signed into law on June 2, 2011. Under the law, "inquiries regarding firearm ownership or possession should not be made by licensed health care practitioners or health care facilities"; the law made it illegal for a physician to ask about or discuss with patients gun ownership, storage, or safe use unless there were concerns about the safety of the patient or others. Violation would incur disciplinary action, including suspension or revocation of license or a fine of up to $10,000.

Shortly after passage, several medical groups sought to overturn the law and, in *Dr. Bernard Wollschlaeger, et al. v. Governor, State of Florida* (http://op.bna.com/hl .nsf/id/mapi-92vmu9/$File/woll%20state's%20brief.pdf) (holding that the law prohibiting practitioners from asking patients if they own guns or have guns in their home should be barred as it is not supported by government interest and that the case is a First rather than Second Amendment issue), the U.S. Southern District Court of Florida ruled the law unconstitutional because it burdened physicians' First Amendment rights by censoring their speech. In July 2012, the ruling was appealed to the 11th Circuit U.S. Court of Appeals and, on November 5, 2012, the appellate court affirmed the lower court's finding that the statute burdens physicians' speech for reasons unrelated to health care, thereby interfering with patients' ability to freely discuss health matters with their providers and access to the full range of their doctors' clinical judgment and guidance. Five other states—Alabama, Minnesota, North Carolina, Oklahoma, and West Virginia—subsequently passed similar legislation, which died when their respective state legislative sessions ended. Like the Florida law, they were heavily promoted by the National Rifle Association (NRA).

Health Care Reimbursement

The shifting of responsibility for treatment decisions was the focus in the first cost containment-related malpractice ruling in *Wickline v. State of California*, 228 Cal. Rptr. 661 (Cal.App. 1986) (www.law.uh.edu/faculty/jmantel/health-law/Wicklinev State239CalRptr810.pdf) (holding that discharge decisions are the responsibility of the physician rather than the insurer). A patient sued the California state Medicaid program for injuries allegedly resulting from a premature hospital discharge following the program's refusal to authorize additional hospital days. The court held against the treating doctor for not challenging Medicaid's refusal to fund the necessary further hospitalization. Because the court did not specifically address the issue of how cost containment does or should affect medical judgment, this decision presented little guidance for physicians struggling with the balance of patient care and economics.

In the early years of the HIV/AIDS epidemic, when no effective therapy was available, the arguments against mandatory universal testing focused on the potential burdens of confidentiality breaches, stigmatization, and discrimination, which were considered to significantly outweigh the limited potential benefits of identifying persons who were HIV-positive. An approach, known as "HIV exceptionalism" (Bayer 1991) addressed these conditions differently in the interests of patient confidentiality and privacy. By the early twenty-first century, however, effective therapeutic and prophylactic interventions were available, reversing the benefit-burden-risk calculus.

In 2006, the Centers for Disease Control (CDC) revised its HIV testing guidelines and recommended testing as part of routine health care for everyone ages 13 to 64. New York City responded with Health Code sect.13.04, which proposed simplified and streamlined testing procedures, including oral rather than written consent, and abbreviated pretest discussion about risks of discrimination and the need for safer behavior; and authorizing the state health care officials to communicate positive test results to health care providers to link patients to care. The city was forced to omit a provision that would have identified patients who had stopped taking their HIV meds or were not responding to treatment and shared this information with the patients and health care practitioners. In response to the diabetes epidemic, the New York City Board of Health (NYCBOH) did require mandatory reporting of test results and other information about diabetes that would only be disclosed to the tested individual and her health care provider.

SUPREME COURT RULING ON PATIENT PROTECTION AND THE AFFORDABLE CARE ACT

Before the ink had dried on President Obama's signature on the Patient Protection and Affordable Care Act (PPACA) (http://housedocs.house.gov/energycommerce /ppacacon.pdf) in 2010, opponents were vowing to repeal the legislation, beginning with a challenge to the constitutionality of its key provisions, the individual mandate and the Medicaid expansion. As discussed in chapter 11, the individual mandate requires most Americans to have "minimum essential" health insurance coverage, obtained through an employer or government program, or purchased through a private company. After a specified date, those who have not complied with the mandate will be required to make a "shared responsibility payment" to the federal government. This penalty is to be paid with an individual's taxes to the Internal Revenue Service, just as tax penalties are paid. The other key provision expands scope of the Medicaid program, which is run jointly by the federal and state governments, and increases the number of persons that states must cover.

In 2011, *National Federation of Independent Business et al. v. Sebelius, Secretary of Health and Human Services, et al.*, 567 U.S. (2012) (www.supremecourt.gov /opinions/11pdf/11-393c3a2.pdf) (upholding individual mandate to buy health insurance because it accords with Congress's taxing power) was argued before the U.S. Supreme Court. The ruling was eagerly anticipated by supporters and opponents of the PPACA as a bellwether indicator of the law's future. A 5-4 majority, surprising because it included Chief Justice John Roberts, upheld the constitutionality of the individual mandate as a tax penalty rather than the violation of interstate commerce law envisioned in legislative intent. A larger 7-2 majority rejected the Medicaid expansion provision as a federal intrusion into the sovereign power of states.

Gene Patenting

In May 2009, the American Civil Liberties Union (ACLU) and the Public Patent Foundation (PUBPAT) filed a lawsuit against Myriad Genetics, the U.S. Patent and Trademark Office (USPTO), and other defendants. The lawsuit claimed that that the patents held by Myriad Genetics on two human genes (BRCA1 and BRCA2) were invalid and unconstitutional.

The Southern District Court of New York broke Myriad's patent claims into (1) composition of matter claims related to isolated DNA sequences and (2) process claims related to methods of gene sequence analysis or comparison to identify mutations that correspond to a predisposition to breast or ovarian cancer (SDNY, p. 2). The court rejected both sets of patents as not meeting the criteria for patentable subject matter. The federal circuit appeals court subsequently overturned the lower court decision and the plaintiffs appealed to the U.S. Supreme Court, which agreed in November 2012 to review the case.

In June 2013, the Supreme Court ruled unanimously in *Association for Molecular Pathology, et al. v. U. S. Patent and Trademark Office, et al.* that (1) isolated genomic DNA (gDNA) is not eligible for patent status because it is simply separated from its natural environment and not distinguishable from DNA found in the human body; but (2) synthetic DNA (cDNA) is patent eligible because the process of omitting portions of the DNA renders it significantly different from naturally occurring DNA. Given its implications for gene-based medical therapies, as well as the overall biotechnology industry, this decision is attracting close scrutiny by ethicists, geneticists, researchers, clinicians, and legal scholars.

REFERENCES

Annas GJ, Law SA, Rosenblatt RE, Wing KR. 1990. *American Health Law*. Boston: Little, Brown and Company.

Bayer R. 1991. Public health policy and the AIDS epidemic: An end to HIV exceptionalism? *New England Journal of Medicine* 324(21):1500–1504.

Becker S. 2004. *Health Care Law: A Practical Guide*. 2nd ed. Chicago: LexisNexis.

Burnwell Secretary of Health and Human Services, et al. v. Hobby Lobby Stores. 2014. www .supremecourt.gov/opinions/13pdf/13-354_olp1.pdf (accessed August 30, 2014).

Burnwell v. Hobby Lobby case timeline, www.hobbylobbycase.com/the-case/case-timeline/ (accessed August 30, 2014).

Curfman GD, Morrissey SM, Greene MF, Drazen JM. 2008. Physicians and the First Amendment. *New England Journal of Medicine* 359(23):2484–85.

Dresser R. 2007. Protecting women from their abortion choices. *Hastings Center Report* 37(6):13–14.

Fine RL. 2001. The Texas Advance Directives Act of 1999: Politics and reality. *H.E.C. Forum* 13(1):59–81.

Fleegler E.W, Monuteaux MC, Bauer SR, Lee LK. 2012. Attempts to silence firearm injury prevention. *American Journal of Preventive Medicine* 42(1):99–102.

Furrow BR, Greaney TL, Johnson SH, Jost TS, Schwartz RL. 2001. *Bioethics: Health Care Law and Ethics*. 4th ed. St. Paul, MN: West Group.

Furrow BR, Johnson SH, Jost TS, Schwartz RL. 1991. *Health Care Law: Cases, Materials and Problems*. 2nd ed. St. Paul, MN: West Publishing Co.

Gostin LO. 2014. Legal and ethical responsibilities following brain death: The McMath and Munoz cases. *Journal of the American Medical Association* 311(9):903–4.

Guttmacher Institute. Requirements for ultrasound. State Policies in Brief, October 1, 2014. New York, NY. www.guttmacher.org/statecenter/spibs/spib_RFU.pdf.

Hobby Lobby. Forbes.com. www.forbes.com/lists/2011/21/private-companies-11_Hobby -Lobby-Stores_ZGO2.html (accessed August 30, 2014).

Kim HC. 2010. Physicians and the First Amendment: The right not to speak. *Journal of Legal Medicine* 31:423–32.

Lazzarini Z. 2008. South Dakota's abortion script—threatening the physician-patient relationship. *New England Journal of Medicine* 359(21):2189–91.

Mears B. 2014. Justices to hear "Hobby Lobby" case on Obamacare birth control rule, www.cnn.com/2014/03/21/politics/scotus-obamacare-contraception-mandate/ (accessed August 30, 2014).

Menikoff J. 2001. *Law and Bioethics: An Introduction*. Washington, DC: Georgetown University Press.

Morse R. 2003. *Grimes v. Kennedy Krieger Institute*—nontherapeutic research with children. *Virtual Mentor* 5(11). http://virtualmentor.ama-assn.org/2003/11/hlaw1-0311.html (accessed August 29, 2014). Morse quotes a study jointly funded by the Environmental Protection Agency and Maryland Department of Housing and Community Development: "Evaluation of Efficacy of Residential Lead Based Paint Repair and Maintenance Interventions," www2.epa.gov/sites/production/files/documents/r95-012.pdf.

Murtagh L, Miller M. 2011. Censorship of the patient-physician relationship: A new Florida law. *Journal of the American Medical Association* 306(10):1131–32.

Pence GE. 2004. *Classic Cases in Medical Ethics: Accounts of Cases That Have Shaped Medical Ethics with Philosophical, Legal and Historical Backgrounds*. 4th ed. Boston: McGraw-Hill.

Quill TE. 2005. Terri Schiavo—a tragedy compounded. *New England Journal of Medicine* 352:1630–33. www.nejm.org/doi/full/10.1056/NEJMp058062 (accessed August 29, 2014).

Superior Court of New Jersey, Appellate Division. Jacqueline BETANCOURT, Plaintiff-Respondent, v. TRINITAS HOSPITAL, Defendant-Appellant. 2010. http://caselaw.findlaw.com/nj-superior-court-appellate-division/1535060.html (accessed August 29, 2014).

Tracy EE. 2011. Three is a crowd: The new doctor-patient-policymaker relationship. *American College of Obstetricians and Gynecologists* 118(5):1164–68.

PART V

AN ETHICS COMMITTEE MEETING

The ethical principles, concepts, and strategies discussed in the preceding sections of this handbook can be seen in action during meetings of institutional ethics committees. Whatever the size and sophistication of your committee's membership, the frequency of its meetings, the scope of its responsibilities, and the complexity of the issues on its agenda, the utility of its work depends on the quality of committee deliberation. The effectiveness with which clinical and organizational matters are addressed is determined by the content and process of the committee meeting, including the engagement of its members and the expertise of its leadership.

This final section of the book illustrates how a committee might apply ethical theory and skills, awareness of organizational and legal imperatives, and sensitivity to group dynamics. What follows is an account of what a committee might sound like as it reviews a hypothetical clinical case and an institutional policy. As you listen in on this meeting, pay particular attention to the following:

- how the issues are introduced and given context
- how the members are provided with information and encouraged to consider different perspectives
- how the group interacts
- how the committee chair and vice chair clarify and reframe the issues, refocus the discussion, summarize the key points, and identify how the deliberations will inform future committee work

LEVIN: Because we have some guests at today's meeting, let's go around quickly and introduce ourselves. I'm Josh Levin, bioethicist in the Division of Bioethics.

KELLER: Dr. Sam Keller, physician liaison for medical center management. We're putting together a new initiative on end-of-life care for hospitalized patients, and we're looking at some of the ethical issues.

NORMAN: Dr. Peggy Norman, medical director of the Home Health Agency.

ROWAN: Gail Rowan, attorney.

SILVER: Ellen Silver, director of education.

POWELL: Dr. Eric Powell, Pediatrics.

MARTINEZ: Reva Martinez, social worker in Palliative Care.

CARRELTON: Rev. Ben Carrelton, chaplain.

BARNETT: Dr. Greg Barnett, Nuclear Medicine.

DOYLE: Barbara Doyle, nurse manager, Oncology.

RICE: Dr. Harriet Rice, Medicine and Hematology.

PRINCE: Abby Prince, community member.

WALTERS: Carol Walters, director, Division of Bioethics.

SEEGER: Dr. Michael Seeger, Cardiology.

LEVIN: Okay, I thought we would start with a case that Jill Carver called to discuss with me a couple of weeks ago. She is clinical director of nursing for Oncology and I hope she will join us during the meeting.

Jill called about a patient and a clinical situation that I thought raised some interesting ethical questions. Even though I understand that the problems have been resolved, it would be useful to think through some of the ethical issues and some of their implications.

Let me ask Barbara Doyle to present the case. And Dr. Barnett, maybe you could add anything you feel is pertinent, and then we could open it up for discussion.

DOYLE: We called Bioethics because we had a 68-year-old patient with metastatic thyroid cancer who was receiving radioactive therapy. He had undergone spinal fusion and radiation, and then presented with spinal cord compression and paraplegia. The only treatment Endocrinology felt would have any impact on his disease was radioactive iodine.

Prior to the patient's admission to our unit, we had a meeting with the head of nuclear medicine, Dr. Sandler, Dr. Rogers from Endocrinology, the nurse manager, the nurse taking care of the patient, Jill, and myself.

We met for one reason. We were concerned about giving radioactive iodine to a patient who wasn't able to take care of himself. He was dependent for all ADLs [activities of daily living]. Because of his disease, he was on a bowel regimen, had a Foley [catheter to collect urine], was immobile, and had a stage II pressure ulcer. In short, he needed full care for all his medical and personal needs. We were going to give him radioactive iodine and this would expose nursing staff to radioactive material in the course of their caring for the patient. We were concerned about the safety of the staff because there is an exposure limit, which, at that time was between 6 and 10 minutes per person per shift.

WALTERS: Could you say more about why you were concerned?

DOYLE: Because spending any amount of time with a patient who has ingested radioactive iodine exposes you to the radioactive material.

LEVIN: Tell us a little bit more about the nature of the risk.

DOYLE: Our concern was about both the risk to staff and the possible effect on patient care. Jill called the bioethics committee because we thought, if staff are worried enough about the risk that they refuse to take care of the patient, then what happens? We weren't at that point yet, but we had to think ahead about possible problems.

LEVIN: This is how I saw the issue: the right of staff to decline to participate in the care of a patient out of concern for their own well-being or threats to their own health, when declining could jeopardize the patient's care. So there were two parts to the issue—the rights of staff and the well-being of the patient—that could be in conflict.

CARRELTON: Can I ask why he needed the treatment? Was it so that he wouldn't be paralyzed anymore?

DOYLE: No. His paralysis could not be changed. He will remain paralyzed.

NORMAN: So it wasn't curative?

DOYLE: It wasn't curative, but palliative, intended to slow down the progression of the disease. That was the only reason that he was getting the therapy.

LEVIN: In what way was it palliative?

DOYLE: Because the growth of the tumor eventually could lead to his death. So by slowing it down—this man wanted to live.

LEVIN: That's not really palliative, but aimed at arresting or slowing the disease. Palliative treatment is focused on managing pain and other symptoms, even while the disease progresses, which is very different.

BARNETT: We did refer to palliation, but probably incorrectly. We really questioned the efficacy of this plan. We gave him one of the highest doses we've ever given. We questioned whether what we were doing would really help him. But it was the only option left to him and he knew it. This is what he and his doctors wanted to do. This was his one shot. We knew we would not repeat it, and we wanted to make it count, so we gave the highest dose we felt we could give.

SEEGER: These are technical issues. We accept risk as caregivers in many different ways, some of which are better defined than others. There is a risk of blood contamination in any patient who has a transmissible disease in the blood. There is a risk of aerosol transmission from respiration. Even if you have gowns and masks, errors occur. People get stabbed with their own needles in the cath [cardiac catheterization] lab.

[TECHNICAL QUESTIONS ABOUT RADIATION DOSAGES]

BARNETT: First, Dr. Seeger, you're educated in dealing with radiation in the cath lab, so you're taking an educated risk. Your physicians and nurses are as well. The nurses on the medicine floors who don't deal with this every day are at an in-between level. They're knowledgeable, but they certainly don't have the risk-benefit understanding of radiation that you all have. That's why we spent time talking with them.

[TECHNICAL ANSWERS ABOUT RADIATION DOSAGES AND PROTECTIONS]

SILVER: Are we asking our nursing staff to expose themselves beyond the 10-minute recommendation?

DOYLE: We actually set the limit at six minutes. I got authorization to hire additional staff because of our concern that the patient is bed-bound and not able to do anything for himself. So we hired additional aides, who knew what was going on, to be on every shift and we clocked everyone to be sure no one exceeded six minutes.

[TECHNICAL DISCUSSION ABOUT THE RATE AT WHICH RADIOACTIVE MATERIAL IS ELIMINATED FROM THE BODY]

LEVIN: Barbara, let me say two things just to clarify the issue that was presented to me. First, if the patient were not turned and given other routine care by the nurses, his care would be compromised. I was told that a number of the nurses were very uneasy about doing this. The second point is that giving the radiation in the first place was something that was thought to have some benefit for the patient. I don't think we've yet clarified what that benefit was expected to be. Then we can look at the benefit-risk analysis.

DOYLE: We had one nurse who was breast feeding. A lot of nurses on my staff are in childbearing years, one who is actively seeking to get pregnant. I told them all that I didn't want them on that side of the hall. Anybody else who felt uncomfortable, I gave the option of not being assigned to care for the patient.

POWELL: Was there actually a risk to someone who is breast feeding or potentially pregnant? Is that risk real?

DOYLE: I wasn't willing to take it. One woman has been trying to get pregnant for a couple of years. I didn't want to put her in that position.

POWELL: But if you're telling them not to go to one side of the hall, what about all the other patients on that side of the hall? You're setting up parameters that may disadvantage other patients whose care may suffer if there is not enough staff.

DOYLE: I don't disagree with you.

[TECHNICAL DISCUSSION COMPARING RISKS AND PROTECTIONS WHEN PATIENTS RECEIVE OUTPATIENT TREATMENT FOR HYPERTHYROIDISM]

MARTINEZ: What about breast feeding?

[TECHNICAL DISCUSSION ABOUT RADIATION EXPOSURE AND THE LACK OF RISK TO BREAST-FEEDING WOMEN]

BARNETT: A breast-feeding nurse takes out a Foley bag full of urine with the hottest iodine there is, she's going to lactate pure breast milk. Being around the patient is not going to put radiation into her milk.

POWELL: So telling someone not to be in the room if she's lactating is more a comfort matter. It's not based on scientific evidence.

BARNETT: No, that's something that I didn't say.

KELLER: Just one more question. What's the medical evidence that this treatment was appropriate?

[TECHNICAL DISCUSSION OF THE MEDICAL JUSTIFICATION FOR THE TREATMENT, INCLUDING EVIDENCE THAT IT IS EFFECTIVE IN SLOWING THE DISEASE]

LEVIN: Was this symptom control? Was the patient in pain?

DOYLE: He was not in pain.

WALTERS: How old is this patient?

BARNETT: Sixty-eight.

WALTERS: Did he make the decision to have this treatment?

DOYLE: He did. He wanted the treatment.

WALTERS: You mean as debilitated as he was, he was still capable of making this choice?

DOYLE: Absolutely.

WALTERS: You've just defused all the arguments I was going to make. That's really interesting. What did the patient expect to get from this treatment?

DOYLE: He wanted to live and he thought this would enable him to live longer. He understood very clearly that he would remain paraplegic and that the treatment might have no effect on his cancer, but he wanted to take the chance. For that reason alone, I believe my staff was so supportive of the treatment.

KELLER: And you're saying that this kind of dose does prolong survival in studies.

BARNETT: Yes. But I don't know yet its effectiveness in this particular patient.

PRINCE: But for his stage of disease it was an appropriate option for him to consider and choose?

MARTINEZ: Perhaps the only option.

BARNETT: I think it *was* his only option.

POWELL: So it would possibly affect survival, but not quality of life. He's going to remain bed-bound, paralyzed, all those things.

DOYLE: Yes.

POWELL: Who determines the quality of the benefit and whether it justifies the risk? Is that what we're asking?

SEEGER: What I was going to raise was his capacity to participate in a decision about a Hail Mary therapy, a treatment of last resort. We take risks at our end, for example, radiation exposure in the cath lab, knowing that there is a concrete benefit for our patients.

SILVER: Sometimes. Sometimes we discover later that there might not be a benefit.

SEEGER: But we don't know that initially. We operate on our best information at the time. We're educated, but so is the staff. What often determines the difference is that some people are willing to take that risk. That's why they're in the cath lab and not up on the floors. I think what counts ethically about their participation is their perspective and their values as to the risk they take and why they choose to take it when they're in this profession.

LEVIN: Could you say more?

SEEGER: Because radiation injury or damage is a cumulative insult over a lifetime depending on tissue and type of radiation, any exposure is an increase in risk.

Now if it's a particularly small risk, then some staff are able to say, "That is a risk I'm willing to take for the concrete benefit of this patient." But I view the professional integrity and commitment of the caregiver as highly as I do the autonomy of the patient. I think we have to value the professional's commitment to a specific situation when it is outside normal practice, which, by all standards, this is.

WALTERS: I want to pick up on what Michael just said. I have argued that caregivers don't have autonomy, they have standards of professional conduct. Within those standards, they may disagree with or opt out of something. I would suggest that within professionalism there isn't a total lack of self-interest. But the professional cannot have the same degree of self-interest as the patient with full autonomy to consent or refuse or act in ways that are appropriate for him or her. I don't think professionals have that unlimited option to put their interests first because their professional obligations may conflict with what they personally would choose.

LEVIN: But you can make the point another way. If a patient is given a high dose of radioactive iodine and then has a cardiac arrest, that patient is going to be resuscitated. That's the training that nuclear medicine people and EMS and ER staff and other caregivers get. They are still required to take care of patients regardless of the risk. If that's what you're saying, then I understand.

WALTERS: I agree and I wondered if this therapy was so out of the line of general practice that it was exempt from caregiver obligations.

LEVIN: I think the question of whether, given this patient's particular medical condition, this was an appropriate treatment is a medical question. But the ethical question concerns the risk to the health professionals taking care of him. We might frame the question in terms of a benefit-risk analysis. Now, we usually talk about benefit, burden, and risk in terms of what the *patient* will experience.

Here, we are asking whether the treatment is one whose benefit to the patient is sufficient to justify the risk it poses to the *professionals*.

I know a number of the nurses had questions and misgivings about the plan and were reluctant to participate in this patient's care. We should be clear, however, that these concerns were prospective. Despite their reluctance, none of the nurses actually refused and the patient's care was not compromised.

PRINCE: Outside the medical context, individuals are free to say, "No, I'm not going to endanger my health or safety by doing things that might harm me." But as a health professional, that right seems limited by obligations. One of the things that occurred to me in this case is what if most of the nurses had refused? What if they said, "Even though it's only a six-minute exposure, we're not going to do it"? What would you do then?

WALTERS: I'm just wondering if there are some other cases in the history of health care that are useful analogies. I'm thinking of two. For principled reasons, a nurse refuses to be involved in abortion cases.

ROWAN: Conscience clause cases.

WALTERS: Yes. And in the early 1980s, some health care providers didn't want to take care of AIDS patients because of what we didn't know about the disease and the risks. Is it useful to look back historically and find analogies?

KELLER: Actually, TB is a better example.

POWELL: SARS.

CARRELTON: Leprosy—the nuns used to put themselves at risk to care for people with leprosy.

MARTINEZ: Six or seven years ago, we had a family with two kids who had malaria. It was during the Ebola scare. There were some decisions made in our ER as far as who did and did not go to the floor because the care of patients in the ER would be compromised if the kids would have been quarantined there. So this isn't that far away.

PRINCE: Yes, and I would even expand the analogy to different professions, as Michael suggested. People who work with asbestos or wash those windows on the outside of skyscrapers are taking those risks, knowing that they come with the job they signed up for.

KELLER: The argument, I guess, is there are some people who said, "Yes, I want to be a nurse, but I didn't sign up for this one."

LEVIN: I'm not sure where this discussion is going. Perhaps someone can refocus us.

SILVER: Let me try. I think it's critical to educate the people involved in patient care about just what risks they face. I find that when nurses or doctors are exposed and they feel that people are giving them facts, they make informed decisions and they're more apt to cooperate. And when they feel they're not getting enough information and the issues are not being dealt with, then they feel that people are holding out on them and that's when rumors start and bad decisions are made.

LEVIN: For me, the central question here is, "What are the limits of professional obligation to take care of patients in light of what is thought to be risk to self?" Now this is a question we've visited before. It's not new, although it presents a bit differently here.

This was not actual caregiver refusal to give care. It wasn't based on religious values or ethics. It was reluctance based on concern about threat to self that seems, under the circumstances, to have been unfounded. I mean, there was no real threat to self, right? I guess that's a question, not a statement.

WALTERS: Can I just summarize? I think Josh clearly framed the issue. We've had certain analogous situations. Caregivers who have principled, philosophical, and religious objections to abortion do not participate in that procedure. When we started to withdraw and withhold life-sustaining treatment more than 30 years ago, people who had principled objections did not participate.

This case falls into a different category where the refusal or reluctance has to do with protecting one's health and safety rather than protecting one's values and principles. Here, there is an analogy to the AIDS epidemic, when we were very clear that the obligation was to care for patients and that the answer to caregiver risk was universal precautions, not opting out. It's worth noting that, as Reva pointed out, this is not confined to the past. When SARS patients in Toronto were intubated, 100% of the staff who were in the room during intubation got SARS. *100%*. We're going to face these situations and these issues in the future. We thought that this case presented an interesting variation on a familiar issue: the limits of professional choice in the face of risk and professional obligations.

LEVIN: So, Dr. Barnett, could you clarify whether there really was a risk to the nurses under these circumstances?

[TECHNICAL DISCUSSION EXPLAINING THAT STAFF HAD BEEN EXPOSED TO A VERY LOW LEVEL OF RADIATION]

[TECHNICAL DISCUSSION ABOUT HOW LEVELS OF EXPOSURE WERE MONITORED]

LEVIN: This is Jill Carver. Jill, I'm glad you're here. In light of the fact that the nurses were ultimately found not to have been at significant risk, do you feel that their reluctance to participate was reasonable?

CARVER: We had quite a few meetings with the nurses. Our approach was to give them all the information we had. If somebody was uncomfortable with the care plan, we had no problem saying, "We'll make sure you don't take care of the patient." Essentially, we asked for volunteers.

Many of the senior nurses were quite funny. They said, "Well, my ovaries don't work anymore anyway, so it's not a problem." We had staff on the floor volunteer to work overtime and then we got approval to hire extra staff.

PRINCE: What if your extra staff was not available?

DOYLE: They were available because we had them booked in advance. My fear was that everybody's six minutes would be up and there would be nobody to care for the patient.

WALTERS: Let me see if I can reframe the ethical question. First of all, I think you guys did a terrific job in taking a difficult circumstance and planning so that patient care would not be compromised.

But now I want to look at this in terms of bioterrorism, which we haven't talked about much in this committee but which is one of the big ethical debates. It seems inevitable that we will face a bioterror attack or an epidemic of avian flu. So, going forward, there are going to be situations in which staff will be asked to do things that may make them uncomfortable. It seems to me that this example of one patient in a difficult circumstance that was handled sensitively and effectively may not be a very good precedent for the uncertain times ahead.

POWELL: It sounds like the people part was handled beautifully. But if you're analyzing it in terms of a major disaster, I have questions about the decisions.

WALTERS: Because of their implications for other similar and not-so-similar circumstances?

POWELL: Yes. For example, in a mass attack, we would not have the luxury of planning ahead, asking for volunteers, or letting people who were uncomfortable opt out.

KELLER: Exactly. The concern with biochemical and nuclear terrorism is that it won't be one person coming into the hospital for elective treatment. The problem will be the masses of injured people who will need immediate and unanticipated attention. So it's easy to see how we'd deplete our staff very quickly, especially if they're only allowed 10 minutes in a protective suit where the temperature gets up over 120 degrees. That type of training in those mock disasters is really very important.

WALTERS: I think that questioning the obligations of health care professionals to deal with very difficult circumstances that require personal sacrifice is high up on the list of things we need to do. I think we have to do this because hospitals will be the first responders.

KELLER: Just one last point about this case. Wouldn't it be useful to share this information with Janet Mandel in Occupational Health so that, if this ever comes up again in a similar or even different way, they don't have to rewrite the whole chapter? They'll already know.

WALTERS: That's a terrific suggestion.

KELLER: Janet probably wouldn't know more than you guys know about this, but at least she and her staff should learn from the body of information that you've developed.

WALTERS: This has been a very useful discussion. Thank you. I think the structural note that Sam just brought in of always involving Dr. Mandel in decisions about staff is an excellent one.

LEVIN: Let me bridge now to Sophia Lawrence, office of the medical director. As you know, many of the requests for bioethics consults are triggered by end-of-life issues. We've had numerous discussions recently in this committee about our DNR order. But it's become clear that the larger context of the discussion really is our policy about forgoing life-sustaining treatment. Because Sophia is about to begin work on revising this policy, we thought we'd bring the matter to the ethics committee and ask her to open up the discussion.

LAWRENCE: The issue that I have been running up against—we've all been running up against—is the inconsistencies between the policy and the clinical situations it's intended to address. It's a very elegant policy but I think it does not always apply to the straightforward clinical situations.

As I've been thinking about the policy, it appears that we have two issues to address—one having to do with technology and the other, perhaps more challenging, having to do with decision-making authority. First, the cases that many of us get called on involve recent technologies, like ventricular assist devices and pacemakers, which are not addressed here because they were not in use when the original policy was drafted. A lot of things that we're able to do now were not included in the category of "life-sustaining treatment." Moving forward, it seems important to be organizationally consistent in how we counsel a care team. It's not helpful to say, "It's okay to do this with this equipment, but not okay to do that with that equipment." At the very least, we should have some consensus on the definition of life-sustaining treatment.

In terms of decision-making authority, I think we also need to step back and look at whether the policy provides useful guidance. It seems that, during the past several years, we have responded to constraints in the law and increasingly complicated cases by adding layers to our decision-making process. We now have a fairly elaborate and cumbersome protocol, involving the clinical team, the family, and administration. The result is somewhat counterproductive from a bedside perspective. When you're looking at a patient who is actively dying and we're intervening with seemingly complicated administrative steps, it's just not useful. So that's some of the context. I would appreciate feedback.

KELLER: I went through this policy last night. For the past three months, I have been looking at patients who have been in the hospital for more than three weeks. Many of the problems in those cases are end-of-life issues. Having had that experience, I find that it's very difficult to take what's in this policy, as Sophia said, and try to apply it to real-life situations. I think it has to be totally revised to make it a little more user-friendly.

I think that the average physician dealing with a difficult situation wouldn't know where to go with this policy and what to do with it. One way of reading it is that patients can't simply die anymore without having a medical director involved. I mean, I read that and I thought to myself, "Well, can't people just die, or do I have to call a medical director to discuss whether I have to intubate every single patient who is actively dying?"

LAWRENCE: That is the heart of the problem.

MARTINEZ: Is there something specific that you can point to in the policy that leads you to think that?

KELLER: Let's see. I highlighted something on page 5D. "The medical director's staff (or a member of the bioethics service) must be contacted to coordinate the necessary steps in assisting the family and the health care team if the family/surrogate wishes to forgo ventilatory support, dialysis, artificial nutrition, and/or hydration." Why is that necessary?

WALTERS: From an ethics perspective, I don't think the law requires that strict a reading because you need to look at the context in which the law was developed and how it is customarily applied in the clinical situation. A most narrow reading, I would argue, is unnecessarily restrictive to physicians when patients are actively dying. A good example would be a patient in the pulmonary care unit. Let's say that he's in multi-organ system failure with end-stage AIDS. His kidneys are failing, and the decision is made not to start him on dialysis because he's dying. He has no advance directive and he's either alone in this world or he's never discussed his care wishes with his family. The fact that we don't know what he would want about dialysis is irrelevant because he's dying.

KELLER: I hear you saying we have no medical, legal, or ethical obligation to offer a treatment if it's not medically indicated.

RICE: How do you decide that something is not medically indicated?

KELLER: Because, in this hypothetical situation, it's not life-sustaining. That's one of the things that I find is difficult with this policy. Some of the terms that you guys use and are comfortable with, the average clinician finds confusing. "Capacity" I understand, but "life-sustaining" or "medically indicated," I don't know what those mean.

CARRELTON: Is there a difference between keeping alive and life-sustaining?

ROWAN: They are the same thing.

NORMAN: Are they? I don't know. I'm trying to think about a patient who is dying. It seems to me that there is a life that could be sustained versus a person who is dying. I guess I'm also thinking of ventricular assist devices. I'm thinking about what Sophia said. And it's going to get worse, not better. There are going to be more expensive, high-tech, invasive ways of postponing death.

SILVER: I think it's important to emphasize that we're trying to keep a balance between the requirements of the law and the clinical needs of dying patients. This is not a matter of seeing how we can get around the law. This is a matter of providing guidance to clinicians who want to practice well within the standard of medical care, the requirements of the law, and the ethical imperatives. Somehow, the policy has to convey that.

KELLER: I have to agree. The problem is that "life-sustaining" as a phrase applies to the case we discussed earlier. That radioactive iodine was a life-sustaining therapy. Yet at the other end we have the patient who, without dialysis, would be dead within two or three days. Well, you put him on dialysis and I bet I could stretch that time frame. We can keep tissue going for weeks in people with no viability. That's life-sustaining, but is it rational?

ROWAN: Well, for the legislature and the courts, the presumption is that people would want to be kept alive unless you have evidence of their wishes to the contrary. Because of that presumption, we always err in favor of providing life-sustaining treatment.

SEEGER: But the law also requires an understanding that patients know the burdens of what we're going to do them against the potential benefits. What we do is often abusive and painful and absolutely magnificent at prolonging dying and suffering.

POWELL: What's the difference between prolonging dying and prolonging life?

LAWRENCE: Where I have trouble as a frontline resource person is saying to professionals, who are inherently risk averse anyway, "You have no clinical, ethical, legal obligation to provide care that's not indicated."

RICE: I don't know how to define this, but I think that we are trying to decide whether patients are living or alive. I'm not quite sure about the semantics or whether we're getting too philosophical, but we are sustaining people who really aren't living. I don't know how we make that distinction. We have patients who are almost brain dead and we're forced by technology to sustain them. Is that really a life? Is that really what the patient would want? That's obviously a slippery slope and we're stuck.

WALTERS: What you have done is frame the discussion that usually takes place under a rubric of quality of life. That, I think, is a very different matter about which people of good will and intelligence can disagree.

I think what we're trying to grapple with is that people don't understand what this policy means. What about our pulmonary care unit [PCU] patient? What if he had told his family he would want everything done? At a certain point, the PCU people would say, "His kidneys are going. It would be crazy to dialyze a patient who is moribund, who has all of these other organ system failures and is crashing on 100% oxygen."

LAWRENCE: But the reason he isn't started on dialysis is not because he told us he didn't want it. It's because it doesn't make any clinical sense.

KELLER: But for patients who clearly fall into that actively dying category, isn't there a way to interpret the phrase "life-sustaining treatment" that permits us not to provide it?

POWELL: The problem is that, if you specify this in the policy and say that something doesn't make clinical sense, there is a danger that it will be interpreted in a quality-of-life sense, which is something we don't want.

KELLER: I think the real problem we have is not just the law or us or the wording of the policy, but that society hasn't come to grips with the reality of death. We have a nation that can't recognize that death is the inevitable consequence of birth. Sooner or later, it's going to happen. If society wants, we can allocate resources indefinitely. We can put LVADs in every one of the patients who has end-stage heart failure. We can then put them all on transplant lists and we can put them in ICUs and on ventilators.

What I'm saying is that we have to be able to define a group of patients who are actively dying. This is not somebody with COPD who you are going to intubate and prolong life or not, or somebody with end-stage dementia who you're going to feed or not. The patients we are talking about have multi-organ system failure. They are dying and they will be dead within a matter of days to a week.

RICE: Maybe it's like the judge said about pornography, "I can't define it, but I know it when I see it." I know a dying patient when I see one. But what do we or don't we have to do to a patient who is actively dying?

SEEGER: For those patients, I would say that nothing is life-sustaining.

POWELL: It's palliation.

PRINCE: But who decides that?

NORMAN: It's not like a definitive point. It's often a continuum and sometimes we're wrong. I have to tell you, just to humble myself, I made a home visit to a patient with a systolic pressure of 80. His mouth was open, he hadn't eaten in 36 hours. I called the family and said, "I just want to let you know it's going to happen soon." I don't usually say that and I don't say it lightly. Twenty-four hours later he woke up. He was diabetic and his sugars were all over the place. He woke up and two weeks later he is eating and his sugars are fine. I don't know what happened, but I was humbled.

RICE: But that's the slippery slope. That's the problem.

SEEGER: I know, but we've got to start somewhere. If somebody raised the issue in that kind of patient, "Should we intubate?" and we didn't have this policy, we would have a tube in that patient, which I think is not what we're trying to do here.

KELLER: The other thing about the policy is that most of it deals with patients or families wanting to abuse treatment, as opposed to the team's questions about how aggressive to be. The policy doesn't really deal with that issue, which is, I think, much more common.

WALTERS: Say a little bit more.

KELLER: The typical scenario concerns the desperately ill patient whose family wants to continue aggressive measures, usually antibiotics. Again and again recurrent sepsis, resistant organisms, more antibiotics, and it just goes on and on. At some point, the physicians say, "We just can't keep doing this forever," and the family says, "Oh yes you can." Is there some way to address that issue? Does that fall under the rubric of life-sustaining?

WALTERS: That falls under the rubric of futility and, if we ever solve this problem, we'll get to that problem.

KELLER: Well, we have a patient in the hospital for five months now. That's our current long stay. Recurrent infections, different antibiotics, round and round—it's just very difficult to watch.

MARTINEZ: The only reason that we're doing this is because the family wants it, not because it makes clinical sense.

KELLER: The son, who is having a very difficult time with his father's illness, keeps insisting that we need to go forward. The attending physician is finding the situation hard to negotiate, and the hospital is stuck.

CARRELTON: Would it be helpful for me to spend some time with the family? Sometimes a new face who just wants to listen can be comforting.

KELLER: It's certainly worth a try.

WALTERS: Sam, if you think it would be helpful to have the bioethics committee consult on your case, let us know.

We haven't explicitly addressed the futility issue, which is lurking at the edges of these cases. Other states accord families more authority to make treatment decisions for their dying relatives, which makes a significant difference in how these situations are handled.

LEVIN: That's a great segue into something that I hope will be useful in our discussion. Because states differ, sometimes significantly, in how they deal with end-of-life issues, I thought it might be worth looking at how forgoing life-sustaining treatment is handled elsewhere. Keeping in mind that this is an ethics discussion, not a legal one, it seemed useful to look at policies in some other states to enrich our thinking about the ethical issues involved. We've said many times here that we don't want policy to drive the ethical analysis, but reflection on how other institutions deal with these issues might reveal ways of thinking about end-of-life issues that could benefit us.

In that spirit, I asked four committee members to do a little research and give us a brief sketch of what happens in four states: California, New York, Oregon, and Texas. To keep the discussion moving and prevent us from getting bogged down, I've asked that these summaries focus just on the key issues that have the greatest relevance to our policy discussion, with the understanding that the statutes and the policies reviewed are much more detailed. So, Abby, please start us off with a picture of what happens in Texas.

PRINCE: I reviewed the relevant Texas statute and one hospital's policy on forgoing life-sustaining treatment. They both clearly lay out the decision-making process and the underlying philosophy, beginning with an acknowledgment of the right of patients to consent to or refuse any treatment, and the recognition that, under certain circumstances, life-sustaining treatment may impose more burden than benefit.

The Texas structure authorizes health care decision making under a wide range of circumstances. Decisions, including the withholding or withdrawing of life-sustaining treatment, may be made in any of the following ways:

- by a competent adult after consultation with a physician
- by a written or verbal advance directive, previously executed by a competent patient
- by a spokesperson designated by the competent patient in an advance directive
- by the attending physician and either the patient's legal guardian or agent under a medical power of attorney, the latter previously designated by the competent patient
- in the absence of patient competence or ability to communicate, advance directive or appointed medical power of attorney, by a spokesperson selected from the following in order of priority:
  o the patient's spouse
  o the patient's reasonably available adult children
  o the patient's parents; or
  o the patient's nearest living relative

MARTINEZ: What about the patient who is incompetent, has not left an advance directive, and has no family or friends to act as decision maker?

PRINCE: In that case, a treatment decision can be made by the responsible physician as long as it is concurred in by another physician who has not been involved in the patient's care.

SEEGER: Well, that pretty much covers all the possibilities in a clear and orderly manner.

PRINCE: Let me tell you a few other noteworthy features of this policy.

- It focuses attention on two categories of patients especially likely to need decisions made about life-sustaining treatment: those in terminal conditions and those in irreversible conditions.
- The policy makes a point of addressing the broader issues of deciding about any and all life-sustaining treatment, rather than specific interventions.
- Physicians are strongly and repeatedly encouraged to initiate timely discussions with patients about advance care planning, including life-sustaining treatment.
- Decisions on behalf of an incapacitated patient are to be based on the patient's wishes, if known, or on an assessment of the patient's best interest.
- The institutional ethics committee is either encouraged or required to be involved in several parts of the process, especially when conflict exists.
- Decisions about life-sustaining treatment for children have additional safeguards, but I imagine that's pretty standard in all states.

WALTERS: Does the policy address futility?

PRINCE: Not directly, but the law and the policy have one really interesting and detailed section dealing with decisions that physicians consider inappropriate. These are decisions by or for patients that either request or refuse life-sustaining treatment. When the patient or surrogate refuses treatment the doctor considers medically indicated, the policy lays out a process for review, discussion, and, if consensus is not possible, transfer of the patient's care to another provider. When the patient or surrogate insists on life-sustaining treatment that the doctors consider not medically indicated, the policy sets up an even more elaborate eight-step process, including medical review, mediation, efforts to transfer the patient, and extensive ethics committee review.

All told, the Texas law, reflected in this policy, seems to provide consistent and helpful guidance for clinicians dealing with a set of difficult issues.

LAWRENCE: It certainly provides a useful model, assuming it would be consistent with law in this state.

LEVIN: Next up, let's look at California. Eric, did you research that?

POWELL: Yes. California has a specific Health Care Decisions Law, which includes several of the same features that Abby just described. The statute also begins by affirming the patient's right to refuse treatment, the inappropriateness of prolonging the dying process when treatment will not benefit the patient, and the importance of keeping health care decision making out of the courts when there is no controversy.

Like Texas state law, the California law lists several ways in which health care decisions, including the withholding or withdrawing of life-sustaining treatment, may be made, including

- by a competent adult;
- by an individual health care instruction, previously written by a competent adult;
- by an agent authorized by a power of attorney for health care, previously designated by a competent adult;
- by a surrogate designated by a competent patient only for the duration of current treatment, illness, or stay in the health care institution, or 60 days; or
- by a court-appointed conservator with the authority to make health care decisions.

KELLER: Except for decisions by the competent patient, all of these require advance authorization, usually by the patient when competent. What happens if that hasn't been done? Is there a default priority list that includes family, as in Texas?

POWELL: I found that curious, too. Neither the statute nor the policy I reviewed specifically mentions family. Yet the statute does say that a domestic partner can make decisions with the same authority as a spouse, although the authority of spouses is not described. Fact sheets about the decision-making law, however, explain that, when a patient lacks capacity and has not delegated decision-making authority, care professionals do what they do in most of these situations—turn to close family or friends who are most likely to know the patient's wishes and values. This informal appointment of a decision maker has apparently been customary in California for years, even though it does not appear in the statute.

NORMAN: What are the criteria for decision making on behalf of incapacitated patients?

POWELL: As in Texas, the agent or surrogate bases decisions on the patient's instructions or wishes, if known, or on an assessment of the patient's best interests, considering personal values.

LEVIN: Any other questions about California? Thanks, Eric. Sam, what can you tell us about Oregon?

KELLER: You might expect that a state that has worked through an assisted suicide law has given a lot of thought to end-of-life issues, and it shows in the legislation and the policy that I reviewed. As in Texas and California, Oregon provides several ways that treatment decisions, including those about life-sustaining treatment, can be made, including

- by a competent adult;
- by a written health care instruction; or
- by a health care representative, who can be one of the following:
  o an attorney-in-fact for health care, designated by a previously competent adult
  o a person who has authority to make health care decisions for the patient, selected from a priority list when the patient is in specified clinical conditions
  o a guardian or other person appointed by a court to make health care decisions for a patient

As in Texas and California, when a patient lacks capacity, the health care representative must base decisions on the patient's wishes, if known, or an assessment of the patient's best interest. But Oregon goes further and builds in additional safeguards. For example, the health care representative may only make decisions about life support or tube feeding in the following circumstances:

- the capable patient had expressly initialed the relevant permission sections in the directive, or
- the patient has been medically confirmed to be in one of the following conditions:
  o a terminal condition
  o permanent unconsciousness
  o a condition in which life-sustaining treatment would not benefit the patient and would cause severe and permanent pain
  o the advanced stages of a progressive, debilitating illness that will be fatal, prevents the patient from swallowing nourishment or water safely or recognizing family, and it is extremely unlikely that this condition will improve

An additional list of safeguards covers the withholding or withdrawing of artificial nutrition and hydration, which can only be done by a statement of the capable patient, an authorized health care representative, or the confirmation that the patient is in one of the specified conditions that I just listed.

The instructions section of the advance directive described in the statute is very specific in explaining conditions under which decisions about life support can be made. These conditions include close to death, permanently unconscious, advanced progressive illness, and extraordinary suffering, all of which are defined. The instructions even explain the phrase "as my physician recommends" to mean that the patient wants the physician to try life-sustaining treatment as long as the physician believes it will be beneficial, after which it should be discontinued. This level of explanation would seem to address concerns about people consenting to things in advance directives without knowing what they mean and care professionals misinterpreting what directives intend. I know I would find clear definitions like this helpful, as I indicated earlier in the discussion about our policy.

NORMAN: You mentioned a priority list for selecting a health care representative. Is that similar to the ones in Texas and California?

KELLER: Yes, thanks for reminding me. If the patient has been confirmed to be in one of the four specified conditions and has not appointed a health care representative or left an advance directive, a representative is named in order from the following list:

- a guardian authorized to make health care decisions
- the patient's spouse
- an adult designated and agreed to by the other people on the list
- a majority of the patient's adult children
- either parent of the patient
- the patient's adult siblings
- an adult relative or friend

And, if none of those people is available, life-sustaining treatment can still be withheld or withdrawn under the direction of the attending after consultation with appropriate people, such as the patient advocate or another physician who is not involved in the patient's care.

The bottom line seems to be that, in Oregon, decisions to forgo life-sustaining treatment can be made in most circumstances, but specified conditions and safeguards have to be met.

LEVIN: Thanks, Sam. Any other questions about Oregon? Ellen, I think you looked at New York.

SILVER: New York's situation is more similar to what we have in this state. Because no decision-making law governs these issues, there is no clear statutory structure for making health care decisions, including those regarding life-sustaining treatment, on behalf of patients without capacity. The legislature has provided some targeted regulation and laws, including a statute authorizing the appointment of health care proxy agents and a statute creating a hierarchy of surrogates who may consent to do-not-resuscitate orders for incapacitated patients. The legislature has also authorized surrogate health care decision making on behalf of specific vulnerable patient populations, including incompetent adults who may have court-appointed guardians, the mentally ill and developmentally retarded, residents of mental hygiene facilities, and minors.

The lack of a surrogate decision-making statute in New York means that health care decision making is governed almost entirely by case law. A line of New York cases has held that, when a patient lacks capacity, a decision to withhold or withdraw life-sustaining treatment requires "clear and convincing evidence" that the patient would have chosen to forgo the treatment in question in the patient's current circumstances. Missouri also requires this rigorous evidentiary standard in the clinical setting. Because the clear and convincing standard is very demanding, it is often very difficult for families to provide the level of evidence necessary when patients may not have explicitly articulated their wishes about life-sustaining treatment. A statement of patient wishes, such as a written living will or oral instructions, is considered to meet the clear and convincing standard.

The fact is that most patients without capacity are not part of specified vulnerable populations, have not appointed health care agents, and may not have articulated their wishes orally or in writing. They are vulnerable just because they need decisions made for them. As Eric pointed out, common practice is for care professionals to turn to family or close friends to make decisions for incapacitated patients. Unlike most states, however, there is no clear surrogate authority in New York for those who can provide insight into their wishes and values. As a result, the customary but informal practice in New York is for family members to consent to treatment but, unless they have clear and convincing evidence of a patient's wishes about life-sustaining treatment, they are unable to make decisions about withholding or withdrawing these measures. The legislature is considering a family health care decision-making bill, which would create a hierarchy of surrogates, similar to the ones in Texas and Oregon.*

MARTINEZ: So what happens now in most cases when the patient lacks capacity and has not appointed a proxy agent or left clear instructions? How do policies deal with that?

SILVER: The policy I reviewed focused on the right to reject unwanted treatment, authority of appointed surrogates, the importance of initiating early discussions with patients and families about care wishes, and the process for eliciting and documenting clear and convincing evidence of the patient's wishes. It is my understanding that most institutions have mechanisms for addressing cases that don't meet these criteria, including exhaustive review by the clinical team, medical director, legal office, and bioethics.

LEVIN: Thanks to all of you for researching and presenting this material. Let's return to discussing our own policy.

LAWRENCE: We have another important resource that we haven't mentioned. The integration of palliative care is an important fact for bioethics, critical care, geriatrics, pediatrics—clinical care in general. So if we have questions about whether a patient is dying, we have this other valuable resource—a team of people who are experts in determining when a patient is dying and how best to arrive at the most appropriate plan of care. In these situations, we should routinely bring in those experts and try to get some kind of consensus that we're

* The New York State legislature enacted the Family Health Care Decision Act in March 2010.

dealing with a patient in the process of dying, a patient who would be appropriate for palliative or hospice care.

WALTERS: Excellent point. If a patient moves from curative treatment to hospice care, my argument is that we're not withdrawing or withholding care from the patient. Although we are withholding what may be life-sustaining care, we're providing appropriate aggressive palliative care for a patient who is dying.

LEVIN: I think part of the problem with the policy is that it defines life-sustaining treatment in terms of specific interventions, rather than the broader context that we heard about in other policies. Specific interventions in some cases may indeed be life-sustaining, but in your example, the very same intervention would not be life-sustaining. So I wonder if there is a way to address the fact that we're not just focusing on the intervention in isolation from the patient's overall prognosis, but that it has to be looked at in context.

LAWRENCE: What would that mean? How would you frame it?

LEVIN: Well, we would have to frame it without actually getting into the slippery slope problem. Without talking about the dying patient, how do we define that category? How do you do it clinically? I don't know.

POWELL: Something like an APACHE or an Apgar score, something that gives specific and clear criteria?

MARTINEZ: I think that might be too specific. But can we leave it nonspecific and yet have something that's meaningful? I'm sorry, I interrupted you.

LAWRENCE: No, just one possible thought. As I was looking at these procedures, the palliative care medicine consult seemed helpful. It seemed to me in some cases, there should be a presumption when you're considering forgoing life-sustaining treatment that a palliative care consult would automatically be part of the plan. Maybe that would help to convince families that you're not abandoning the patient. It's just a different kind of care. I don't know if that's practical.

KELLER: Can I just point out on page 4, that C2 already acknowledges the point that we're making about the importance of palliative care? But somehow that gets lost when we focus on specific interventions.

[TECHNICAL DISCUSSION OF HOW AND WHEN VARIOUS INTERVENTIONS ARE LIMITED OR WITHDRAWN]

LAWRENCE: Clinically also in terms of palliative care, it's not a yes/no thing. I mean, it's often a time line where we say, "Let's try one course of antibiotics," thinking of your patient at home. We'll do that once or twice. Then after twice we'll stop because we'll know we're in the territory where nothing is working. It's a process, not an event.

WALTERS: Just let me make one comment and then Michael, you've been very patient again. One of the things we do in bioethics when we negotiate plans is time-limited trials, similar to what Sophia is describing. We say, "For the next 36 or 48 hours, we're going to do X. Then we'll come back and reevaluate whether X is right, or X plus 1 or X minus 1." I like the idea of having a policy that reflects a process, rather than specifics. Maybe that would help. Michael?

SEEGER: That's actually a very interesting concept. Then it puts in something that could be defined in the documentation—that we have a process of testing a therapy and determining whether it was effective, promising, or futile. We set a parameter and define by these criteria, and at the end of X we will evaluate it accordingly. Thus, we can determine that it's futile.

MARTINEZ: Isn't that similar to the section of the Oregon statute that Sam mentioned? Something about the advance directive providing for the attending physician to try life support as long as it was beneficial and then, when it was no longer helping the patient, being able to discontinue it. That sounds like the policy is able to build in the idea of trials.

WALTERS: This is what people argue in the ethics literature. You try something and see if it works. If it doesn't work, you are justified in stopping it.

RICE: While I agree with what you said about people, families, and the world thinking, "Oh, life will go on forever," I think that in the hospital, it's more a sense of, "You're going to abandon me because I'm dying." Patients and families fear that. So this approach, this process really mitigates that fear. It says, "No, you're involved with me. You're dying, but we're in this together."

CARRELTON: I think you're on to something. There are a lot of problems coming to terms with clinical reality. But I do find that often what's necessary is helping people realize that they're still part of the process.

KELLER: I want to go back to your palliation concept. When you have an engaged family with an active dialogue and an understanding of the situation, you don't even need to go through the palliative care consult. They're already on board. They get it.

The problem with palliation as required policy for this is that it's most useful for the families that are either not understanding the clinical situation or not dealing with it in a way we view as rational. We say, "Difficult family, difficult doctor." Palliative care is for dying patients whom we are not able to treat adequately within the limits of what society allows. If you want to go to hospice, you have to specifically say, "I accept the following limits on the kinds of treatments that will be available to me."

PRINCE: Not any longer. Under new hospice interpretations, patients can continue to receive some kinds of care that used to be considered strictly curative and not appropriate for hospice. You don't have to make the same kinds of stark decisions about treatment.

LEVIN: Could I bring us back to a suggestion on the policy? I find an inconsistency in it. There are all these really good things here, like principle 1, the very first bullet on page 2. "Physicians and other providers have no medical, legal, or ethical obligation to offer or provide treatment(s) that are not medically indicated." Then there is that other statement, C2 on page 4, which repeats the same thing. That, I think, is all fine and should remain.

WALTERS: Yes, I understand what you're saying. When I sat down to read this policy for the first time in a long time, I thought, "What a lot of words!" By the time you get through it, you don't know where you've been. The first thing I'd like to see is a two-page policy. You've got to get it in two pages or it's not helpful in the trenches.

Second, I think it should have a different starting point. I love this discussion we've been having. It's been very clarifying. When patients are actively dying, the focus should be on their physical, emotional, and spiritual comfort, and the comfort of their families. When a patient is not clearly dying—when there is potential for clinical improvement—we have a different discussion and different decisions. But, in the presence of active dying, we want to focus on what will benefit this patient most at this time. Then we need a process that gets us to that decision and a policy that speaks to that goal.

LEVIN: I would argue ethically and legally that we need a policy that helps caregivers figure out what they're supposed to do.

Unfortunately, we are just about out of time. We knew when we began this discussion that we couldn't hope to resolve these difficult issues in one session. But we've made a start and I know that this matter will come back to this committee again. Sophia, as the point person on this policy, you had the first word and now you get the last.

LAWRENCE: Someone asked before what the purpose of the policy is. My understanding is that hospital policies are intended to provide structure, information, and guidance to help clinicians and administrators through a set of consistent processes. This is an especially difficult policy because it deals with hard issues, which are made harder by the constraints of state law.

My goal—and this discussion has been enormously helpful—is to develop a policy that reflects the clinical realities of end-of-life care, the professional and ethical obligations we have to dying patients, and the legal realities that shape to some extent what we do. I will take my notes of this meeting and try to do a first draft of a revised and simplified policy that captures what has been said here. Again, thank you so much for your thoughtful comments and suggestions.

Index

214–15; meeting example, 383–402; membership of, 215–17; models for, 7; organizational, development of, 206–9. *See also* education by ethics committees

Ethics Consultation (Fox et al.), 227, 234

Ethics for Health Care Organizations (Blustein et al.), 208

ethics grand rounds, 245–46

ethnicity: health disparities and, 188–89; nondiscriminatory care and, 202–3; role of, in health care, 11–12

eugenics movement, 123–24

euthanasia, 172

evaluation of ethics consultation service, 229–32

experiential interests, 114–15

expertise of ethics committees, 217–18

exploitation of elderly, 112–13

family: assisting to come to terms with death, 134–35; conflicts between patients and, 147–48; DNR orders and, 144–45; end-of-life care and, 148–51, 177; as interpreters, 38, 52, 176; requests to "do everything" by, 155; sharing decision making with, 152–53; terminology for analgesia and, 169–70. *See also* adolescents; children; minors; parents

Family Care Decisions Act (New York), 399

feminist ethics, 11

fetuses: genetic testing of, 103, 123–25; maternal-fetal issues, 101–3, 374–75; moral status of, 100; viability of, and abortion, 371–72

fidelity: confidentiality and, 58; truth telling and, 47–48

fiduciary relationship, 4, 47–48, 339

firearms, 90, 378

Five Wishes, 29

formulation of ethics question, 235

Fosmire v. Nicoleau, 360

Fox, E., 232

futility. *See* medical futility

gag laws, 378

gamete donation, 95

gender, role of, in health care, 12

genes, human, patents on, 380

genetic diagnosis, pre-implantation, 93–95

Genetic Information Nondiscrimination Act (GINA), 359

genetic testing, prenatal/newborn, 103, 123–25

genomic screening of newborns, 103–4

genomic testing and control of information, 62–63

geriatrics. *See* elderly persons

gestational carriers, 92, 97–98

giving up compared to giving permission, 179–80

goals: of care, 148–51, 153, 301–4; of ethics consultation service, 230–31

Gonzalez v. Carhart, 99, 371–72

grand rounds: ethics committees and, 245–46; organizational ethics service and, 208–9

Green, Chad, 369

Green, David, 373

Grimes v. Kennedy Krieger Institute, 355–56

Griswold v. Connecticut, 357

group physician practice, 197

"Guidelines for Transferring Patients between Services," 270–72

harm prevention: to identified others, 60, 358–59; to unidentified others, 60–61

health, social determinants of, 190

health care ethics: definition and concerns of, 3; role of, in clinical medicine, 4–5. *See also* clinical ethics consultation; ethics committees

health care plans, religious exemptions from, 373

health care proxies/agents, 27, 28, 138–39; decisional capacity for appointment of, 20; living wills and, 140

health care reform, 194–95. *See also* Patient Protection and Affordable Care Act

Health Insurance Portability and Accountability Act of 1996 (HIPAA), 59

Hispanics, 12

history of ethics committees, 5–7, 213

"HIV exceptionalism," 379

Hobby Lobby, 373

hope, redefining, 52, 180

hospices, 162, 176–79, 401

hospitals: palliative care services in, 162; place of ethics committees in governance structure of, 219–22; prospective payment for, 187; teaching, and confidentiality, 59; transition from, 117–18

"iatrogenic loneliness," 116

ICDs (implantable cardiac defibrillators), 267–70

ICU beds, allocation of, 250–55

identity and disability, 123

immigrants, unauthorized, access to health care, 184, 187–88

implantable cardiac defibrillators (ICDs), 267–70

implicit rationing, 192

Improving Competencies in Clinical Ethics Consultation (American Society for Bioethics and Humanities), 216, 225